Frontiers in Anti-Infective Drug Discovery
(Volume 9)

Edited By

Atta-ur-Rahman, *FRS*
Kings College,
University of Cambridge,
Cambridge,
UK

&

M. Iqbal Chaudhary
H.E.J. Research Institute of Chemistry,
International Center for Chemical and Biological Sciences,
University of Karachi,
Karachi,
Pakistan

Frontiers in Anti-Infective Drug Discovery

Volume # 9

Editor: Prof. Atta-ur-Rahman, *FRS* and M. Iqbal Chaudhary

ISSN (Online): 1879-663X

ISSN (Print): 2451-9162

ISBN (Online): 978-1-68108-829-7

ISBN (Print): 978-1-68108-830-3

ISBN (Paperback): 978-1-68108-831-0

need for a court order if at any point you breach any terms of this License Agreement. In no event will any delay or failure by Bentham Science Publishers in enforcing your compliance with this License Agreement constitute a waiver of any of its rights.

3. You acknowledge that you have read this License Agreement, and agree to be bound by its terms and conditions. To the extent that any other terms and conditions presented on any website of Bentham Science Publishers conflict with, or are inconsistent with, the terms and conditions set out in this License Agreement, you acknowledge that the terms and conditions set out in this License Agreement shall prevail.

Bentham Science Publishers Ltd.
Executive Suite Y - 2
PO Box 7917, Saif Zone
Sharjah, U.A.E.
Email: subscriptions@benthamscience.net

BENTHAM SCIENCE

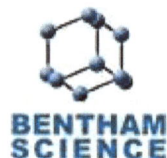

CONTENTS

PREFACE

Infections caused by viruses, bacteria, fungi, and parasites have caused death and suffering to humans and other life forms since their existence. Discoveries of antibiotics in 1928 and the development of vaccines were two important landmarks in our fight against harm caused by these unseen enemies. However, various infection-causing agents soon developed resistance against almost all available antibiotics, making the treatment an ever-growing challenge. Similarly, many fast mutating viruses have rendered many vaccines ineffective. The COVID-19 pandemic has posed an extensional threat to the human race, and it is a stark reminder of our vulnerabilities against infections. To meet these re-emerging challenges, it is imperative to constantly understand the molecular basis of infections and drug resistance, identify new drug targets and develop new chemotherapeutic agents. Unfortunately, till recently, pharmaceutical research for anti-infective agents has been given a low priority due to "economic feasibility" considerations. Only in the last decade, the topic has received global attention and vigorous research pursued in academic and pharmaceutical laboratories.

The book series *"Frontiers in Anti-infective Drug Discovery"* has been publishing review articles on key aspects of this field. Volume 9 is not different from the previous well-received volumes. It contains 5 carefully selected reviews on various key stages of drug development and approaches against infections caused by bacteria and parasites. The Review by Samatani *et al* is focused on a critically important aspect of drug development *i.e.* optimal choice of dose regimen. They explain the use of *in vitro* data against pathogens, animal PK/PD, clinical pharmacokinetics, and Monte Carlo simulations in this process. The chapter by Fadauloglou *et al* is focused on the role of post-translational modifications (PTMs) of microbial and host proteins during a successful bacterial and viral invasion in host cells. As a result, PTMs have recently emerged as novel and promising targets for the discovery of new anti-infective therapies.

Jean Michael Brunel has contributed an article on the potential of hydrazine-based agents as novel drug candidates against resistant bacteria and fungi, as well as their structure-activity relationships. The development of drugs against the second most important neglected parasitic disease, leishmaniasis, is the focus of the chapter by Roy and Mazire. They have reviewed the literature on various new therapeutic options and their current stages of development against this debilitating poor man's disease. Dengue viral hemorrhagic fever is also an important health challenge for the developing world. Leowattana *et al.* have commented on various re-purposed drugs currently in various stages of development against dengue virus infection and its various forms.

The 9th volume of this important book series comprises scholarly contributions from several leading experts to whom we are indebted. "Team Bentham" also deserves our appreciation for a job very well done. Among them, Ms. Asma Ahmed (Senior Manager Publications), and Mr. Mahmood Alam (Editorial Director) of Bentham Science Publishers have played a key role in the timely completion of the volume in hand. We sincerely hope that the efforts of authors and the production team will help readers to better understand and appreciate the importance of vigorous research and development activities currently underway against infections that cause tremendous suffering to humanity.

Atta-ur-Rahman, *FRS*
Kings College
University of Cambridge
Cambridge
UK

M. Iqbal Choudhary
H.E.J. Research Institute of Chemistry
International Center for Chemical and Biological Sciences
University of Karachi
Karachi
Pakistan

List of Contributors

Amarnath Sharma Clinical Pharmacology and Pharmacometrics, Janssen Research & Development LLC, New Jersey, USA

Amit Roy Department of Biotechnology, Savitribai Phule Pune University, Ganeshkhind Road, Pune-411007, India

Anastasia Tomatsidou Howard Taylor Ricketts Laboratory, Argonne National Laboratory, Lemont, Illinois, USA
Department of Microbiology, University of Chicago, Chicago, Illinois, USA

Dimitra Paliogianni Institute of Molecular Cell and Systems Biology, College of Medical, Veterinary & Life Sciences, University of Glasgow, Glasgow G12 8QQ, USA

Jean Michel Brunel Aix Marseille University, INSERM, SSA, MCT, Marseille, France

Mahesh N. Samtani Clinical Pharmacology and Pharmacometrics, Janssen Research & Development LLC, New Jersey, USA

Maria Amprazi Institute of Molecular Biology and Biotechnology, Foundation of Research and Technology-Hellas, Heraklion, Crete, Greece
Department of Biology, University of Crete, Heraklion, Crete, Greece

Pathomthep Leowattana Tivanon Medical Clinics, 99 Tivanon Road, Muang, Nonthaburi 11000, Thailand

Priyanka H. Mazire Department of Biotechnology, Savitribai Phule Pune University, Ganeshkhind Road, Pune-411007, India

Tawithep Leowattana Department of Medicine, Faculty of Medicine, Srinakharinwirot University, 114 Sukhumvit 23, Wattana District, Bangkok 10110, Thailand

Vasiliki E. Fadouloglou Department of Molecular Biology and Genetics, Democritus University of Thrace, Dragana University Campus, Alexandroupolis 68100, Evros, Greece

Wattana Leowattana Department of Clinical Tropical Medicine, Faculty of Tropical Medicine, Mahidol University, 420/6 Rajavithi road, Rachatawee, Bangkok 10400, Thailand

Use of Preclinical and Early Clinical Data for Accelerating Antimicrobial Drug Development

Mahesh N. Samtani[1,*], **Amarnath Sharma**[1] and **Partha Nandy**[1]

[1] *Clinical Pharmacology and Pharmacometrics, Janssen Research & Development LLC, New Jersey, USA*

Abstract: Antimicrobial drug development over the last two decades suggests that the choice of dose and dosing regimen can be selected at a very early stage. This is achieved by optimizing several key factors that are properties of the drug, the bug, and the host species. Drug exposure metrics, relative to the potency of the drug, are computed during the early stages of anti-infective drug development. These metrics serve as predictors of efficacy in the animal models of infection. Drug exposure relative to its potency can be expressed using a few metrics such as AUC/MIC, T>MIC, or C_{max}/MIC. The class of drugs that the anti-infective belongs to often determines the optimal choice of the metric for a given anti-microbial (and is empirically chosen based on pre-clinical data). There are various anti-microbial drug classes available on the market. Despite a large number of drug classes, there is reasonable consensus that the PK/PD target, *i.e.* metric of relative drug exposure described above, obtained from *in vitro* and animal experiments can predict the efficacy of specific drugs in humans. The steps involved in the derivation of this crucial PK/PD metric and dosing regimen in humans are as follows: (a) First, the metric is chosen and then the magnitude of the metric is computed using *in vitro* and animal PK/PD experiments; (b) Next, drug properties such as plasma protein binding are included as correction factors for the PK/PD target; (c) Finally, the non-clinical information is combined with early clinical pharmacokinetic data to estimate which dosing regimen has the greatest probability of attaining the PK/PD metric. This methodology of computing the dosing regimen and estimating the probability of successful target attainment accounts for two key sources of variability. These are between-patient variation in clinical pharmacokinetics and the gamut of MIC values that reflect the susceptibility of pathogens to the anti-microbial drug. These sources of variability are incorporated by running Monte Carlo simulations that are population-based in nature *i.e.* they account for variability in both the pathogen and the host. These sophisticated simulations answer the critical question around the rate of target attainment for dosing regimens of the new antibiotic drug. In summary, combining *in-vitro* data, animal PK/PD, early clinical pharmacokinetics, and Monte Carlo simulations expedites decision making in antimicrobial drug development. These efficiencies

* **Corresponding author Mahesh N. Samtani:** Clinical Pharmacology and Pharmacometrics, Janssen Research & Development LLC, New Jersey, USA; Tel.: +1-908-704-5367; E-mail: msamtani@ its.jnj.com

can lead to earlier and faster entry into full development for anti-microbials and aid optimal choice of dose regimen for phase 2/3 studies.

Keywords: Antimicrobial, Drug-development, MIC, Modeling, Monte-Carlo, PK/PD, Probability, Protein-binding, Simulation, Target-attainment.

INTRODUCTION

Drug development of antimicrobials over the last 2 decades has been revolutionized by the pragmatic selection of dose and dosing regimens driven by limited but well defined and validated factors that are characteristics of the drug, the pathogen and the host [1]. A robust predictor of anti-microbial efficacy is achieving the pharmacokinetic/pharmacodynamic (PK/PD) target *i.e.* a drug exposure metric such as area under the curve (AUC) or % time above minimum inhibitory concentration (%T>MIC) or peak concentration (C_{max}) relative to the susceptibility of the organism. Despite a large number of classes of antimicrobial agents, there is increasing consensus that PK/PD targets from *in-vitro* and *in vivo*. preclinical studies are predictive of efficacy in humans [1].

One way of utilizing the PK/PD target is to examine whether the free plasma drug concentrations required for anti-microbial efficacy based on preclinical data, can be safely achieved in early human trials. The technique of examining the adequacy of different regimens to treat a myriad of pathogens is based on Monte Carlo simulation methods that allow assessment of how frequently specific doses of the new drug are expected to achieve therapeutic targets. This methodology has the potential to help with study design for subsequent phases of drug development whereby only those doses with a high probability of success are selected. The antimicrobial development process starts off with assessing antimicrobial activity of an agent *in vitro* against several different laboratory strains of microbes, followed by *in vivo* studies in appropriate animal models with microbes of interest where the right PK/PD target is established. The pathogens causing the infection stay the same across species and this allows translation of efficacy from animals to humans. The PK/PD target is also species independent because the pathogen is susceptible in any species as long as the PK exposure is achieved. The PK/PD target is both a drug and bug property since it allows tailoring the exposure relative to the pathogen's susceptibility *e.g.* exposure should increase with decreasing susceptibility [2]. This is followed by assessing pharmacokinetic characteristics of the drug in healthy human volunteers. Utilizing the totality of such information and reinforcing the knowledge surrounding susceptibility and prevalence of antibacterial strains of interest in the community, extensive Monte-Carlo simulations are undertaken to ascertain the right dose and dosing regimen for a given indication. The objectives of the Monte-Carlo analysis are to (i) describe the population pharmacokinetic (PK) behavior of a novel anti-microbial in development by capturing the absorption and disposition properties using plasma concentrations collected during Phase 1 studies; (ii) to assess the expected performance of various doses and dosing regimens in clinically attaining PK/PD target measures associated with *in-vivo* efficacy in animal models over a range of pathogen susceptibilities using Monte Carlo simulations; and (iii) utilize the results of the Monte Carlo simulations to identify the optimal dose and dosing regimen for subsequent stages of drug development. The magnitude of the PK/PD target is generally obtained from the murine thigh infection model (but the animal model can vary depending on the infection being treated) and correction factors such as plasma protein binding are incorporated to adjust for species differences. Human PK data are usually obtained from early Phase 1 clinical studies. The pre-clinical efficacy information is then combined with the human PK data to determine which clinical dose has the highest probability of achieving the desired PK/PD target. These dosing computations and the calculation of the probability of successful target attainment explicitly account for inter-subject variability in human PK parameters during simulations, the relative natural prevalence of pathogens for target attainment, and the variability in pathogen susceptibility to allow dual individualization of pathogen and humans to the drug. The results from such exercise aids decision making for the development of novel antimicrobials. These decisions encompass the transition of a novel drug entity into full clinical development and the selection of dosing regimens for future phase II/III trials or making a "no-go" decision if PK/PD target attainment is lower than 90%.

Drug, Bug and Host Interactions: Five Critical Factors

Infections caused by multidrug-resistant bacteria are a serious threat to the general population and continue to cause significant morbidity and mortality worldwide. Application of bio-simulations that allow integration of prior information about the variability in human PK and pathogen susceptibility for assessing the likelihood of success for clinically chosen dose and dosing regimens has increased tremendously in the last 2 decades. The utility of Monte Carlo simulations for dose optimization of anti-microbials was first illustrated in 1998 to the FDA anti-infective drug products advisory committee for the antibiotic evernimicin [3]. Monte Carlo simulation allows integration of the knowledge about the PK profile of the drug and the differences in pathogen susceptibility to the drug to evaluate the expected likelihood of success of a given treatment in a particular disease during future clinical trials.

These bio-simulations are driven by five critical factors that describe the interaction between the drug, pathogen, and host [1]. These five factors include (i) the PK/PD target; (ii) distribution of pathogen susceptibility to the drug; (iii) variability in human PK; (iv) the drug's protein binding characteristics; and (v) the natural frequency of pathogen occurrence within a given infection type (Fig. **1**). The PK/PD target is a drug exposure metric normalized to the susceptibility of the organism and it serves as a predictor of drug efficacy [1]. The degree of pathogen susceptibility is obtained from *in-vitro* experiments that measure the minimum inhibitory concentration (MIC) required to suppress bacterial growth. Thus, drug exposure normalized by pathogen susceptibility is represented by PK/PD target metrics such as the area under the curve over MIC (AUC/MIC), peak concentration over MIC (C_{max}/MIC), or percent time during a dosing interval when plasma drug concentrations are above the MIC (%T>MIC).

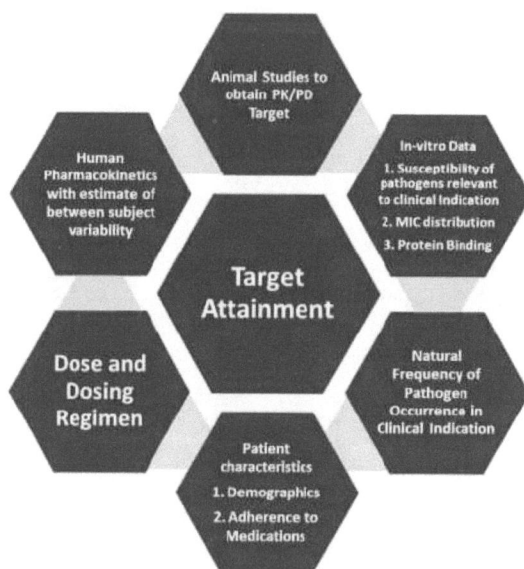

Fig. (1). Sources of information for a model-based estimation of target attainment using Monte Carlo Simulations. The sources of information are represented as interconnected pieces in the outside hexagons which are necessary for computing target attainment.

The choice of the three main PK/PD targets used in this analysis (C_{max}/MIC, AUC/MIC, and %T>MIC during a dosing interval) varies by drug class and depends on whether the drug of interest has time-dependent or concentration-dependent killing. For concentration-dependent drugs, the antimicrobial activity depends on peak drug concentrations. Either C_{max} or AUC drives the PD for these anti-infective agents, and this property is often associated with drug classes such as aminoglycosides and fluoroquinolones. They exhibit bacterial growth suppression even after limited exposure to the drug. These drugs can therefore be administered using a dosing interval that is somewhat longer than what is predicted by the PK half-life. This attribute offers fewer doses per day or per treatment and may improve adherence to antibiotics [4]. In contrast, for time-dependent killing, optimal drug effects are obtained as long as concentrations are maintained above the MIC during each dosing interval. Moreover, since sustained concentrations are required during an entire dosing interval, these drugs are often dosed intravenously as infusions and require repetitive dosing. The repetitive or continuous dosing is often not an issue for adherence since these drugs are used in critically ill patients suffering from life-threatening infections in intensive care units. Antibiotics that belong to this class include beta-lactams, carbapenems, cephalosporins *etc.*

PK/PD targets, as indicated above, are drug-class specific and are assumed to be similar across species because they reflect the drug's mechanism of action responsible for the *in-vivo* interaction between the drug and the pathogen [1]. Therefore, during preclinical development, the PK/PD target is usually obtained from dose-fractionation experiments in the murine infection models [1]. Pathogens reside in the interstitial space between cells, and the fraction of drug that is accessible to this effect site is the free concentration in plasma [5]. Drug PK is therefore corrected for differences in protein binding between mice and humans. It is recognized that in the clinical setting, there exists between-subject variability in human PK and there is a range of MICs for pathogen susceptibility to the drug. Variability in pathogen susceptibility and PK are accounted for in a simulation model, and each factor is described by a distribution of values. Even though the PK/PD target is fixed, the target exposure to be achieved at each MIC changes. As an example, with each doubling of MIC, the target AUC needed for successful treatment also has to double so that the established target is met. This is commonly referred to as dual individualization, which means that as the pathogens become less susceptible, greater drug exposure is needed to suppress their growth [6].

The degree of variability in drug PK that produces differences in drug exposure metrics (AUC, C_{max}, *etc.*) across individuals is obtained through drug disposition studies in the human population. If the drug hasn't entered the clinic yet, then the pre-clinical PK can be scaled to estimate human PK using either simple allometry or physiologically based PK modeling. These estimates are then used to create an exposure metric distribution for several thousand subjects using simulations and the between-subject variability in all PK parameters, which is generally inflated to 40% coefficient of variation (CV) to reflect higher variability that is generally observed in patient populations. Similar to the PK variability in the human population, the pathogen of interest also displays variability in its susceptibility to the drug (PD variability). The probability of being inhibited at a certain MIC is therefore obtained from a large collection of bacterial isolates (usually several 100s to 1000s isolates).

Generally, a population PK model is developed using plasma concentration-time data from single and multiple ascending dose studies from healthy subjects in early clinical development. The modeling strategy delineated in this chapter helps to assess the utility of different dose and dosing regimens. The mean parameter estimates and inter-subject variability obtained from the population PK model are utilized as inputs for a series of Monte Carlo simulations. These simulations are carried out for various dose and dosing regimens to estimate the probability of attaining different PK/PD targets. These computations are performed across target disease pathogens with wide-varying susceptibilities and a diverse frequency of natural occurrence. Finally, the appropriateness of the dose and dosing regimens is judged based on the probability of attaining projected efficacious drug exposure metrics described above. Thus, these analyses are aimed at assessing the expected performance of various dosing regimens in attaining PK/PD target measures associated with *in vivo* efficacy over a range of MICs using Monte Carlo simulations and providing quantitative/integrated support in identifying optimal dose and dosing regimens for subsequent stages of drug development.

METHODOLOGICAL ASPECTS

Skin infection is used only as an example for illustration purposes to explain the computation process in the sections below, and the methodology consists of 4 steps:

1. *In vitro* susceptibility testing
2. *In vivo* testing in the animal model of choice to define the choice of the PK/PD metric and PK/PD target threshold
3. Obtaining human PK data usually from normal healthy volunteers
4. Monte Carlo simulations and incorporation of susceptibility and prevalence information from surveillance data

These methods take the exposure-response relationship into consideration and allow examination of what-if scenarios such as the effect of administering a dose not studied during development. Monte Carlo computations are fairly rigorous and explicitly accounts for sources of variability that can impact the possibility of successful treatment with a new drug entity, which include: (i) inter-subject PK variability; (ii) formulation (and food effect if available for early phase 1 studies) on relative bioavailability; (iii) pathogen sensitivity and drug potency reflected by the PK/PD target; (iv) variability in pathogen susceptibility to the drug; and (v) natural occurrence of pathogens relevant to the clinical scenario.

Model for *In-vitro* MIC Distributions and Pathogen Frequency of Natural Occurrence

Based on the target product profile and susceptibility of pathogens for a given infection to the drug, target indications are chosen. For this exercise, we will consider complicated skin and skin structure infection (CSSI) as the main target indication. CSSI and pneumonia are used as example infections throughout the text and they are used only for illustration purposes. The computations illustrated for CSSI as an example are also applicable to other infections as well. The pathogens primarily responsible for CSSI are *Enterobacteriaceae spp.* (13.1%), *Enterococcus faecalis* (4.2%), *Pseudomonas aeruginosa* (8.0%), *Staphylococcus spp.* (65.4%), *and Streptococcus spp.* (9.3%). The percentages in brackets represent the natural frequency of occurrence of these pathogens in CSSI, and these were obtained from the literature [7]. Moreover, the *in-vitro* activity was represented as the entire distribution of MICs against *Enterobacteriaceae spp.* (n=101), *Enterococcus faecalis* (n=101), *Pseudomonas aeruginosa* (n=98), *Staphylococcus spp.* (n=249), *and Streptococcus spp.* (n=149). The MIC distribution used here is the susceptibility of CSSI pathogens to an antibiotic ceftobiprole based on frequencies reported in the literature [8]. The natural frequency of occurrence is a disease-specific parameter, while the MIC distribution is a drug-specific parameter obtained *in-vitro* from a collection of bacterial isolates for each new anti-bacterial agent under development.

Model for *In-vivo* PK/PD Target

The choice of *in-vivo* animal model depends on (a) the PK of the drug in the animal species of interest; (b) the type of infection that will be the target indication in the clinic; and (c) the pathogen under study. Infections are studied in their respective organ sites in the animal model *e.g.* lung infection models are used to evaluate pneumonia. Other such examples of specific body site animal infections include pyelonephritis, peritonitis, meningitis, osteomyelitis, and endocarditis. However, by far the most common model for studying *in-vivo* antimicrobial activity of new drug candidates is the murine neutropenic thigh infection model [9]. Immunocompromised neutropenic mice were infected with the pathogen of interest in the posterior thigh muscles. After bacterial inoculation, various incremental and fractionated doses of the drug are administered in different groups of mice. One day after drug administration, the mice are sacrificed and the thigh muscles are collected for quantitative cultures. PK is usually established in a separate group of neutropenic mice infected with the same pathogens used in the dose-fractionation studies.

An inhibitory sigmoid model is used to characterize the *in-vivo* antimicrobial activity. Various PK/PD metrics (AUC/MIC, Cmax/MIC, %T>MIC) are used as the independent variable, while the microbial load characterized by the logarithm of colony forming units per gram of tissue ($\log_{10}$ CFU/g) is the dependent variable. The model is used to determine (i) which PK/PD metric best captures the sigmoidal relationship; and (ii) the magnitude of the best-chosen PK/PD metric associated with bacterial stasis (when the bacteria have reached the same $\log_{10}$ CFU/g as inoculated). Bacteriostasis is generally sufficient because once the drug achieves static effect in humans, the immune system can clear the infection [2]. The PK/PD threshold obtained from the murine infection model is essential for guiding clinical dose selection because it is correlated with clinical outcome [1, 3] *i.e.* the PK/PD metric is identical across species once corrected for protein binding since this is a drug-specific property that is not dependent on the species that is infected with the bug and in which the PK is measured. The estimated PK/PD target is often derived from multiple strains of pathogens and the average is taken across the strains to get a refined PK/PD target [10]. Assuming the plasma free fraction in mouse and man are 0.75 and 0.65, respectively, the PK/PD target is corrected for protein binding difference as follows:

$$\text{Human AUC}\!\Big/\!\text{MIC} = \text{Mouse AUC}\!\Big/\!\text{MIC} \bullet \frac{\text{Mouse Plasma Free Fraction} (0.75)}{\text{Human Plasma Free Fraction} (0.65)} \qquad \textbf{(1)}$$

Population PK Parameters Representing Human Variability

At the earliest stages of drug development, a representation of the population PK parameters characterizing human variability in drug absorption and disposition can be obtained from (a) allometrically scaled PK parameters and between-subject variability of ≥40% in all PK parameters, which is generally observed in patients; or (b) a population PK model that is used to describe the earliest human plasma concentrations data collected from Phase 1 single and multiple ascending dose studies in healthy subjects (between-subject variability from Phase 1 may need to be inflated as well to reflect inter-patient variability and accommodate other uncertainties).

As an illustration, we consider an oral drug whose efficacy (PD) is driven by AUC at steady-state. The drug had a CL of 0.05 L/hr/kg in humans with a between-subject variability that is log-normally distributed with a 40% CV. Similarly, body weight was assumed to have a mean of 70 kg with a log-normal distribution and 30% CV for Monte Carlo simulations. The drug formulation was assumed to have a high relative oral bioavailability of 90% with low variability, which was simulated using a beta distribution having shape parameters of 900 and

100 (this parameter can be tweaked to assess formulation effects on PK and target attainment). The R code is shown in the appendix, it also illustrates how the computations could be performed if the PD was driven by peak concentrations rather than the area under the curve.

All calculations were performed for a drug with AUC/MIC as the PK/PD target. However, to complete the illustration, a second antibiotic was considered that is dosed intravenously as a 1-hour infusion, whose PD is driven by %T>MIC. For this illustration, the appendix (**1b**) with the R code shows calculations that compute fractional target attainment *i.e.* just the Monte Carlo simulation part for the PK. Computations after fractional target attainment are identical regardless of the PK/PD metric of interest. To illustrate %T>MIC computations, the PK parameters of an antibiotic [11] that follows 2-compartment disposition with zero-order input and first-order elimination are considered. The PK parameters and covariate effects obtained using data mostly from Phase 1 and 2 studies (and limited sparse data from Phase 3) and a population PK model are reported in Table **1**.

Target Attainment Computation

The population PK parameters were used as the basis for randomly generating a dataset of 5000 subjects. The AUC for each of these virtual subjects was computed from the ratio of dose over CL multiplied by the relative bioavailability for the simulated scenario for assessing dose and formulation effects. Calculated in this manner, the AUC represents the anticipated drug exposure at steady state during the 24-hour dosing interval. Residual variability was not introduced into the calculations of simulated AUC. The randomly generated AUCs that exceed the PK/PD target scaled by the MIC (Table **2**) were tallied and referred to as fractional target attainment. It is recognized in these simulations that even though the PK/PD target is fixed, the target exposure is needed to be attained at each MIC changes.

Table 1. **The PK parameters of an antibiotic used to illustrate %T>MIC computations.**

Parameters [a]	Estimate	Interindividual Variability (% CV) [f, g]	Inter-occasion Variability (% CV) [g]
CL (liters/h) [b]	13.6	19.24	14.90
V_c (liters) [c]	11.6	19.13	18.55
V_p (liters) [d]	6.04	24.82	30.18
Q (liters/h) [e]	4.74	41.59	-
Power	-	-	-

(Table 1) cont.....

Parameters [a]	Estimate	Interindividual Variability (% CV) [f, g]	Inter-occasion Variability (% CV) [g]
CL - CRCL	0.659	-	-
V_c - weight	0.596	-	-
V_p - weight	0.840	-	-
Q - weight	1.06	-	-
V_p - age	0.307	-	-
V_p - CRCL	0.417	-	-
The proportional shift in CL for race	-	-	-
Black	0.0204	-	-
Hispanic	0.163	-	-
Other	−0.0445	-	-

[a] CL is the drug's clearance, CRCL is creatinine clearance, CL_{race} is the race effect on CL, V_c and V_p are central and peripheral distribution volumes, and Q is distributional clearance.

[b] $CL=13.6 \cdot (CRCL/98 \text{ ml} \cdot \text{min}^{-1})^{0.659} \cdot (1+CL_{race}[0$ for white, 0.0204 for black, 0.163 for Hispanic, -0.0445 for other]).

[c] $V_c=11.6 \cdot (weight/73 \text{ kg})^{0.596}$

[d] $V_p= 6.04 \cdot (CRCL/98 \text{ ml} \cdot \text{min}^{-1})^{0.417} \cdot (weight/73 \text{ kg})^{0.840} \cdot (age/40 \text{ years})^{0.307}$

[e] $Q=4.74 \cdot (weight/73 \text{ kg})^{1.06}$

[f] Off-diagonal elements of covariance matrix: $covariance_{CL,Vc}=0.0349$ and $covariance_{Q,Vp}=0.0924$.

[g] For simulations interindividual variability was inflated with interoccasion variability to reflect patient variability.

Table 2. Estimate of the overall attainment of the microbiological target by the drug at 1000 mg dose for *Staphylococcus spp.*

MIC (mg/L)	Target AUC (mg.h/L)	Number of *Staphylococcus* Strains	Fraction of Pathogen Distribution	Fractional Target Attainment (%)	Product of Fractions
0.06	6	3	0.012	100.0	1.2
0.12	12	10	0.040	100.0	4.0
0.25	25	83	0.333	100.0	33.3
0.50	50	77	0.309	99.9	30.9
1.00	100	49	0.197	97.3	19.1
2.00	200	22	0.088	69.6	6.1
4.00	400	5	0.020	20.1	0.4
8.00	800	0	0.000	1.2	0.0
16.00	1600	0	0.000	0.0	0.0
	-	-	-	-	Σ 95%

For example, if the AUC/MIC target is 100 hours, then with each MIC doubling, the target AUC must also double. This underscores the fact that as bacteria become more virulent, greater drug exposure is needed to suppress their growth. The variability in pathogen susceptibility is presented as the probability of being inhibited at a certain MIC. This probability of pathogen susceptibility for every species at each MIC was calculated by computing the fraction of strains inhibited at that MIC. The probability of attaining the PK/PD target for the virtual population of patients infected by a specific pathogen species was obtained by multiplying the fractional target attainment at each MIC by the proportion of pathogen strains with that MIC. The product of fractions at each MIC was added and the probability of achieving the PK/PD target was derived and reported in tabular format. This computation addresses the question about the probability of attaining a specific target at a specific dose against a specific pathogen species causing a particular disease such as CSSI. The process was repeated for each pathogen species and the target attainment for each pathogen species was weighted by the pathogen's frequency of natural occurrence in CSSI. The weighted products across all pathogen species were summed to compute the final target attainment rate or TAR. The results can be plotted as a final target attainment probability as a function of relevant treatment variables such as dose, formulation, *etc.* This procedure is described schematically in Fig. (**2**). Calculation of AUCs and PK/PD target attainment computations are performed using R. A representative R script for Monte Carlo simulation for one of the dosing scenarios is provided in the Appendix.

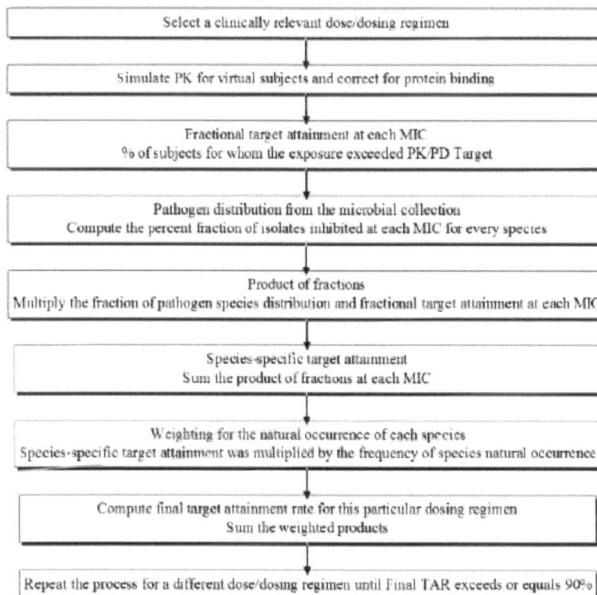

Fig. (2). Flow chart depicting the Monte Carlo optimization of trial success.

Assumptions Adopted During Modelling And Simulation

It is important to pay close attention to model assumptions because simulation outcomes can be quite sensitive to underlying assumptions about model components. The modeling and simulation strategy delineated in the sections above utilized the following assumptions:

a. The PK model and the formulation effect on drug absorption are often derived from the earliest single ascending dose clinical studies. The simulations are designed to predict drug exposure at steady state upon multiple dosing and therefore, PK stationarity was assumed.
b. Stationary PK was assumed for the intravenous antibiotic (Appendix **1b**) which implies that target attainment determined from single-dose simulations apply to steady state multiple dosing scenarios. This assumption was permissible because the accumulation factor for this drug was close to one.
c. Stationary PD was also assumed wherein time-dependent phenomena such as post-antibiotic effect and resistance development were not incorporated during the simulation process.
d. The PK models are derived from healthy volunteer data and the PK parameters are assumed to remain unaffected in the patient population. However, inter-subject variability was inflated to reflect higher variability in patients.
e. Inter-subject variability in protein binding was not incorporated.
f. No formal model was developed to describe dropouts and complete compliance was assumed when simulating virtual populations. This is a fair assumption because adherence to antibiotics for life-threatening infections during acute treatment is expected to be high.
g. The *in-vitro* pathogen distributions obtained from a collection of clinical isolates were assumed to be representative of the general widespread microbial population occurring in the clinical situation.
h. The natural occurrence of pathogens was obtained from the literature. The distribution of organisms observed in this one trial was assumed to be representative of the general widespread microbial population occurring in CSSI.
i. The uncertainty and analytical error in MIC determinations was not added as a source of variation in the Monte Carlo simulations.
j. The PK/PD threshold derived from the murine thigh infection model is based on the bacteriostatic endpoint. Dose selection based on a bacteriostatic threshold does not apply to clinical situations involving serious or severe infections where the host immune system is compromised. For these infections, a greater magnitude of drug exposure (and dose) maybe needed to eliminate the infection.

k. These target attainment results are often applicable to pilot formulations used in early development. However, if solid dosage formulations used in later development have a lower extent of drug absorption, then the high level of target attainment achieved with formulations may not be applicable to the solid dosage forms tested in late development.

CASE-STUDY RESULTS: APPLICATION OF MONTE-CARLO APPROACH

Target Indication and Patterns of *In-vitro* Killing

The antibacterial spectrum of the new anti-infective agent is studied *in-vitro*. The appropriate indication for the drug is based on the pathogen species that are susceptible to the drug. As an example, if the drug has activity against Pseudomonas aeruginosa then a potential indication could be ventilator associated pneumonia. For adding more indications, the activity of the drug would have to be tested against additional species. These bacterial species would have to be true pathogens for indications under consideration. Importantly, the clinical pathogens tested *in vitro* not only have to belong to the clinical indication under consideration but should also be obtained from various geographic regions to get pathogen distributions from different countries [12]. The isolates are used to obtain the variability in pathogen susceptibility to the drug as MIC distributions. These isolates are then also used for *in-vivo* testing in animal models to obtain the right PK/PD target for the drug under study. *In vitro* experiments also demonstrate patterns of kill curves where drug effects are either concentration-dependent (higher concentration leading to more efficient killing) *vs.* time-dependent effect (killing occurs as long as concentrations exceed MIC). This pattern helps design the right dose fractionation experiments in animal models of infection to determine the type and extent of PK/PD target (*e.g.* AUC/MIC) needed for efficacy.

Pathogen Susceptibility and Natural Occurrence

The natural pathogen frequency in CSSI (as an example) is reported in Fig. (**3**), which shows that Staphylococcus is the most prevalent species responsible for this infection. The entire MIC distributions against these five classes of pathogens are provided in Fig. (**4**). If new data become available and are deemed to be quite different than the prior knowledge of pathogen susceptibility and natural occurrence, the target attainment computations must be updated to obtain the most appropriate estimate of the probability of clinical success. This update process is not illustrated, but it simply requires rerunning the codes with the updated pathogen information.

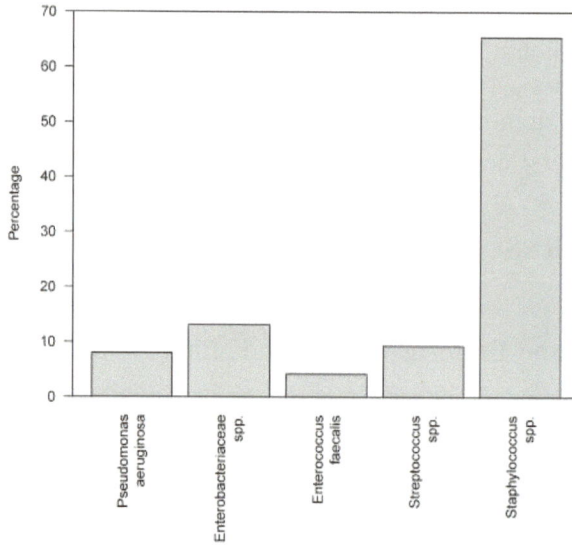

Fig. (3). Natural frequency of occurrence of pathogens in CSSI.

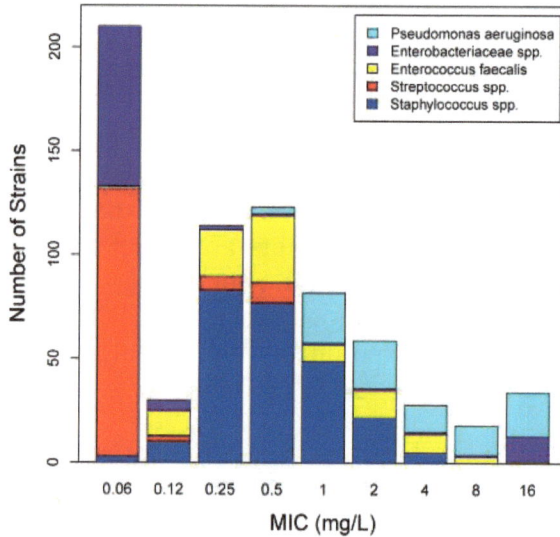

Fig. (4). MIC distribution of relevant clinical pathogens in CSSI for one example antibiotic.

PK/PD Target Based on The Murine Thigh Infection Model

The results from the murine study are shown in Fig. (**5**) and AUC/MIC was the PD-linked variable for drug efficacy. The total mouse (AUC_T/MIC) target related to bacterial stasis was 87 hours and after protein binding correction, the human PK/PD target was estimated to be about 100 hours.

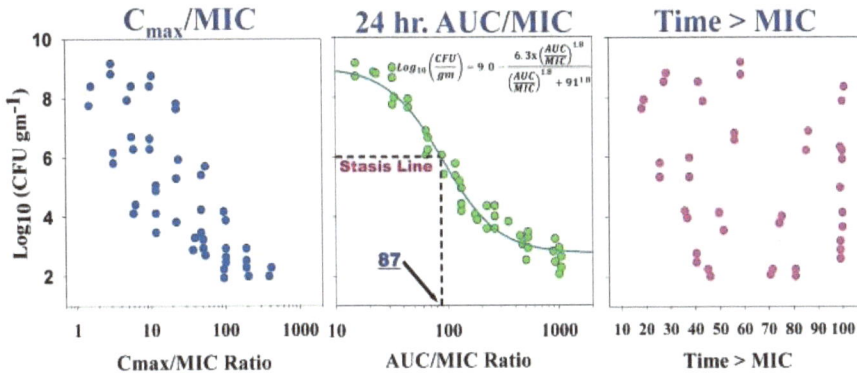

Fig. (5). Murine PK/PD - Solid line represents the fit to the data. 87 hours is the murine AUC/MIC target.

Clinical PK

The number of subjects available for PK model development is usually small and the underlying population model is often derived from healthy subjects. PK/PD target attainment however, reflects what to expect for a patient population. Thus, as Phase 2/3 study data become available, the target attainment computations are constantly updated to obtain the most appropriate estimate of the probability of clinical success. This update process is not illustrated here, but it simply requires rerunning the codes shown here with the updated PK model.

Monte Carlo Simulation Results

Simulation of one virtual trial with 5000 subjects is illustrated in the Appendix. The computations displayed in Table **2** provide an illustration of the methodology for the estimation of microbiological target attainment against *Staphylococcus spp.* by the drug at the 1000 mg dose. Fig. (**4**) represents the magnitude of variability in the pathogen susceptibility to the drug. The estimate of fractional target attainment based on the Monte Carlo simulation shown in Fig. (**6**) takes into account the variability in drug absorption and disposition in the population. Integration of these two distributions (pathogen variability and fractional target attainment), is obtained in a straightforward manner by multiplying the two to obtain the product of fractions across MIC values. To take an expectation over the entire MIC distribution, a sum of the product of fractions in the final column of Table **2** was performed to obtain a point estimate of species-specific target attainment of 95%. This value of 95% is informative because it indicates that for *Staphylococcus spp*, which is the most prevalent pathogen in CSSI, 95% of the patients inflicted with this pathogen are likely to achieve successful target attainment at the chosen dose and regimen. It is noteworthy that this species-specific target attainment of 95% is pertinent only to 1 dosing scheme (1000 mg daily with a formulation having high relative bioavailability), one pathogen species (*Staphylococcus spp.*), the PK/PD target of 100 hours, and the PK parameter estimates outlined in Table **1**.

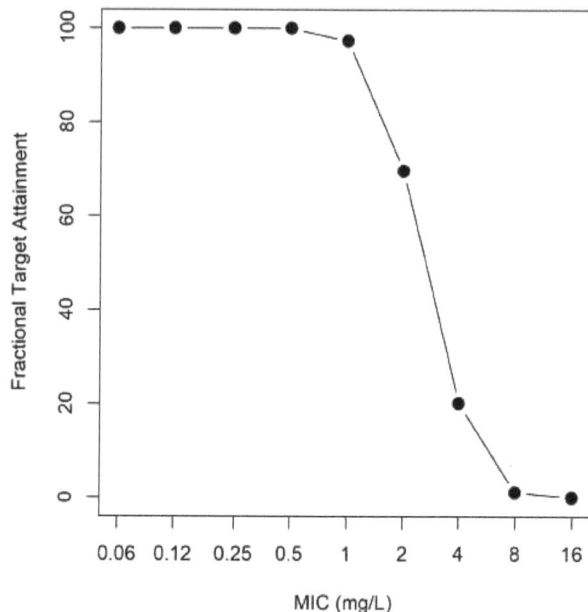

Fig. (6). Fractional target attainment at each MIC.

The next important step was to evaluate the expected attainment rates across each target pathogens for CSSI to obtain target attainment for the other 4 species (see Appendix **1a**). As the last step, by accounting for the frequency of natural occurrence of pathogens (Fig. **3**), a final TAR of 90% was obtained for this scenario. If the target attainment was lower than 90% then the entire process could be repeated at higher dosage strength and/or using data from other potential formulations.

SUMMARY

This work summarizes state-of-the-art data analysis of information gained from *in vitro* experiments, *in vivo*. animal studies, first in human PK profiles, Monte-Carlo methods and susceptibility/prevalence data from surveillance studies that are critical for accelerating antibiotic drug development.

The target attainment approach integrates the population PK variability (Fig. **6**) with the population distribution of the MICs (Fig. **4**). It is used to determine the probability of target attainment given the PK properties of the drug in the human population and the susceptibility of various microorganisms to the drug. Since the intended clinical indication is defined, and more than one bacterial species is known to cause the particular type of infection, the cumulative fraction of response in the population is based on the relative frequency of occurrence of each species. Thus, the probability obtained from the exercise illustrated in Table **2** was weighted by relative frequency of occurrence from (Fig. **3**). This weighted probability is the Final TAR and the entire computation is illustrated using a sample R code (Appendix **1a**).

Under- or inappropriate dosing of antibiotics is dangerous and unethical because it can lead to the emergence of resistant pathogens. Understanding the relationship between antibiotic concentration and the antimicrobial effect is essential for eradicating the pathogen and preventing the emergence of resistant pathogens. The Monte-Carlo approach represents a highly sophisticated methodology in anti-infective research for dose-selection of new drug entities. This approach maximizes %T>MIC, AUC/MIC or Cmax/MIC with the targets for stasis derived from pre-clinical models and PK parameters obtained from population PK models to compute the likelihood of target attainment for dosage regimens that may not have been studied in clinical trials with patients [13 - 16]. Recently mechanism-based models have been derived that assess (i) antibiotic combinations (ii) antibacterial resistance (iii) effects of the immune system (iv) bacterial cultures that contain susceptible and resistant sub-populations [13, 15]. These mechanism-based models are based on *in vitro* PK/PD data collected using hollow-fiber infection models [13, 15] to derive the relationship between patient PK profiles and resistance development for further *in-vivo* evaluations.

By taking into account sources of biological variability and by recognizing the pharmacological interaction between the pathogen, host and drug, an educated decision can be made regarding a dosing regimen that is most probable of succeeding in a future clinical trial.

As such, modeling and simulation provide a powerful, objective and transparent tool to support key decision points in the drug development program. These key decisions include the transition of a new molecular entity into full development (go/no go decision), dose selection for future clinical trials in patient populations and establishing appropriate susceptibility breakpoints for antibiotics. Simulations of this nature are also useful in devising post-marketing strategies by comparing target attainment for the new drug *vs.* marketed competitors in the same class or antibiotics of a different class used in the same indication. Such comparisons offer very objective criteria for deciding whether the new drug entity has merit for commencement into full development and if the product will be competitive in the market landscape. Such inferences could be based upon (i) a superior microbiological profile (ii) a more convenient dosing schedule (iii) lower cost of goods for a highly potent antibiotic that is effective at lower doses. As an example, once daily dosing will offer better compliance *versus*-marketed comparators that may require administration twice daily in clinical practice to obtain a similar level of target attainment. This framework is thus a general model-based drug development scaffold for the rapid advancement of drugs in the antimicrobial pipeline.

The success of this approach in antibiotic development has led to similar methodology being adopted for direct anti-viral therapy as well [17, 18]. In contrast, the investment in antibacterial research and development is hampered by less favorable returns and lack of economic incentives due to several reasons such as (a) short course of treatment for antibiotics *vs.* long-term therapy for chronic illnesses; (b) resistance to the antibiotic limiting the use of the antibacterial agent; (c) saturated market and significant competition from generics; (d) Conserving antibiotic use of novel agents to prevent the emergence of resistance [19, 20]. This has slowed down antibiotic drug development, while the incidence of antibiotic treatment resistant strains is on the rise [19, 20]. Antibiotic resistance poses a global threat to public health and the animal infection models can be used to identify PK/PD targets that suppress resistance emergence as well. For example, in the murine thigh infection model, the AUC/MIC target of levofloxacin against P. aeruginosa had to be increased 2-fold to suppress the emergence of resistant subpopulations [21, 22]. This suggests that we can identify PK/PD targets that prevent bacterial resistance. These exposure metrics are larger than the targets needed for typical clinical efficacy. Once these target exposures are identified, simulations can be utilized to (a) identify dosing regimens in patient populations that prevent resistance development and (b) accelerate the development of drugs targeting resistant pathogens such as Methicillin-resistant *Staphylococcus aureus* (MRSA).

In summary, a Monte-Carlo based bio-simulation tool is presented that allows evaluation of the expected clinical success of antibiotics on the basis of preclinical and early clinical PK information. This methodology allows the utilization of information from early development studies for facilitating late-phase drug development decisions. The results of this exercise may aid decisions such as transition of a novel anti-microbial into full development and the selection of dosing regimens with a high probability of success in larger Phase II/III trials. Methodology was utilized by the authors, and their collaborators in the development of the antibiotic doripenem and the readers are referred to the literature for further details [11, 23 - 26].

CONSENT FOR PUBLICATION

Not applicable.

CONFLICT OF INTEREST

All authors are employees and stockholders of Janssen Research and Development.

ACKNOWLEDGEMENTS

Declared none.

APPENDIX 1A

The R Code for Monte Carlo Simulation based on a drug with %T>MIC as the PK/PD metric. Code illustrates how the equations can be modified if Cmax/MIC was the PK/PD metric of interest.

```
#~~~~~~~~~~~~~~~~~~~~~~~~~~~~~~~~~~~~~~~~~~~~~~~~~~~~~~~~~~~~~~~~~~~~~~~~~~~~~~~~~~~~~~~
#~~~~~~~~~~~~~~~~~~~~~~~~~      GENERAL SETTINGS    ~~~~~~~~~~~~~~~~~~~~~~~~~~~~~~~~~~~~~~~~~~~~
#~~~~~~~~~~~~~~~~~~~~~~~~~~~~~~~~~~~~~~~~~~~~~~~~~~~~~~~~~~~~~~~~~~~~~~~~~~~~~~~~~~~~~~~
rm(list=ls(all=TRUE))# Clean up WD
set.seed(555)       # Will allow simulation to be regenerated in future
nSubj         =5000   # Number of Subjects
AUCMICTarget =100    # TARGET AUC/MIC FROM A MOUSE THIGH INFECTION MODEL # REPLACE WITH CMAXMICTarget IF CMAX DRIVE PD
DOSE         =1000   # mg
MIC          =c(0.06,0.12,0.25,0.5,1,2,4,8,16) # mg/L
#~~~~~~~~~~~~~~~~~~~~~~~~~~~~~~~~~~~~~~~~~~~~~~~~~~~~~~~~~~~~~~~~~~~~~~~~~~~~~~~~~~~~~~~
#~~~~~~~~~~~~~~~~~~~~~~~~~~   BUG FREQUENCY: DATA ENTRY   ~~~~~~~~~~~~~~~~~~~~~~~~~~~~~~~~~~~~~~
#~~~~~~~~~~~~~~~~~~~~~~~~~~~~~~~~~~~~~~~~~~~~~~~~~~~~~~~~~~~~~~~~~~~~~~~~~~~~~~~~~~~~~~~
freq1 = c(3  ,10, 83, 77,  49, 22, 5 ,0 , 0 ); freqa=freq1/sum(freq1) #Staph
freq2 = c(129, 3, 7 , 10,  0,  0, 0 ,0 , 0 ); freqb=freq2/sum(freq2) #Strep
freq3 = c(1  ,12, 22, 32,  8,  13, 9 ,3 , 1 ); freqc=freq3/sum(freq3) #Enterococcus
freq4 = c(77 ,5 , 2 , 1 ,  1,  1, 1 ,1 , 12); freqd=freq4/sum(freq4) #Enterobacteriaceae
freq5 = c(0  ,0 , 0 , 3 , 24,  23, 13,14, 21); freqe=freq5/sum(freq5) #Pseudomonas
nat.occ     =c(65.4, 9.3,4.2, 13.1,8.0)/100        # CSSI
freq.all    =cbind(freqa, freqb, freqc, freqd,freqe)   # all bugs
bug.types   =length(freq.all[1,])                  # bug types
#~~~~~~~~~~~~~~~~~~~~~~~~~~~~~~~~~~~~~~~~~~~~~~~~~~~~~~~~~~~~~~~~~~~~~~~~~~~~~~~~~~~~~~~
#~~~~~~~~~~~~~~~~~~~~~~~~~    CREATE VIRTUAL PATIENT PK   ~~~~~~~~~~~~~~~~~~~~~~~~~~~~~~~~~~~~~
#~~~~~~~~~~~~~~~~~~~~~~~~~~~~~~~~~~~~~~~~~~~~~~~~~~~~~~~~~~~~~~~~~~~~~~~~~~~~~~~~~~~~~~~
TVCL = 0.05
ETA1 = rnorm(nSubj,sd=0.4)
WT   = 70*exp(rnorm(n = nSubj,mean = 0, sd=0.3))
CL=TVCL*WT*exp(ETA1)
Bioavailability = rbeta(n = nSubj,shape1 = 900,shape2 = 100)
auc=Bioavailability*DOSE/CL
#~~~~~~~~~~~~~~~~~~~~~~~~~~~~~~~~~~~~~~~~~~~~~~~~~~~~~~~~~~~~~~~~~~~~~~~~~~~~~~~~~~~~~~~
#~~~~~~~~~~~ UPDATE EQUATION TO CMAX IF PEAK CONCENTRATIONS ARE THE DRIVER FOR PD ~~~~~~~~~~~~~~~~~~~
#~~~~~~~~~~~~~~~~~~~~~~~~~~~~~~~~~~~~~~~~~~~~~~~~~~~~~~~~~~~~~~~~~~~~~~~~~~~~~~~~~~~~~~~
#~~~~~~~~~~~  EQUATION FOR Cmax,ss FOR 1 CMT PK MODEL IF CMAX IS THE PD DRIVER ~~~~~~~~~~~~~~~~~~~~~~~
#~~~~~~~~~~~~~~~~~~~~~~~~~~~~~~~~~~~~~~~~~~~~~~~~~~~~~~~~~~~~~~~~~~~~~~~~~~~~~~~~~~~~~~~
```

```
# ke     <-  function(cl,v)      cl/v
# acr.ka <-  function(ka,tau)    1/(1-exp(-ka*tau))
# acr.ke <-  function(cl,v,tau)  1/(1-exp(-ke(cl,v)*tau))
#  css<-function(cl,v,ka,tau,dose,time) ((dose*ka)/(v*(ka-ke(cl,v))))*((exp(-ke(cl,v)*time)*acr.ke(cl,v,tau))-(exp(-ka*time)*acr.ka(ka,tau)))
# tmax<-function(cl,v,ka,tau) log((ka*(1-exp(-ke(cl,v)*tau))/(ke(cl,v)*(1-exp(-ka*tau))))/(ka-ke(cl,v))
# cmaxss<-function(cl,v,ka,tau,dose,...) css(cl,v,ka,tau,dose,tmax(cl,v,ka,tau))
#~~~~~~~~~~~~~~~~~~~~~~~~~~~~~~~~~~~~~~~~~~~~~~~~~~~~~~~~~~~~~~~~~~~~~~~~~~~~~~~~~~~~~~~~~~~~~~~~~~~~~
#~~~~~~~~~~~~~~~~~~~~~~~~~   FRACTIONAL TARGET ATTAINMENT   ~~~~~~~~~~~~~~~~~~~~~~~~~~~~~~~~~~~~~~~~~~~
#~~~~~~~~~~~~~~~~~~~~~~~~~~~~~~~~~~~~~~~~~~~~~~~~~~~~~~~~~~~~~~~~~~~~~~~~~~~~~~~~~~~~~~~~~~~~~~~~~~~~~~~
AUC=AUCMICTarget*MIC          # AUC target at each MIC # REPLACE WITH CMAXMICTarget Target IF CMAX DRIVE PD
MIC.length=length(MIC)        # Number of MIC values
FTAR<-numeric(MIC.length)  # Store FTARs at each MIC in a numeric vector
for (q in 1:MIC.length)       # FTAR at each MIC is calculated
{FTAR[q]=(sum(auc >= AUC[q]))*100/nSubj} # % of AUCs >= Target @ each MIC
#~~~~~~~~~~~~~~~~~~~~~~~~~~~~~~~~~~~~~~~~~~~~~~~~~~~~~~~~~~~~~~~~~~~~~~~~~~~~~~~~~~~~~~~~~~~~~~~~~~~~~~
#~~~~~~~~~~~~~~~~~~~~~~~~   PLOT FRACTIONAL TARGET ATTAINMENT   ~~~~~~~~~~~~~~~~~~~~~~~~~~~~~~~~~~~~~~~
#~~~~~~~~~~~~~~~~~~~~~~~~~~~~~~~~~~~~~~~~~~~~~~~~~~~~~~~~~~~~~~~~~~~~~~~~~~~~~~~~~~~~~~~~~~~~~~~~~~~~~~~
par(pty="s")
plot(MIC,FTAR,axes=F,xlab="MIC (ug/mL)",ylab="Fractional Target Attainment",log="x",cex=1.5, type="b", pch=16)
axis(2); axis(1, at=MIC, labels=as.character(MIC));box()
#~~~~~~~~~~~~~~~~~~~~~~~~~~~~~~~~~~~~~~~~~~~~~~~~~~~~~~~~~~~~~~~~~~~~~~~~~~~~~~~~~~~~~~~~~~~~~~~~~~~~~~
#~~~~~~~~~~ CALCULATE TARGET ATTAINMENT RATE ACROSS BUG VARIABILITY ~~~~~~~~~~~~~~~~~~~~~~~~~~~~~~~~~
#~~~~~~~~~~~~~~~~~~~~~~~~~~~~~~~~~~~~~~~~~~~~~~~~~~~~~~~~~~~~~~~~~~~~~~~~~~~~~~~~~~~~~~~~~~~~~~~~~~~~~~~
POF=NULL                      # Reserve a name for product of fractions
for (y in 1:bug.types)     # Loop for 5 Bug types
{POF2<-FTAR*freq.all[,y]; POF<-cbind(POF,POF2)}       # POF=FTAR*bug.freq
(SUM.FOR.EACH.BUG<- apply(POF, 2, sum))  # Sum of POFs
(SUM.CORRECTED.NAT.OCCURANCE<-SUM.FOR.EACH.BUG*nat.occ) # Nat.Occurrence
(FINAL.TAR<-sum(SUM.CORRECTED.NAT.OCCURANCE))          # Sum for 5 Bugs
#~~~~~~~~~~~~~~~~~~~~~~~~~~~~~~~~~~~~~~~~~~~~~~~~~~~~~~~~~~~~~~~~~~~~~~~~~~~~~~~~~~~~~~~~~~~~~~~~~~~~~~
#~~~~~~~~~~ RERUN THE CODE (OR PUT IT IN A LOOP) FOR A DIFFERENT DOSE, REGIMEN, FORMULATION, OR PK/PD TARGET ~~~~~~~~~~
#~~~~~~~~~~~~~~~~~~~~~~~~~~~~~~~~~~~~~~~~~~~~~~~~~~~~~~~~~~~~~~~~~~~~~~~~~~~~~~~~~~~~~~~~~~~~~~~~~~~~~~
```

APPENDIX 1B

The R Code for Monte Carlo Simulation based on a drug with %T>MIC as the PK/PD metric. The computations are performed to calculate fractional target attainment. Computations beyond fractional target attainment are identical to those illustrated in Appendix 1a (See Section "calculate target attainment rate across bug variability" in the code shown above). These simulations illustrate how fractional attainment can be computed across various thresholds of 25 to 35% T>MIC as well.

```
################################################################################
#                   Anti-Infective Code - 2 CM IV Infusion
#                         Clean-up & Set Seed
#                          GENERAL SETTINGS
################################################################################

rm(list=ls(all=TRUE))# Clean up WD
set.seed(555)        # Will allow simulation to be regenerated in future

################################################################################
#                    Constants and Dosing Regimens
################################################################################

nSubj       <-    5000             # Number of Subjects
Period      <-    8                # Interdosing interval in hours
nObs        <-    Period/0.1       # Number of Observations
Div         <-    500              # Dose in mg for IV infusion
Inf.time    <-    1                # Duration of the infusion
KO          <-    Div/Inf.time     # Infusion time in hour
TIME        <-    seq(0.1,Period,length=nObs)   # SAMPLING TIMES (HRs)
TAU         <-    TIME             # Switching variable for PK function
SUBSET      <-    TAU>Inf.time     # Find time when to switch off Infusion
TAU[SUBSET] <-    Inf.time        # TAU=Time if t.le.Inf.time else TAU=Inf.time
fup         <-    (100-8.5)/100    # Free fraction in plasma
MIC         <-    c(0.0625,0.125,0.25,0.5,  1,2,4,8,16)
```

```
############################################################################################
#                                    OMEGA MATRIX
############################################################################################

   symmat<-function(a) {
   npar <- round((sqrt(8*length(a)+1)-1)/2)
   sel <- 0
   b <- matrix(0,ncol=npar,nrow=npar)
   for (i in seq(npar)) {
     for (j in seq(i)) {
       sel <- sel+1
       b[i,j] <- a[sel] } }
   for (i in seq(npar-1)) {
     for (j in seq(npar-i)) {
       sel <- j+i
       b[i,sel] <- b[sel,i] } }
   b }


 omega=symmat(c(3.70E-02,
               3.49E-02,  3.66E-02,
               0.00E+00,  0.00E+00,  1.73E-01,
               0.00E+00,  0.00E+00,  9.24E-02,  6.16E-02,
               0.00E+00,  0.00E+00,  0.00E+00,  0.00E+00,  2.20E-02,
               0.00E+00,  0.00E+00,  0.00E+00,  0.00E+00,  0.00E+00,  3.44E-02,
               0.00E+00,  0.00E+00,  0.00E+00,  0.00E+00,  0.00E+00,  0.00E+00,  9.11E-02      ))

############################################################################################
#                      Simulate Demographics and Individual PK
############################################################################################
# Preferably sample from a database of covariates and sample rows of covariates to maintain
# correlation between covariates. This is an example code for sampling rows of covariates
  # demographics=Nonmem.Data[!duplicated(Nonmem.Data$ID),c("CRCL","AGE","RACE","WT")]
  # mix.it.up=sort(sample(1:nrow(demographics), nSubj, replace=T))
  # demographics=demographics[mix.it.up,]
  # list2env(setNames(split(as.matrix(demographics),
  #                    col(demographics)), names(demographics)), envir=.GlobalEnv)
# Split the dataset by column after converting to matrix, set the names (setNames)
# and use list2env to assign the objects in the global environment
# http://stackoverflow.com/questions/28221755/how-to-split-a-r-data-frame-into-vectors-unbind
############################################################################################

   repeat{ CRCL=100+rnorm(nSubj,mean=0,sd=30)
   if ((length(which(CRCL<0)))==0){break} }      # Simulate only positive values of CRCL
   AGE=runif(n=nSubj,min=20,max=80)              # Uniform Distribution for AGE
   RACE=sample(1:4,size=nSubj,replace = T,prob = c(0.8,0.05,0.1,0.05))
   WT       =70*exp(rnorm(n = nSubj,mean = 0, sd=0.3)) # Log normal distribution for weight

   CLRACE=RACE
   SUBSET1 <- CLRACE==1
   SUBSET2 <- CLRACE==2
   SUBSET3 <- CLRACE==3
   SUBSET4 <- CLRACE==4
   CLRACE[SUBSET1]     <-       0
   CLRACE[SUBSET2]     <-       0.0204
   CLRACE[SUBSET3]     <-       0.163
   CLRACE[SUBSET4]     <-      -0.0445

   CLCOV=(1+CLRACE)
   TVCL1=13.6*((CRCL/98)^0.659)
   TVCL=TVCL1*CLCOV
   TVV1=11.6*((WT/73)^0.596)
   TVQ =4.74*((WT/73)^1.06)
   TVV2=6.04*((WT/73)^0.84)*((AGE/40)^0.307)*((CRCL/98)^0.417)

   THETA.IND <- matrix(rep(0,nSubj*4), nrow=nSubj)
   CONC      <- matrix(rep(0,nSubj*nObs), nrow=nSubj)
   library(mvtnorm)
   eta <- rmvnorm(nSubj, mean=rep(0,7), omega)
   BSV =eta[,1]
   ISV =eta[,2]
   IKV =eta[,4]
   BOV =eta[,5]
   IOV =eta[,6]
   IGV =eta[,7]
```

```
CLVAR=BSV+BOV
VCVAR=ISV+IOV
VPVAR=IKV+IGV
QVAR=eta[,3]

THETA.IND[,1]=TVCL*exp(CLVAR)
THETA.IND[,2]=TVV1*exp(VCVAR)
THETA.IND[,3]=TVV2*exp(VPVAR)
THETA.IND[,4]=TVQ *exp(QVAR)

for(I in 1:nSubj) {
    CL   <- THETA.IND[I,1]
    VC   <- THETA.IND[I,2]
    VP   <- THETA.IND[I,3]
    Q    <- THETA.IND[I,4]
    K10 <- CL /VC
    K12 <- Q/VC
    K21 <- Q/VP
    Beta <- 0.5*(K12+K21+K10-((K12+K21+K10)^2-4*K21*K10)^0.5)
    Alfa <- 0.5*(K12+K21+K10+((K12+K21+K10)^2-4*K21*K10)^0.5)

    TERM1=KO/(VC*(Alfa-Beta))
    TERM2=(K21-Alfa)/Alfa
    TERM3=1-(exp(Alfa*TAU))
    TERM4=(Beta-K21)/Beta
    TERM5=1-(exp(Beta*TAU))
    TERM6=exp(-Alfa*TIME)
    TERM7=exp(-Beta*TIME)
    CONC[I,] <-  (TERM1*TERM2*TERM3*TERM6+TERM1*TERM4*TERM5*TERM7)*fup   }
yquantiles = apply(CONC,2,quantile, probs=c(.025, .5, .975))

par(pty="s",tck=-0.01)
plot(1,1,axes=F,log="y",type="n",xlab="Time (hr)",ylab="Free Conc. (mg/L)",xlim=range(TIME),ylim=c(.06,64))
    lines(TIME,yquantiles[1,],lwd=2, col=2, lty=3) ; lines(TIME,yquantiles[2,],lwd=4, col=1); lines(TIME,yquantiles[3,],lwd=2, col=2,
            lty=3)
    axis(1, cex=.8, at=seq(0,Period,1), labels=as.character(seq(0,Period,1)));
    axis(2, at=c(MIC,32,64), labels=as.character(round(c(MIC,32,64),2)), cex=.8,las=2)

    mtext(side=3, "Median & 95% Prediction Interval" , at=Period/2, cex=1)
    box()

#########################################################################################
#                                  %Time > MIC
#########################################################################################

    MIC.length=length(MIC)
    Tper       <- matrix(rep(0,nSubj*MIC.length), nrow=nSubj)

    for (q in 1:MIC.length)
    {for (m in 1:nSubj) {
        Tper[m,q] <- length(CONC[m,][CONC[m,]>=MIC[q]])/(nObs)*100       # % Time when conc > MIC
    }}

#########################################################################################
#                            FRACTIONAL TARGET ATTAINMENT
#########################################################################################

    Threshold=c(25,30, 35)
    Threshold.length=length(Threshold)
    FTAR      <- matrix(rep(0,Threshold.length*MIC.length), nrow=MIC.length)

    for (s in 1:Threshold.length)     {
      for (r in 1:MIC.length) {
        FTAR[r,s]= length(Tper[,r][Tper[,r]>=Threshold[s]])/nSubj
      }     }

    plot(1,1, axes=F,xlab="MIC (mg/L)", ylab="Fractional Target Attainment ", xlim=range(MIC), ylim=c(0,1), log="x", type="n")

    for (tt in 1:Threshold.length)
    {lines(MIC,FTAR[,tt],pch=tt,cex=1.2,col=tt, type="b")}
    axis(2, cex=.8,at=seq(0,1,.1), labels=as.character(round(seq(0,1,.1),1)))
    axis(1, at=MIC, labels=as.character(round(MIC,2)), cex=.8)

    threshkey=paste0("PD Threshold ",as.character(Threshold),"%")
    legend ("bottomleft",legend =threshkey,bty="n", cex=.9,pch=1:3,col=1:3)
    box()
```

REFERENCES

[1]   Drusano GL, Preston SL, Hardalo C, *et al.* Use of preclinical data for selection of a phase II/III dose for evernimicin and identification of a preclinical MIC breakpoint. Antimicrob Agents Chemother 2001; 45(1): 13-22.
[http://dx.doi.org/10.1128/AAC.45.1.13-22.2001] [PMID: 11120938]

[2]   Drusano GL. Antimicrobial pharmacodynamics: critical interactions of 'bug and drug'. Nat Rev Microbiol 2004; 2(4): 289-300.
[http://dx.doi.org/10.1038/nrmicro862] [PMID: 15031728]

[3]   Ambrose PG. Monte Carlo simulation in the evaluation of susceptibility breakpoints: predicting the future: insights from the society of infectious diseases pharmacists. Pharmacotherapy 2006; 26(1): 129-34.
[http://dx.doi.org/10.1592/phco.2006.26.1.129] [PMID: 16506354]

[4]   Liu P, Allaudeen H, Chandra R, *et al.* Comparative pharmacokinetics of azithromycin in serum and white blood cells of healthy subjects receiving a single-dose extended-release regimen *versus* a 3-day immediate-release regimen. Antimicrob Agents Chemother 2007; 51(1): 103-9.
[http://dx.doi.org/10.1128/AAC.00852-06] [PMID: 17060516]

[5]   Craig WA. Pharmacokinetic/pharmacodynamic parameters: rationale for antibacterial dosing of mice and men. Clin Infect Dis 1998; 26(1): 1-10.
[http://dx.doi.org/10.1086/516284] [PMID: 9455502]

[6]   Sánchez-Navarro A, Sánchez Recio MM. Basis of anti-infective therapy: pharmacokinetic-pharmacodynamic criteria and methodology for dual dosage individualisation. Clin Pharmacokinet 1999; 37(4): 289-304.
[http://dx.doi.org/10.2165/00003088-199937040-00002] [PMID: 10554046]

[7]   Kimko H, Xu X, Nandy P, *et al.* Pharmacodynamic profiling of ceftobiprole for treatment of complicated skin and skin structure infections. Antimicrob Agents Chemother 2009; 53(8): 3371-4.
[http://dx.doi.org/10.1128/AAC.01653-08] [PMID: 19528285]

[8]   Farrell DJ, Flamm RK, Sader HS, Jones RN. Ceftobiprole activity against over 60,000 clinical bacterial pathogens isolated in Europe, Turkey, and Israel from 2005 to 2010. Antimicrob Agents Chemother 2014; 58(7): 3882-8.
[http://dx.doi.org/10.1128/AAC.02465-14] [PMID: 24777091]

[9]   Dudley MN, Griffith D. Animal models of infection for the study of antibiotic pharmacodynamics. In: Nightingale CH, Murakawa T, Ambrose PG, Eds. Antimicrobial Pharmacodynamics in Theory and Clinical Practice. New York: MacGraw Hill 2002; pp. 67-97.

[10]   Craig WA. Draft report of the pharmacodynamic activities of RWJ-416457. Internal Report 2006.

[11]   Nandy P, Samtani MN, Lin R. Population pharmacokinetics of doripenem based on data from phase 1 studies with healthy volunteers and phase 2 and 3 studies with critically ill patients. Antimicrob Agents Chemother 2010; 54(6): 2354-9.
[http://dx.doi.org/10.1128/AAC.01649-09] [PMID: 20385854]

[12]   European Agency for the Evaluation of Medicinal Products, Committee for Proprietary Medicinal Products 2011. http://www.ema.europa.eu/docs/en_GB/document_library/Scientific_guideline/2009/09/WC500003417.pdf

[13]   Landersdorfer CB, Ly NS, Xu H, Tsuji BT, Bulitta JB. Quantifying subpopulation synergy for antibiotic combinations *via* mechanism-based modeling and a sequential dosing design. Antimicrob Agents Chemother 2013; 57(5): 2343-51.
[http://dx.doi.org/10.1128/AAC.00092-13] [PMID: 23478962]

[14]   Das S, Li J, Riccobene T, *et al.* Dose selection and validation for Ceftazidime-Avibactam in adults with complicated intra-abdominal infections, complicated urinary tract infections, and nosocomial pneumonia. Antimicrob Agents Chemother 2019; 63(4): e02187-18.
[http://dx.doi.org/10.1128/AAC.02187-18] [PMID: 30670413]

[15]   Bulitta JB, Hope WW, Eakin AE, *et al.* Generating robust and informative nonclinical *in vitro* and *in vivo.* bacterial infection model efficacy data to support translation to humans. Antimicrob Agents Chemother 2019; 63(5): e02307-18.
[http://dx.doi.org/10.1128/AAC.02307-18] [PMID: 30833428]

[16]   Rizk ML, Bhavnani SM, Drusano G, *et al.* Considerations for dose selection and clinical pharmacokinetics/pharmacodynamics for the development of antibacterial agents. Antimicrob Agents Chemother 2019; 63(5): e02309-18.
[http://dx.doi.org/10.1128/AAC.02309-18] [PMID: 30833427]

[17]   Preston SL, Piliero PJ, Bilello JA, Stein DS, Symonds WT, Drusano GL. *In vitro-in vivo.* model for evaluating the antiviral activity of amprenavir in combination with ritonavir administered at 600 and 100 milligrams, respectively, every 12 hours. Antimicrob Agents Chemother 2003; 47(11): 3393-9.

[http://dx.doi.org/10.1128/AAC.47.11.3393-3399.2003] [PMID: 14576093]

[18]   Gomeni R, Xu T, Gao X, Bressolle-Gomeni F. Model based approach for estimating the dosage regimen of indomethacin a potential antiviral treatment of patients infected with SARS CoV-2. J Pharmacokinet Pharmacodyn 2020; 47(3): 189-98.
[http://dx.doi.org/10.1007/s10928-020-09690-4] [PMID: 32435882]

[19]   So AD, Gupta N, Brahmachari SK, *et al.* Towards new business models for R&D for novel antibiotics. Drug Resist Updat 2011; 14(2): 88-94.
[http://dx.doi.org/10.1016/j.drup.2011.01.006] [PMID: 21439891]

[20]   Årdal C, Lacotte Y, Ploy MC. Financing Pull mechanisms for antibiotic-related innovation: opportunities for Europe. Clin Infect Dis 2020; 71(8): 1994-9.
[http://dx.doi.org/10.1093/cid/ciaa153] [PMID: 32060511]

[21]   Jumbe N, Louie A, Leary R, *et al.* Application of a mathematical model to prevent *in vivo.* amplification of antibiotic-resistant bacterial populations during therapy. J Clin Invest 2003; 112(2): 275-85.
[http://dx.doi.org/10.1172/JCI200316814] [PMID: 12865415]

[22]   Sumi CD, Heffernan AJ, Lipman J, Roberts JA, Sime FB. What antibiotic exposures are required to suppress the emergence of resistance for gram-negative bacteria? A Systematic Review. Clin Pharmacokinet 2019; 58(11): 1407-43.
[http://dx.doi.org/10.1007/s40262-019-00791-z] [PMID: 31325141]

[23]   Bhavnani SM, Hammel JP, Cirincione BB, Wikler MA, Ambrose PG. Use of pharmacokinetic-pharmacodynamic target attainment analyses to support phase 2 and 3 dosing strategies for doripenem. Antimicrob Agents Chemother 2005; 49(9): 3944-7.
[http://dx.doi.org/10.1128/AAC.49.9.3944-3947.2005] [PMID: 16127078]

[24]   Samtani MN, Flamm R, Kaniga K, Nandy P. Pharmacokinetic-pharmacodynamic-model-guided doripenem dosing in critically ill patients. Antimicrob Agents Chemother 2010; 54(6): 2360-4.
[http://dx.doi.org/10.1128/AAC.01843-09] [PMID: 20385857]

[25]   Samtani MN, Vaccaro N, Cirillo I, Matzke GR, Redman R, Nandy P. Doripenem dosing recommendations for critically ill patients receiving continuous renal replacement therapy. ISRN Pharmacol 2012; 2012: 782656.
[http://dx.doi.org/10.5402/2012/782656] [PMID: 22888451]

[26]   Perez-Ruixo JJ, Cox E, De Ridder F, *et al.* Simulation in clinical drug development. In: Bertau M, Mosekilde E, Westerhoff H, Eds. Biosimulation in Drug Development. Weinheim: Wiley-VCH 2007; pp. 1-24.
[http://dx.doi.org/10.1002/9783527622672.ch1]

CHAPTER 2

Post-Translational Modifications: Host Defence Mechanism, Pathogenic Weapon, and Emerged Target of Anti-Infective Drugs

Maria Amprazi[1,2,#], **Anastasia Tomatsidou**[3,4,#], **Dimitra Paliogianni**[5,#] and **Vasiliki E. Fadouloglou**[6,*]

[1] *Institute of Molecular Biology and Biotechnology, Foundation of Research and Technology-Hellas, Heraklion, Crete, Greece*

[2] *Department of Biology, University of Crete, Heraklion, Crete, Greece*

[3] *Howard Taylor Ricketts Laboratory, Argonne National Laboratory, Lemont, Illinois, USA*

[4] *Department of Microbiology, University of Chicago, Chicago, Illinois, USA*

[5] *Institute of Molecular Cell and Systems Biology, College of Medical, Veterinary & Life Sciences, University of Glasgow, Glasgow G12 8QQ, UK*

[6] *Department of Molecular Biology and Genetics, Democritus University of Thrace, Dragana University Campus, Alexandroupolis 68100, Evros, Greece*

Abstract: Post-translational modifications are changes introduced to proteins after their translation. They are the means to generate molecular diversity, expand protein function, control catalytic activity and trigger quick responses to a wide range of stimuli. Moreover, they regulate numerous biological processes, including pathogen invasion and host defence mechanisms. It is well established that bacteria and viruses utilize post-translational modifications on their own or their host's proteins to advance their pathogenicity. Doing so, they evade immune responses, target signaling pathways and manipulate host cytoskeleton to achieve survival, replication and propagation. Many bacterial species secrete virulence factors into the host and mediate host-pathogen interactions by inducing post-translational modifications that subvert fundamental cellular processes. Viral pathogens also utilize post translational modifications in order to overcome the host defence mechanisms and hijack its cellular machinery for their replication and propagation. For example, many coronavirus proteins are modified to achieve host invasion, evasion of immune responses and utilization of the host translational machinery. PTMs are also considered potential targets for the development of novel therapeutics from natural products with antibiotic properties, like lasso peptides and lantibiotics. The last decade, significant progress was made in understanding the mechanisms that govern PTMs and mediate regulation of

---

[*] **Corresponding author Vasiliki E. Fadouloglou:** Department of Molecular Biology and Genetics, Democritus University of Thrace, Dragana University Campus, Alexandroupolis 68100, Evros, Greece; Tel: +302551030640; E-mail: fadoulog@mbg.duth.gr
[#] These authors have equal contribution.

Atta-ur-Rahman, *FRS* and M. Iqbal Choudhary (Eds.)
All rights reserved-© 2021 Bentham Science Publishers

protein structure and function. This urges the identification of relevant molecular targets, the design of specific drugs and the discovery of PTM-based medicine. Therefore, PTMs emerge as a highly promising field for the investigation and discovery of new therapeutics for many infectious diseases.

Keywords: ADP-ribosylation, Antimicrobial drugs, Antiviral drugs, Bacterial effector proteins, Bioengineering, Biopharmaceuticals, Coronavirus, Deamidation, Drug target, Elimination, Glycosylation, Host invasion, Innate immunity, Lantibiotics, Lipidation, Natural antimicrobial peptides, Palmitoylation, Pathogenic bacteria, RiPPs, Secretion systems, Spike protein, Thiopeptides, Ubiquitination, Vaccine design.

INTRODUCTION

After translation at the ribosome, proteins may undergo chemical changes on their amino acids. These changes are called post-translational modifications (PTMs); they display a high diversity and enumerate several hundreds of different kinds [1]. It is expected that their number will be substantially increased in the future along with the advances in technology such as the development of mass spectrometry and proteomics. PTMs can be reversible or irreversible, enzymatically or non-enzymatically catalyzed additions of diverse chemical groups ranging from small moieties to full proteins. These groups are usually added to the side chains, even though they can be linked to main chain atoms as well. Moreover, PTMs include the formation or cleavage of chemical bonds. Again, the new bonds may link side-chain or side-chain to main-chain atoms. Proteolysis is the most trivial example of chemical bond cleavage and disulfide bonds the most common, post-translational, side-chain cross links.

On the molecular level, PTMs may have multiple roles influencing the protein function, the structural stability, or the interaction network of the modified molecule. It has been shown that the addition of small, polar moieties such as hydroxyl-groups in the active site or around the active site of enzymes may increase their catalytic activity by, for example, stabilizing the transition state [2 - 4]. On the contrary, such an addition can cause the opposite effect and inactivate an enzyme if the new group of atoms is located in a place that blocks accessibility of the active site. Likewise, modification of a residue, crucial for the catalysis, will probably result in attenuation or full inactivation of the enzymatic catalysis. The formation of cross-links between different parts of a molecule or alterations to the backbone stereochemistry may increase the molecular rigidity and consequently affect structural stability and flexibility. Often, PTMs result in changes in physicochemical properties [5]. For instance, phosphorylations and deamidations usually add negative charges, Lys acylations eliminate positive charges, hydroxylations increase the hydrophilicity, while lipidations increase the hydrophobicity of the modification site. These alterations may affect the interaction network of the protein either by introducing constraints that block existent interaction interfaces or by creating novel sites for interactions.

On the cellular level, PTMs are widely used as regulatory factors during multiple physiological processes [6]. Phosphorylation/dephosphorylation is a text-book paradigm of how a PTM may undertake a major regulatory role in signaling pathways. Likewise, histone modifications, primarily through Lys methylation and acetylation, is an essential regulatory mechanism, which controls gene-transcription activation and inactivation. Glycosylation is another well-known PTM which plays a fundamental role in molecular recognition and activation of immune response. In line with well-established knowledge, research in the last decade has discovered novel aspects of PTM biology and has demonstrated its significance and implication in more processes than it was originally expected. There are three properties that render PTMs an ideal control-switch for biological regulation. First, PTMs are usually reversible and therefore highly dynamic. Second, they do not necessarily affect the whole molecular population but just a part of it. Last, they are produced directly on site, where they are needed. This enables the cell to respond quickly and on-demand to many stimuli. We know today that this mechanism is involved in cell homeostasis, adaptation to environmental or intracellular changes including cell stress, as well as cell defence, beyond the typical glycosylation.

Not surprisingly, many pathogens, including bacteria and viruses, use PTM-based strategies to subvert eukaryotic defense and dominate their hosts [7 - 10]. Several recent studies, based on proteomics and mass spectrometry assays, indicate substantial differences in post-translationally modified proteome upon pathogen-host interactions and during infection. Pathogens can post-translationally modify their and their host's proteomes. It has been shown for example, that *Leptospira* is adapted to the host during infection by modulating both protein expression and protein PTMs, including methylation and acetylation [11]. On the other hand, the *Listeria* toxin Listeriolysin induces changes to the host proteome *via* PTMs [12]. In particular, extensive alterations of components of the host ubiquitin machinery were observed in response to the toxin. Last, a proteome comparison of virulent and attenuated *Ehrlichia* demonstrates important differences in phosphorylation and glycosylation [13]. These differences are indicative of dependence on the host interactions.

During invasion, pathogens translocate an arsenal of effectors inside the host cytosol [14 - 16]. A subset of them, in some organisms a noteworthy subset, is related with PTMs. Once within the host, these proteins can either cause modifications to the eukaryotic proteins or undergo modifications as substrates of the host PTM-network [17]. In any case, the induced alterations work for the pathogen's advantage and result in subverting eukaryotic mechanisms and promoting microbial survival and replication. Obviously, they are complicated procedures which involve many protein partners, and often a single effector is implicated and regulate more than one processes. In many cases, pathogen virulence depends on a multitude of PTMs, as for example phosphorylation, glycosylation, ubiquitination, sumoylation, acylation, lipidation, ADP-ribosylation, AMPylation, deamidation, eliminylation *etc*, (Fig. **1**) [7].

Given the extent and significance of PTMs for virulence, it is obvious that a deep knowledge of the mechanisms underlying PTM-based pathogenic strategies is critical to understand infectious pathogenicity. Hence, PTMs have been considered to be potential drug targets for developing new therapeutics for a wide range of infectious diseases. Especially the significant progress of the last decade, which has shed light to multiple aspects of how PTMs are used to target key regulatory pathways in the host, has significantly strengthen the potential of PTM-based drug design. Such therapeutics would have the advantage of high selectivity since they would probably be able to act not only on a specific molecule but also on a specific time and cellular location, where this molecule would be produced at a specific time-window of the cell cycle. The identification of relevant molecular targets, the design of specific drugs and the discovery of medicine based on PTMs is an exciting and highly promising field.

In this chapter, the significance of PTMs in processes of eukaryotic defence including innate and adaptive immunity and microbial pathogenicity is highlighted. Examples from highly infectious species of bacteria such as the *Yersinia, Pseudomonas, Legionella, Salmonella, Shigella* and others as well as the coronavirus, the causative agent of the new pandemic, are used. The emerging potential of the PTM-based drug design for infectious diseases with particular reference to natural products with antimicrobial activity is also extensively covered. We emphasize on mechanisms and host-pathogen interactions which either have newly emerged or they had a substantial progress during the last decade. Our aim is to point out the complexity, adaptability and sophistication of the mechanisms involved in host-pathogen interactions during infection at the level of PTM-based interactions. Significant progress, covered by extensive literature, has been made in the topic the past decade. We often refer the reader to excellent, recent reviews diving into specific areas of the field.

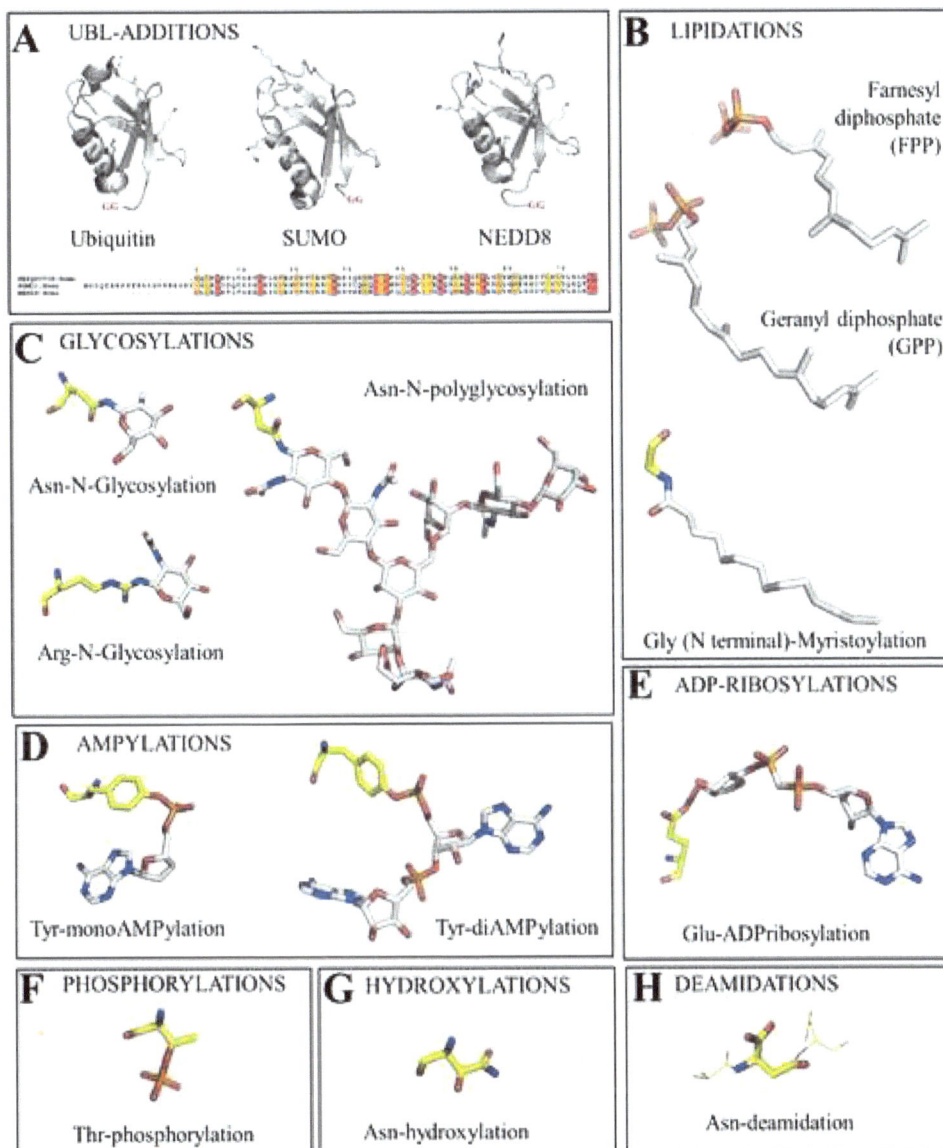

Fig. (1). Overview of the most important modifications that are extensively discussed in this chapter (A-H). Carbon atoms are grey for the modifiers and yellow for the modified residues. Throughout the figure oxygens are red and nitrogens blue. The figure was prepared using PyMOL [18]. The sequence alignment was performed using the program T-COFFEE [19] and the ENDscript server [20].

PTMS IN THE FRONTLINE OF EUKARYOTIC DEFENCE AND PATHOGENIC INVASION

The mammalian immune system comprises of an intricate network of interactions, fine-tuned to avoid various types of invaders. PTMs are in the forefront of these defence mechanisms, taking part in pathogen recognition, protein activation and translocation [21]. Innate and adaptive immunity responses act in synergy to fend off pathogenic threats. Innate immunity is the first line of defence, unleashing a generalized attack upon the invading microbes, while adaptive immunity is specific to the invading pathogen with the help of antibodies [22, 23].

Innate Immunity

Innate immunity is responsible for discriminating against non-endogenous components, which are recognised by pattern-recognition receptors (PRRs). PRRs can sense "non-self" factors by detecting pathogen-associated molecular patterns (PAMPs) and danger-associated molecular patterns (DAMPs) from infectious pathogens and injured host cells, respectively. The main categories of PRRs are toll-like receptors (TLRs), retinoic-acid-inducible gene I (RIG-I)-like receptors (RLRs), nucleotide-binding domain and leucine-rich repeat containing molecules (NLRs), c-type lectin receptors (CLRs) and cyclic GMP/AMP synthase (cGAS) [23, 24].

Upon pathogen detection, two main pathways are activated, the interferon (IFN) regulatory factor (IRF) pathway and the nuclear factor κB (NF-κB) pathway, along with inflammatory responses [25, 26]. It has been demonstrated in earlier reviews that the same pathogenic stimuli can be recognised by more than one receptors and more than two receptors can share the same signalling pathway or lead to the same host effector response [27, 28]. The immune response signalling pathways are so complex and intertwined that there are many ways to categorise their components. PRRs can be distinguished based on their cellular localisation, their pathogen/ligand discrimination, the downstream signalling pathway they are involved in, or the PTMs that govern and guide the immune responses. These all have been studied in previous reviews [10, 21, 27 - 30] and here we will try to present a concise guide of the immune responses triggered upon pathogenic infection and based on PTMs. We will focus on TLRs, NLRs, RLRs and the cGAS sensor as they are the most commonly and extensively studied.

TLRs are membrane bound receptors that recognise a variety of microbial pathogenic patterns and activate both NF-κB and IRF pathways [31]. TLRs are often accompanied by adaptor proteins. All TLRs docked on the cytoplasmic membrane interact with MyD88, which is the signal mediator for the NF-κB pathway [32]. The NF-κB pathway involves mitogen-activated protein kinases (MAPKs) and IκB kinases (IKKs) leading to the production of inflammatory cytokines and subsequently to an increased blood flow and recruitment of phagocytes to the infection sites [21, 25, 33]. The phosphorylated IκB is targeted for degradation allowing for NF-κB translocation to the nucleus and expression of pro-inflammatory molecules [34]. On the other hand, TLRs able to sense viruses, as well as endosomal TLR4, are partnered with the adaptor TRIF, a dual inducer of both NF-κB and IFN pathways [31, 35, 36]. TRIF phosphorylation leads to the recruitment of interferon regulatory factor 3 (IRF3) [37]. IRF3 in turn, gets activated *via* phosphorylation by TBK1, dimerises through the same phosphorylation site and is translocated to the nucleus to induce production of IFNs [37]. Another example of PTMs, present in key signalling positions, involves TLR3 which resides on the membrane of endosomes and binds to dsRNA. The crystal structure revealed that the TLR3 molecule is heavily glycosylated in Asn residues and one of them (Asn413) directly interacts with the dsRNA (Fig. **2**) [38]. Point mutations of Asn413 dampen RNA sensing [39] which was also confirmed by studies on hepatitis viruses [40].

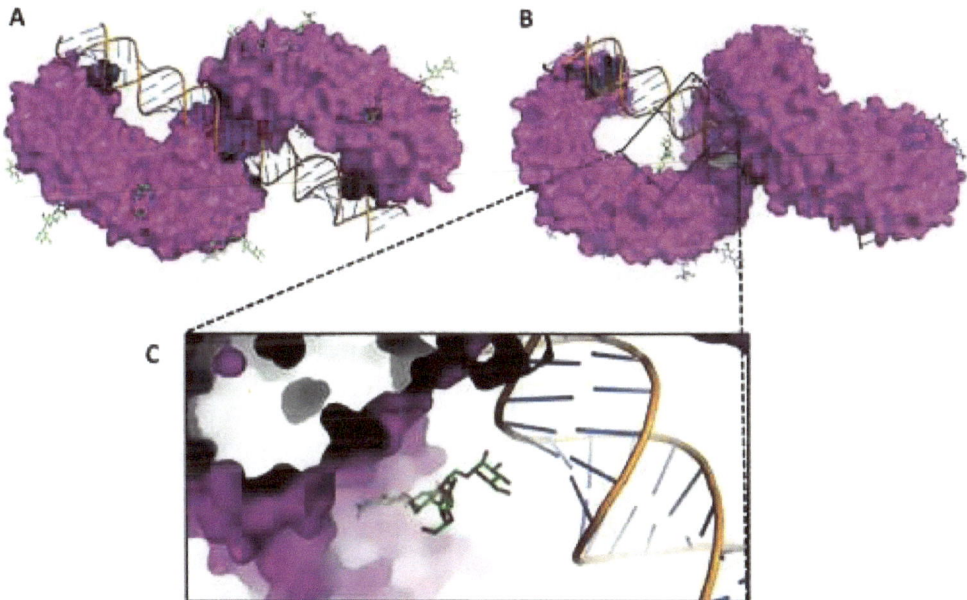

Fig. (2). Crystal structure of the TLR3 receptor/dsRNA complex. **(A)** Surface represention of the dimeric TRLR3 in complex with dsRNA. TLR3 is heavily glycosylated on Asp residues. The glycans are shown in green sticks. **(B)** The TLR dimer is slightly rotated relative to **(A)** to clearly show the Asn413-dsRNA interaction. Mutational analysis of Asn413 revealed diminished RNA sensing. **(C)** Close-up of the glycosylated Asn 413 interaction to dsRNA (PDB 3CIY). The figure was prepared using PyMOL [18].

NOD1 and NOD2 are the main pathogen and damage sensors in the cytoplasm. They induce NF-κB signalling and trigger inflammasome formation and activation of proinflammatory cytokines [41]. While other PRR types can trigger this signalling cascade [42], NRLs are also involved in the formation of the inflammasome complexes, along with other proteins, and mediate the recruitment and activation of caspase-1 *via* proteolytic cleavage [26, 43]. The activated caspase-1 activates proinflammatory cytokines *via* cleavage, leading to inflammation response and apoptosis [28, 44, 45]. Pathogenic PTMs influence PRR-dependent inflammatory responses by targeting innate sensors and downstream signalling molecules. The regulation of inflammatory responses is extremely important as it can cause side effects in human health [46 - 48].

RLRs are cytoplasmic dsRNA receptors that mediate type I IFN production through the adaptor protein MAVS [49]. The two major sensor proteins are RIG-I and melanoma differentiation-associated protein 5 (MDA5) and they detect 5'-tri-/di-phosphates of dsRNA in the cytoplasm through their C-terminal domain [50]. Upon ligand binding, RIG-I is activated *via* K63-ubiquitination, accompanied by conformational change and dimerization with MDA5 and MAVS [51]. Phosphorylation of MAVS leads to IRF3/7 and NF-κB pathway activation as well as to type I IFNs production, in a similar manner as described above for TLRs [37, 50, 52]. It also induces 14-3-3 regulatory proteins which interact with RIG-I in order to promote its ubiquitination and activation [53], proving that both ubiquitination and phosphorylation are essential in initiating RLR signalling. This interaction together with the PTMs that control antiviral responses are mere examples of the vast interactome network that is created upon viral invasion [53 - 55].

cGAS can function as an antiviral signalling component by sensing nucleic acids (dsDNA) in the cytoplasm [56]. It then catalyses the production of 2'-5'-linked cyclic GMP-AMP molecules that act as a second messenger [57]. This messenger is then transferred to neighbouring cells through junctions [58]. There, it activates STING *via* phosphorylation on Ser366 [37] and triggers an antiviral response *via* the type I IFN pathway [52]. In a recent study, the PTMs that decorate cGAS and participate in ligand binding and signal activation were characterized [59]. Acetylation of Lys384 in cGAS was observed in close proximity with the ligand DNA but further biochemical and functional experiments are needed to elucidate its actual role. Additionally, in the same study, acetylated Lys198 was shown to modulate cytokine production in the cGAS signalling pathway. Acetylation levels dropped upon viral infection [59].

Adaptive Immunity: Antibodies

The production of IgG antibodies from B-cells is considered to be a catalyst in adaptive immunity [60]. We will focus on the PTMs of IgG antibodies and not on the signalling pathway that induces their production which has been extensively reviewed elsewhere [61 - 64]. The structure and function of IgG antibodies is a well-established knowledge [65, 66]. An extensive network of disulfide bonds along the whole molecule reinforces structural stability. IgG antibodies are divided into four subclasses, IgG1-4, based on the different patterns of connection between the inter-chain disulfide bonds in the linker sequence between the C_H1 and C_H2 domains of each chain. A disulfide bond inter-connects the C_H1 and C_L domains provides additional stability for the formation of the antigen binding site. Many other intra-chain disulfide bonds are also present in every domain [67].

Another PTM that contributes to the integrity and activity of the IgG molecule is N-glycosylation, that occurs at the highly conserved Asp297 on the C_H2 portion of the Fc region. The glycans linked to the antibodies are initially structures rich in mannose molecules, which are later removed and replaced by specific monosaccharides [68]. Glycosylation also occurs in the Fab fragment of IgG in order to facilitate the identification of bacterial pathogens. Fab glycosylation constitutes the focus of several therapeutic development studies due to its role in regulating antibody function and antigen binding [69, 70].

Eukaryotic Regulatory Processes Are Pathogenic Targets

In order to establish infection, pathogenic bacteria must overcome host defence, inhibit production of antimicrobial factors and subvert fundamental host structures, such as actin cytoskeleton networks and membrane dynamics [71]. To do so, bacteria exploit effector proteins and toxins, which are usually transferred into the host cytosol, and once intracellularly, they are able to inhibit and/or manipulate central signalling pathways as those based on G-proteins, ubiquitin and ubiquitin-like protein modifications [72]. These pathways regulate fundamental cellular processes such as immune response and cell cycle and this explains why many pathogens have developed mechanisms to interfere with and interrupt them.

GTPase-mediated signalling is quite common in eukaryotes and regulates a plethora of processes and responses. For example, it is known that Rho family G proteins regulate actin dynamics and cytoskeletal rearrangement [73]. In particular, different members of this family have been related with different actin responses *i.e.* activation of Rho proteins leads to stress fiber formation, Rac is responsible for membrane ruffling and Cdc42 is involved in filopodia formation. Manipulating the host cytoskeleton is often used by intracellular pathogens to promote their entry, survival and proliferation into the host cell [74].

Ubiquitin (Ub) and ubiquitin-like proteins (Ubl), such as SUMO and NEDD8 (Fig. **1A**), are small, structurally homologous peptides which play major roles as regulatory proteins in eukaryotic organisms [75, 76]. Eukaryotes use these peptides to post-translationally modify substrate-proteins and change their structure, stability (half-life), catalytic activity and/or protein-protein interaction pattern. These modifications also target proteins for proteasome degradation, alter their cellular localization and trigger recognition and signalling networks since they can be recognized by eukaryotic receptor Ub/Ubl binding domains. Typically, ubiquitination involves the formation of a covalent isopeptide bond between the carboxy group of a C-terminal Gly (Fig. **1A**) residue on ubiquitin (Ub-Gly76) and the ε-amino group of a Lys residue on the target protein. Besides Lys, Ub can also be linked to the thiol or hydroxyl-groups of Cys or Thr/Ser residues, respectively or to the N-terminus of the substrate protein [77 - 79].

Moreover, Ub has seven lysine residues (Fig. **1A**) which serve as sites of self-ubiquitination and give rise to the formation of polyubiquitin chains [80]. Consequently, several patterns of ubiquitination are observed *i.e.,* protein substrates can be mono-ubiquitinated simply or multiply, or polyubiquitinated by Ub-chains. Similar to ubiquitination, other types of peptide (Ubl) additions, such as sumoylation and neddylation, can target protein substrates to modify their fate. The different patterns of ubiquitination or Ubl additions have very different effects on the fate of the modified substrate proteins. These proteins are usually involved in several, quite diverse cellular pathways such as the NF-κB pathway, autophagy, cytoskeleton dynamics and transcription factor regulation [75].

Ubiquitination and other Ubl additions are enzymatic, reversible modifications which require the consecutive activity of three different enzymes namely E1, E2 and E3 [75]. First, the carboxy terminal Ub-Gly is activated by ATP-dependent, E1 enzymes (Ub-activating enzymes). A thioester bond is formed between the Ub carboxy terminus and an active site Cys of E1. Then, the activated Ub is transferred to the active site Cys of the E2 enzyme (Ub-conjugating enzymes). Finally, E3 enzymes (E3 ligases) catalyse the bond formation between the carboxy group of the carboxyterminal Ub-Gly and the ε-amino group of a Lys residue on the target protein [81]. E3 ligases could be single-subunit or mutli-subunit complexes. The single-subunit E3 ligases have at least one of the following domains: HECT, RING or U-box, which are responsible for the interaction with the E2 enzymes. Mutli-subunit E3 complexes are for example the skp1-cullin-F-box (SCF) and the cullin-RING (CRL) ligases. Different types of E3 ligases follow a different enzymatic mechanism for Ub transfer to the substrate protein [82, 83].

BACTERIAL PATHOGENICITY EMPOWERED BY PTMS

Pathogenic bacteria display a tremendous ability to exploit PTMs in order to promote virulence. They usually interfere with host defence, signal transduction, cytoskeleton and membrane dynamics as mentioned above. Pathogens have developed three main strategies, based on PTMs, in order to gain control of the host and wreak havoc. First, bacterial effectors are translocated into the host to directly modify host proteins. Common and novel activities which will be discussed later in detail, are (de)phosphorylation, eliminylation, lipidation, deamidation, glycosylation, (de)ubiquitination as well as addition or removal of ubiquitin-like proteins (Fig. **1**). Second, bacterial effectors are translocated into the host and undergo modifications by host proteins, thus achieving their timely activation or correct subcellular localization. Third, bacterial proteins are modified by their own machineries prior to host interaction. In the following paragraphs we present specific examples of how pathogens take advantage of PTMs to subvert the host.

Yersinia Yops Effectors: An Arsenal of Post-Translational Modifiers

Yersinia sp. cause a range of human diseases. *Yersinia enterocolitica* and *pseudotuberculosis* are enteropathogens while *Yersinia pestis* is the causative agent of plague. *Yersinia* uses a type III secretion system (T3SS) to inject six virulence factors, the so-called *Yersinia* outer proteins (Yops), into the cytosol of phagocytic cells [84, 85]. The targets of these proteins are mainly (i) the actin cytoskeleton which results in actin disruption, cytoskeletal rearrangements and inhibition of phagocytosis, and (ii) the host signaling pathways which result in inhibition of the innate immune responses, promoting intracellular survival of *Yersinia*. The cytoskeleton dynamics are modulated by YopT, YopO/YpkA and YopE, which act on monomeric GTPases of the Rho family. Although YopE is the only Yop effector which does not cause PTM, it actually undergoes itself ubiquitination by the host machinery. YopT is a Cys-protease while YopO/YpkA is a GTPase-inhibiting protein, which also exhibits kinase activity. Inhibition of the immune system is achieved by the activity of YopH, which is a Tyr-phosphatase, and YopP/J, which is an acetyltransferase. An enzymatic activity was only recently assigned to YopM, which was a long-lasting enigma.

Under physiological conditions, Rho family G proteins are located on the inner membrane where their interaction partners are found. Anchoring to the membrane is achieved through a prenyl group which is linked at a CaaX motif at their C-terminus ('a' stands for aliphatic and 'X' for any residue). YopT cleaves the peptide bond upstream the prenylated motif and releases the proteins from the membrane. YopT belongs to the same structural family with *Escherichia coli* B toxin, *Pseudomonas syringae* AvrPphB [86] and a module of the *Photorhabdus asymbiotica* multifunctional, virulence-related PaTox toxin [87]. Although the structure of YopT has not been determined yet, the structures of AvrPphB and the homologous PaTox module reveal a papain-like fold (Fig. **3A**).

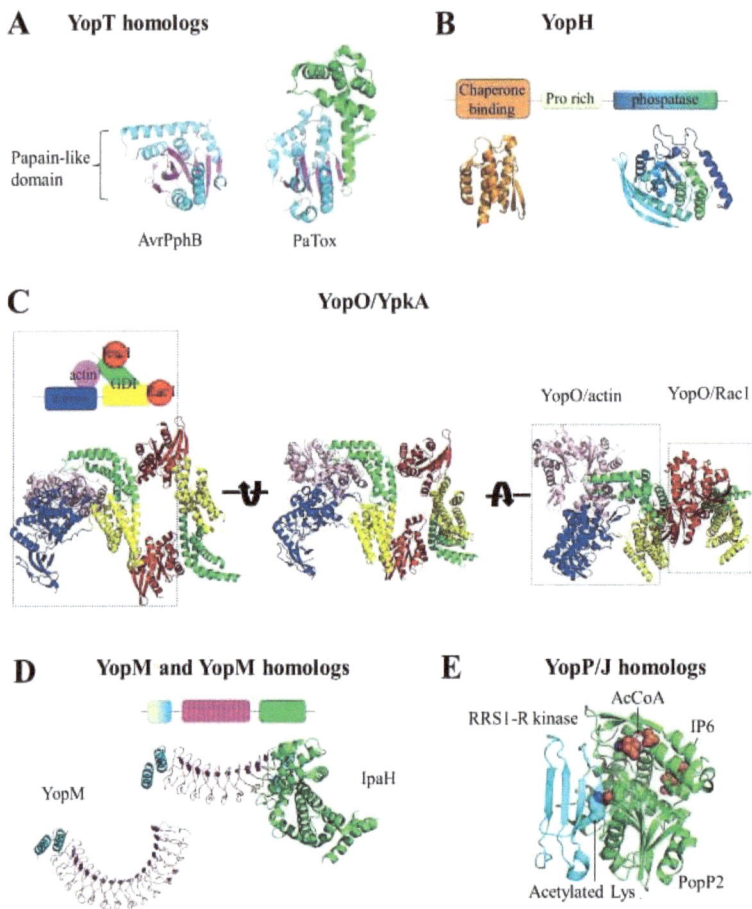

Fig. (3). Crystal structures of Yops and Yops-homologs. **(A)** Ribbon representation of the YopT homologs *P. syringae* AvrPphB (PDB 1UKF) and *P. asymbiotica* PaTox (PDB 6HV6). For comparison the molecules are shown at the same orientation. The papain-like domain is shown in cyan/pink. **(B)** Schematic presentation of the full length YopH. The structures of the N-terminal chaperon binding domain (PDB 1HUF) and the C-teriminal PTPB1 phosphatase domain (PDB 1QZ0) are shown in cartoon. **(C)** Ribbon representation of the YopO structure (blue/yellow/green) in complex with Rac1 (red) and actin (pink). Three views related by rotation are shown. The panel is a composition of the PDB files 2H7V (YopO/Rac1 complex) and 4CI6 (YopO/actin complex). The different complexes are boxed differently in the third view. **(D)** Schematic representation of the full length YopM. The protein comprises three domains: a N-terminal alpha-helical, a middle horseshoe and a C-terminal. Ribbon representation of the structures of YopM (PDB 1JL5) and IpaH3 (PDB 3CVR). For comparison the molecules are shown at the same orientation and the same colour code is adopted for schematic and ribbon representations. **(E)** Ribbon representation of the YopP/J (green) in complex with the WRKY domain of the RRS1-R kinase (cyan), acetylo CoA (spacefill) and IP6 (spacefill). The acetylated Lys in contact with the catalytic Glu are shown in spacefill (PDB 5W3X). The figure was prepared using PyMOL [18].

Y. enterocolitica YopO (YpkA in *Y. pseudotuberculosis* and *Y. pestis*) is an effector with two enzymatic activities which are located in two structurally diverse protein domains. The N-terminal domain of YopO/YpkA (Fig. **3C**) is a Ser/Thr kinase resembling a Hank-type eukaryotic protein kinase and the C-terminal domain is a Rho-GTPase binding domain resembling in structure and function a GDI (GDP dissociations inhibition) [88]. The N-terminus of the protein also includes a secretion/translocation signal, which leads and attaches the protein to the inner surface of the host plasma membrane, while the C-terminus binds actin (Fig. **3C**). Kinase, GDI and actin-binding activities of YopO/YpkA are all orchestrated to achieve manipulation of host actin-dynamics in order to disrupt cytoskeleton and prevent phagocytosis. *Yersinia* strains which abolish any of these activities are non-pathogenic.

YopO/YpkA is activated within the host cell *via* its interaction with actin. This interaction activates YopO autophosphorylation which in turn seems to stimulate YopO kinase activity in the host [89 - 91]. The effector, which in its apo form is highly flexible, binds monomeric actin *via* both kinase and GDI domains forming a 1:1 complex (Fig. **3C**). The interaction induces large conformational changes and sequesters actin from polymerization process due to steric hindrance [92 - 94]. In addition, YopO/YpkA binding to actin not only prevents its polymerization but also recruits polymerization regulators, making their phosphorylation feasible. YopO/YpkA-mediated phosphorylation leads to misregulation of actin polymerization [94, 95]. One such regulator is the recently characterized, gelsolin actin-remodelling protein. YopO/YpkA phosphorylation of gelsolin results in calcium-independent activation of gelsolin. Activated protein severs actin and cripples phagocytosis [96].

Gα subunits of heterotrimeric G-proteins and especially members of the Gαq family have been identified to be another substrate of the YopO/YpkA kinase activity [97]. The effector protein phosphorylates Ser47 which lies on the highly conserved, among the GTPase domain of Gα subunits, diphosphate binding loop. Ser47 plays an important role in GTP binding and magnesium ion coordination and its modification results in inhibition of guanine nucleotide binding, inactivation of G-proteins and consequently inactivation of multiple Gαq signaling pathways. It is believed that the addition of a negative charge is responsible for the reduction of GTP binding affinity [97].

Members of the Rho family of G-proteins known to regulate actin-dynamics and consequently cytoskeletal dynamics and cell motility, are also targets of the YopO/YpkA [91]. This interaction is mediated through the C-terminal domain and sequesters G-proteins from actin-polymerization processes by preventing their activation (Fig. **3C**).

YopH is a very active and versatile Tyr-phosphatase since its activity has been associated with inhibition of both phagocytosis and immune response. YopH has a great range of substrates with most of them associated with contact-dependent signaling [98]. Some of the best characterized YopH substrates are focal adhesion proteins such as p130cas, Fyb and SKAP-HOM. Adhesion of *Yersinia* to integrins of the outer eukaryotic membrane triggers a cascade of phosphorylations inside the cell which promote phagocytosis, inflammation and immune response. Since eukaryotes very often utilize phosphorylations as a signal transduction mechanism, it is vital for pathogens to develop mechanisms for shutting down those signals. YopH belongs to this category of effectors as it is able to inhibit early phosphorylation events, inflammatory response and actually disrupt focal adhesion. For example, it has been shown that upon contact of *Yersinia* with the host cell, the latter phosphorylates SKAP-HOM and Fyb in 30 seconds. However, YopH-mediated dephosphorylation has been observed in less than 2 minutes. The structure of YopH comprises three domains: a N-terminal chaperone binding domain, a proline-rich domain, and a catalytic, C-terminal domain, which resembles the eukaryotic PTPB1 phosphatase family (Fig. **3B**). The active site retains the characteristic HC(X5)R(S/T) motif and the Cys-Arg-Asp catalytic triad ('X' stands for any amino acid).

The sequence of YopM homologs from different *Yersinia* species comprises three major modules: (i) a N-terminal alpha helical domain, where a secretion/translocation signal and an autonomous translocation domain reside, (ii) a horseshoe, middle domain comprising a varying number of leucine-rich repeats, which is believed to be the scaffold for recruiting protein interactors, and (iii) a C-terminal domain (Fig. **3D**). Until lately, YopM was characterized as an enigma because it could not be related with any enzymatic activity and its function remained unclear. Recent data indicate that YopM supresses the pyrin-related, infection-induced inflammasome activation [99]. Pyrin inflammasomes are induced by YopE and YopT proteins when RhoA GTPase is inactivated [100]. YopM is able to limit the immune response against infection by activating host kinases which phosphorylate and inhibit pyrin [101, 102]. This is an example of a bacterial effector which hijacks and regulates host kinases to modulate the physiological PTM pattern of the host in order to promote infection. In addition, a recent study [103] associates the N-terminal domain of YopM with a novel E3 ubiquitin ligase activity which targets the NLRP3 (NOD-like receptor family pyrin domain-containing 3) inflammasome and induces necrotic cell death. In particular, Wei *et al.* report that the N-terminal of YopM resembles the bacterial IpaH E3 ligase family and it is associated with the Lys63 ubiquitination of NLRP3 (Fig. **3D**).

YopJ/P inhibits the NF-κB and the MAPK pathways and dampens inflammatory and innate immune responses [104]. It has been shown that the protein can disrupt kinase activity of multiple substrates including MAPKs, IκB kinases and the TGFβ-activated kinase (TAK1) [105, 106]. The catalytic domain of the protein has structural similarities with the C55 family of cysteine proteases and retains a conserved catalytic triad. Although the family encompasses deubiquitinases and desumoylases, YopJ/P is actually an acetyltransferase (Fig. **3E**). It has been shown that the protein acetylates Ser/Thr residues, crucial for phosphorylation, and Lys residues [107]. Moreover, it has been shown that YopJ/P requires a eukaryotic factor namely inositol hexakisphosphate (IP6) for activation. Binding of IP6 induces conformational changes that increase the binding affinity of protein for acetyl-coenzyme A [108].

Activation of Bacterial Effectors by Host-Mediated Post-Translational Modifications

We have already mentioned two bacterial effectors, *Yersinia sp.* YopO/YpkA and YopJ/P, which need eukaryotic factors for their activation. Indeed, there are many examples of effectors whose function is only activated inside the host, thus ensuring that they will not be harmful for the bacterium itself [109]. Effector activation by eukaryotic factors is achieved either allosterically or by the attachment of post-translational modifications. For example, two out of the four *Pseudomonas aeruginosa* exoenzymes, ExoY and ExoU, require a eukaryotic factor for stimulation or enhancement of their enzymatic activity. ExoY, which alters cytoskeleton dynamics through a yet unknown mechanism, is a nucleotidyl cyclase allosterically activated by F-actin [110 - 112]. On the other hand, ExoU combines both post-translational modification and allosteric activation from ubiquitin. ExoU is a phospholipase A able to cause damage to the host cellular membrane [113]. It consists of a N-terminal patatin-like phospholipase domain, a middle bridging domain and a C-terminal four-alpha- helical bundle [114, 115]. The C-terminal domain is responsible for membrane localization, it is indispensable for catalytic activity and it is required for the double ubiquitination of ExoU at Lys178 [116]. Although the biological impact of this modification remains elusive, it has been shown that another ubiquitin, non-covalently associated, is required for stimulation of ExoU catalytic activity [117 - 119]. This ubiquitin binds to the bridging and the C-terminal domains and its synergistic action with the substrate leads to a conformational rearrangement of the four-alpha-helical bundle [120].

Ubiquitination, phosphorylation, lipidation and sumoylation are the most common host-mediated effector modifications (Fig. **1A, B, F**). Recently, asparaginyl-hydroxylation was identified as a novel modification in this category. In the rest of this section we describe examples of host-mediated activation of bacterial effectors through phosphorylation and asparaginyl-hydroxylation.

Ser/Thr/Tyr-phosphorylation and dephosphorylation are the most common modifications used in a myriad of signalling and regulatory pathways in eukaryotes. From the many examples of bacterial effectors which are phosphorylated by eukaryotic factors, we will describe the case of the T3SS-secreted AvrPto and AvrPtoB effectors from the phytopathogen *Pseudomonas syringae* and the T4SS secreted *Helicobacter pylori* CagA. The effectors AvrPto and AvrPtoB are modular, structural homologs. It has been shown that the AvrPtoB C-terminal domain is an E3 ubiquitin ligase which targets and leads to degradation host factors such as the Fen kinase and the exocyst EXO70B1 [121]. However, other host kinases such as the tomato Ser/Thr kinase Pto and the *Arabidopsis* SnRK2.8 evade degradation and phosphorylate AvrPtoB and AvrPto [122] inducing activation of either effector-triggered immunity or bacterial virulence [123]. Although AvrPto and AvrPtoB share structural similarities, their crystal structures in complex with Pto revealed that each one of the effectors interact with the kinase by a different interface [124, 125] (Fig. **4A**). In addition, different sites of phosphorylation by the eukaryotic factor have been reported for each effector [125 - 127].

CagA is an oncoprotein related to high risk of gastric cancer that dampens chemotherapeutic-induced apoptosis in gastric cancer cells [128]. The protein is phosphorylated by Tyr-kinases of the Src (SFKs) and Abl families, which are involved in signal transduction [129, 130]. Phosphorylation occurs at the EPIYA motif repeats, which are found at the C-terminal domain, and causes effector activation and induction of cytoskeletal rearrangements and morphological alterations of the host cells. It has been shown that phosphorylated CagA interacts with the SHP2 phosphatase (Src homology 2 (SH2) domain-containing Tyr phosphatase 2) through the phosphorylated EPIYA motifs and triggers the SHP2 activity [131] (Fig. **4B**). Activated SHP2 dephoshorylates the focal adhesion kinase (FAK) and activates the Ras/MAPK/ERK signaling pathway. On the other hand, interaction between SHP1 (SHP2 mammalian homolog) and CagA occurs in an EPIYA-Tyr-phosphrylation independent way and activates the phosphatase activity of SHP1. Subsequently, SHP1 dephosphorylates CagA and attenuates its function. Moreover, CagA is involved in its own negative regulation.

Phosphorylated CagA can bind and activate the C-terminal Src kinase (Csk) which, in turn, phosphorylates inhibitory tyrosine residues of SFKs and inhibits SFKs which can no longer phosphorylate CagA.

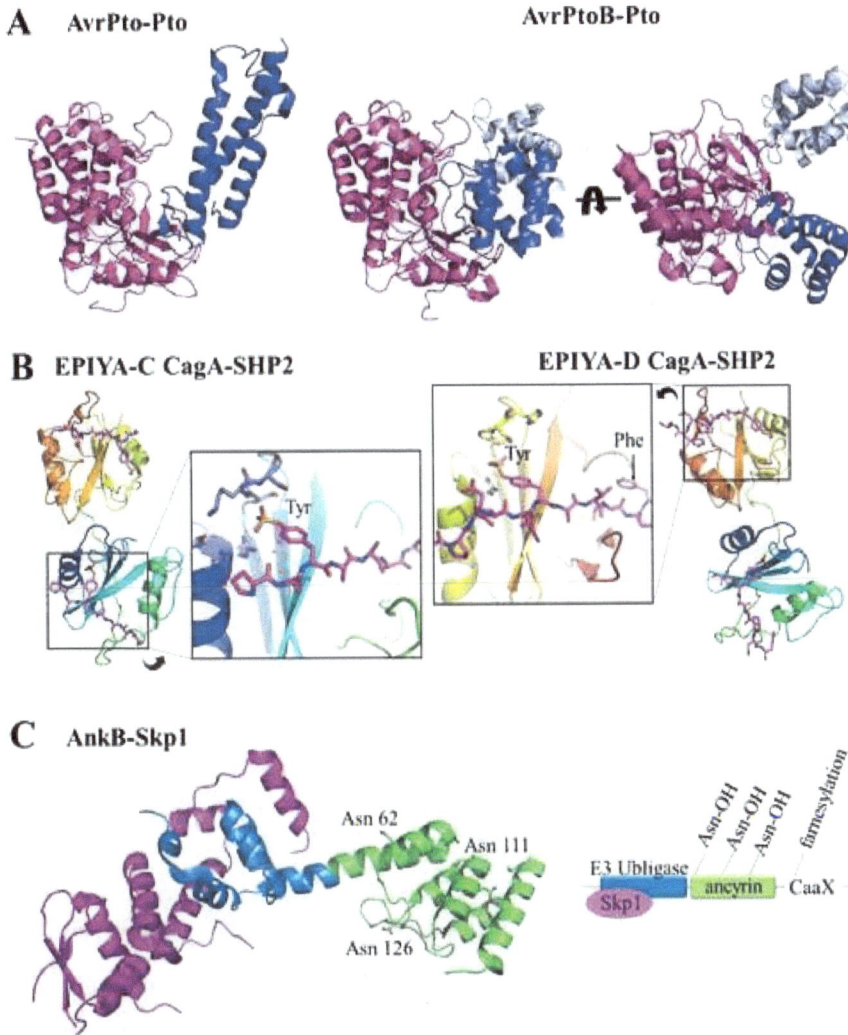

Fig. (4). Crystal structures of bacterial effectors in complexes with host factors. **(A)** Ribbon representation of AvrPto (PDB 2QKW, magenta) and AvrPtoB (PDB 3HGK, magenta) in complex with tomato Pto kinase (blue and light blue). Pto kinase interacts differentially with the effectors using a common (blue) and a unique (light blue) interface. **(B)** Ribbon representation of the SH2 domain of the pro-oncogenic SHP2 phosphatase (coloured blue to orange from N- to C-terminus, PDB 5X7B (left) and 5X94 (right)) in complex with the Western CagA specific EPIYA-C peptide (stick representation, left) and the East Asian CagA specific EPIYA-D peptide (stick representation, right). The closer association of the East Asian CagA with gastric cancer is attributed to a higher binding affinity with SHP2 due to additional interactions of the indicated Phe residue. **(C)** Ribbon representation of the *Legionella* effector AnkB (blue/green) in complex with the eukaryotic factor Skp1 (magenta), PDB 5K35. The schematic representation on the right clarifies the domain organization and highlights PTM sites. The figure was prepared using PyMOL [18].

On the opposite side of phosphorylation, which is a common and well-established modification, is found asparaginyl-hydroxylation which is a relatively rare modification and quite novel as a bacterial pathogenicity factor. *Legionella pneumophila* AnkB is a eukaryotic-like effector protein which has a significant role in intracellular replication. The N-terminus of the protein is a non-canonical F-box domain which is implicated in a Skp1-Cullin-F box E3 ubiquitin ligase complex [132] (Fig. **4C**). The C-terminus is an ankyrin domain comprising three ankyrin repeats and being responsible for recruitment of polyubiquitinated proteins to the vacuole-containing membrane where they are degraded and used as a source of essential amino acids for *Legionella* replication. The last C-terminal residues, downstream the ankyrin domain, encompass a CaaX motif which is farnesylated by the host. Farnesylation leads the protein to the vacuole-containing membrane (host-mediated effector localization is discussed in the next section). Recently, it was shown that the ankyrin domain harbors sites susceptible to Asn hydroxylation *via* the eukaryotic factor inhibiting HIF (FIH) [133]. FIH, is a 2-oxoglutarate dioxygenase which recognises the motif L(X)5[D/E]aNa and hydroxylates the Asn residue at C_β [134]. The modification is considered to be a protein-protein interaction modulator. Three sites are modified (Asn62, Asn111 and Asn126) and it was shown that these hydroxylations are indispensable for function such as the recruitment of polyubiquitinated proteins to the *Legionella*-containing vacuole and the bacterium intra-vacuolar replication (Fig. **4C**). This is the first time that a bacterial effector undergoes asparaginyl-hydroxylation by a eukaryotic factor. Additional effectors from *Legionella* and other pathogens have been identified to possess the FIH consensus including the *Yersinia* YopM and the *Shigella* IpaH4.5. However, their Asn-hydroxylation remains to be experimentally confirmed.

Localization of Bacterial Effectors to Membranes by Host-Mediated Post Translational Lipidations

Membranes are an exceptionally important cell structure at all levels of host-pathogen interaction [135]. A recent study shows that approximately 30% of the T3SS and T4SS translocated effectors are targeted to membranes, including the plasma membrane, intracellular organelles and phagosomes [136]. Moreover, it is known that intracellular pathogens target a significant number of their effectors to the pathogen-containing vacuoles. Consequently, it is not surprising that membranes and membrane-associated proteins are major targets of pathogenic effectors. Pathogens employ two main strategies to promote membrane localization of their proteins after their translocation into the host cell. First, the effectors harbor domains which recognize and bind membrane lipids such as the phosphoinositide (PI) lipids [137]. Subcellular compartments and organelles can be distinct because of their diverse lipid composition. Hence, effectors can recognize and bind different PIs through novel domains as in the case of *Legionella* SidC protein. SidC, inhibitor of a unique family of E3 ubiquitin ligases, encompasses a specific phosphatidylinositol-4-phosphate (PIP/PI4P) binding domain able to anchor the protein on the *Legionella*-containing vacuole [138, 139]. Second, the effectors, similar to many eukaryotic proteins such as the G-proteins we described above, harbor specific motifs which can be suitably post-translationally modified to facilitate membrane targeting. The most common modifications used by a wide range of bacteria and viruses to deliver effectors to host membranes are host-mediated lipidations (Fig. **1B**) such as prenylation, farnesylation, geranylation, palmitoylation and myristoylation [140 - 145]. Lipidations not only activate secreted bacterial toxins but also contribute to adhesion and invasion to host cells. Among the proteins we have already mentioned, *L. pneumophila* AnkB is farnesylated at a C-terminal CaaX motif in order to be transferred and attached to the *Legionella*-containing vacuole. Likewise, the *P. syringae* AvrPto is targeted to the plant membrane *via* myristoylation.

S-palmitoylation is the reversible addition of palmitoyl chains to Cys residues *via* thioester bonds. S-prenylation is the attachment of either farnesyl or geranylgeranyl chains to a Cys residue located in a C-terminal CaaX motif *via* a thioester bond. N-myristoylation is the addition of the 14-carbon long myristic acid to the N-terminal Gly of the MGXXXS/T motif. S-prenylation and N-myristoylation are typically irreversible modifications. All these modifications are catalyzed from host enzymes to specific effector motifs as soon as the later enters the host cytosol.

Similar to *L. pneumophila*, *Salmonella typhimurium* and *Brucella abortus* are intracellular pathogens which ensure their survival and replication inside specific vacuoles, the so-called *Salmonella*- and *Brucella*-containing vacuoles, respectively. *S. typhimurium* SifA and SseI proteins are encoded by the *Salmonella* pathogenicity island 2 (SPI2) and they are mainly responsible for *Salmonella*'s survival inside the host. In particular, SifA has a role in the host membrane dynamics as well as in the organization and maturation of *Salmonella*-containing vacuoles. SifA is mainly organized in two domains. The N-terminal domain binds the host SifA kinesin interacting protein (SKIP), which in turn binds the plus-end-directed microtubule motor kinesin. The structure of the C-terminal domain resembles the structure of SopE *Salmonella* effector which has guanine nucleotide exchange factor (GEF) activity [146] and belongs to the family of WxxxE bacterial effectors. Indeed, SifA shares common properties with GEFs as it binds Rho-family G proteins in their GDP-bound form. It was shown that SifA is prenylated by the host geranylgeranyl transferase I at the C-terminal Cys333 which is located in the motif $C_{331}LC_{333}CFL$ [147]. In addition, SifA is subject to an S-acylation on the Cys331 which resides close to the prenylated residue and it is believed that functions as a second signal which regulates protein association with the membrane. During infection, SifA also interacts with the SseJ *Salmonella* effector, which localizes on the phagosome membrane. SseJ has deacylase and acyltransferase activities and belongs to the family of glycerophosholipid-cholesterol acyl transferases [146]. There is evidence that both domains of SifA together with SKIP, SseJ and small Rho-family G proteins form a complex which cooperatively promotes phagosome tubulation [146, 148]. SifA undergoes a third post-translational modification by Caspase-3. The later cleaves SifA and divides the two domains which are subsequently localized differently and exert their functions independently [149].

On the other hand, the phenotype associated with *Salmonella* SseI is defected host-cell migration. After its delivery into the host cell, SseI is S-palmitoylated at the N-terminal Cys9 by a subset of host palmitoyltransferases resulting in its targeting to specific domains of the plasma membrane [150]. Although there is no plasma membrane targeting motif other than the modified cysteine residue, it has been shown that approximately 100 amino-terminal residues are required for the correct modification. Moreover, the carboxyterminal domain of the protein exhibits deamidase activity on Gαi substrates, resulting in their persistent activation [151, 152]. Deamidation of host G-proteins by bacterial effectors is a known virulence mechanism and will be discussed later in detail.

Recently, it was shown that S-palmitoylation of *Brucella* PrpA effector is also crucial for its function into the host cell. PrpA is involved in the modulation of host immune response [153]. It is translocated from the *Brucella*-containing vacuole to the host cell and targeted to the plasma membrane through S-palmitoylation of two N-terminal Cys residues [154]. The modification is performed by host biochemical processes and it is necessary for PrpA stabilization, accurate localization to the plasma membrane and proper activity into the host cell.

An unusual case of bacterial effector related with post-translational de-lipidation is the *Shigella* IpaJ. Although myristoylation is an irreversible modification in eukaryotes, it was found that the bacterial IpaJ can cleave myristoylated Gly residues from eukaryotic proteins [155]. IpaJ represents an entire family of proteins found in many pathogenic bacteria with a Cys protease activity. Initially, IpaJ was identified as demyristoylase of ADP-ribosylation factor 1 (ARF1), which is a small G protein. IpaJ cleaves the N-terminal myristoylated Gly of ARF1 and inhibits protein trafficking [156]. In particular, ARF1 functions as a regulator of the Golgi apparatus. Myristoylation anchors ARF1 to the Golgi membrane and serves as a "myristoyl switch" between the activated and inactivated forms. In the activated GTP-bound form, the modified N-terminus is exposed and promotes association with the membrane, while in the inactivated GDP-bound form, the modified N-terminus is masked to solvent and the protein is soluble. Accordingly, the "myristoyl switch" allows ARF1 to recruit substrate proteins to the membrane and subsequently is responsible for triggering a wide range of biological cascades. It has also been shown that although IpaJ is generally a promiscuous demyristoylase, it exhibits specificity for members of the ARF/ARL family of G, Golgi associated, proteins [155].

Eliminylation: A Particular Case of Dephosphorylation

Several pathogenic bacteria produce effectors which display an enzymatic activity, different from phosphatase and kinase, called phosphothreonine lyase. Phosphothreonine lyases mediate the irreversible removal of a phosphate group from a phosphorylated Thr residue of a host protein. This enzymatic reaction is called eliminylation and it is different from the phosphoryl transfer mechanism used by phosphatases [157].

S. typhimurium produces the T3SS effector, SpvC, which functions as a phosphothreonine lyase [158, 159]. Once translocated into host cells, SpvC catalyzes the β-eliminylation of the phosphate group at the Thr residue within the dually phosphorylated pThr-X-pTyr motif of MAPKs, leading to their inactivation [157]. Except from the loss of phosphoric acid and H_2O during eliminylation, the phosphorylated Thr residue, essential for MAPK activity, is converted into dehydrobutyrine. Dehydrobutyrine lacks the -OH group and it can no longer be phosphorylated [160]. This explains why this modification is irreversible. Even though it has been indicated that SpvC specifically dephosphorylates c-Jun N-terminal kinase (JNK) and extracellular signal-regulated protein kinase (ERK) *in vitro*, only the inactivation of ERK was demonstrated *in vivo* [161]. Before its enzymatic function was discovered, SpvC was known to be required for *Salmonella* pathogenicity in mice [162, 163]. SpvC contribution in pathogenicity is linked to a mechanism of evading host immune responses. More specifically, an increased IL-8 secretion was detected in HeLa cells infected with a *Salmonella* Δ*spvC* mutant strain [159]. Furthermore, the mRNA levels of inflammatory cytokines and chemokines were significantly induced, during the early stages of *Salmonella* infection, in the intestine of a streptomycin-treated mouse model infected with Δ*spvC* mutant strain [161].

Shigella flexeni also produces a T3SS effector with a phosphothreonine lyase activity named OspF [164]. OspF shares 71% sequence identity with SpvC and as expected, it irreversibly modifies MAPKs of the infected host cells [165]. OspF, similarly to SpvC, dephosphorylates *in vitro* JNK, p38 and ERK diminishing host immune response during infection. In addition, OspF enzymatic activity causes the attenuation of polymorphonuclear leukocytes recruitment at the site of the infection in mouse and rabbit infection models therefore reducing the NF-kB-mediated transcription of inflammatory genes [166].

AMPylation: An Emerging Modification in Bacterial Pathogenicity

AMPylation is the addition of an AMP moiety to the hydroxyl-group of a Tyr, Thr or Ser residue through a phosphodiester bond [167] (Fig. **1D**). The process is catalysed by AMPylases, which use ATP as the source of AMP. AMPylation was first implicated in pathogenicity when effectors from *Vibrio parahaemolyticus* and *Histophilus somni* were found to modulate host GTPases [168, 169]. Since then, GTPases have been established as major targets of AMPylases [170]. Although AMPylation is an emerging modification in bacterial pathogenicity, it has been extensively reviewed recently [171 - 173] and therefore it will not be further discussed here.

ADP-Ribosylation: An Ancient Modification with Huge Potential for Infection

ADP-ribosylation is the reversible addition of an ADP ribose from a nicotinamide adenine dinucleotide (NAD+) to a protein substrate *via* a glycosidic linkage (Fig. **1E**). Arg is one of the commonly ADP-ribosylated residues *via* a N-glycosidic bond. The modification is enzymatic and is catalyzed by ADP-ribosyl transferases (ARTs). The reverse process, the ADP-ribosyl cleavage, is catalysed by the, so called, ADP-ribosyl erasers and ensures a dynamic control of protein ADP-ribosylation [174]. This modification is widespread among all kingdoms of life and controls numerous, diverse and fundamental biological processes [175]. In addition, pathogens often use ADP-ribosylation to modify host proteins in order to promote virulence. Interestingly, the first discovered ARTs were the bacterial cholera and diphtheria toxins, which encompass a catalytic domain responsible for the modification and an additional domain responsible for protein translocation across the membrane. ADP-ribosylation is known for a long time, however, its full potential for regulation and pathogenicity remains to be elucidated. It is believed that targeting the ADP-ribosylation signaling has a great potential as a novel therapeutic strategy [176].

P. aeruginosa exotoxins ExoY and ExoU have been discussed at the section of host-mediated effector modifications. The other two *P. aeruginosa* exotoxins, ExoS and ExoT, are closely related bifunctional effectors with high sequence identity. They both encompass a N-terminal G protein activating domain (GAP) and a C-terminal ADP-ribosyl transferase domain (ART) [177, 178]. Although both proteins perform the GAP activity to the same subset of G-proteins, they exhibit specificity on their ART substrates. Moreover, distinct and coordinated functions have been identified for the domains. The synergistic activity of the domains has been related with changes in cytoskeleton dynamics and impairment of adhesion, migration and phagocytosis of infected host cells. As far as the ART activity is concerned, ExoS ribosylates a broad range of substrates namely Rho, Ras and Rab while ExoT has a restricted number of substrates *i.e.* Crk. Although ART activities of both ExoS and ExoT are related to *P. aeruginosa* keratitis, only ExoS ART is related to filopodium formation and bacteria dissemination during pneumonia [179, 180].

Many recent studies have demonstrated another facet of ADP-ribosylation in bacterial pathogenicity. In particular, ADP-ribosylation may be a prerequisite in order for a non-canonical, ligase-independent, pathogen-controlled ubiquitination to take place. This very exciting aspect of bacterial virulence is discussed in detail later.

Deamidation: From Biological Clock to Virulence Factor

Deamidation is the irreversible modification of Asn and Gln residues to Asp or isoAsp and Glu or pyroGlu, respectively (Fig. **1H**). The consequence is the increase of either the negative charge or the polypeptide rigidity at the site of modification. Early work identified deamidation as a nonenzymatic modification, mainly related with protein aging and functioning as a built-in biological clock [181]. However, recent evidence demonstrates that deamidation is often enzymatically catalyzed and directly related to regulation of cellular functions and pathogenicity [172, 182, 183]. Nowadays, deamidation has been established as a bacterial virulence factor often used to modulate host function. Protein families which have been identified as eukaryotic substrates of deamidation by bacterial effectors include G proteins, elongation initiation factors, and proteins from the ubiquitin and ubiquitin-like signaling pathways.

Bacterial Deamidation of Host G Proteins

Cytotoxic Necrotizing Factors (CNFs) are homologous proteins which exhibit deamidation activity against Rho family G proteins and are expressed by *E. coli* (CNF$_{1-3}$) and *Yersinia* (CNFY). CNF$_1$ deamidates RhoA Gln63, a residue located on the switch II region, trapping the protein in a constitutively activated form. Similarly, CNFY activates the RhoA, Rac and Cdc24 GTPases. Overall, it was shown that CNFY modulates innate immune and inflammatory responses and enhances the delivery of Yops inside phagocytes [184]. A recent study shows that CNFY is thermo-regulated through a thermo-labile RNA structure at the 5' untranslated region [185]. CNFs are organized in two domains: the N-terminal receptor binding and translocation domain and the C-terminal deamidase, papain-like domain. After cellular uptake, the protein undertakes autoproteolysis and the two domains are separated.

VopC toxin is another member of the CNF-like superfamily which is expressed from the *Vibrio parahaemolyticus* and mediates invasion to nonphagocytic cells [186]. Unlike CNFs, VopC is delivered to the host through a T3SS and consequently possesses a different N-terminus. VopC deamidates Rac1 and Cdc42 GTPases but not RhoA [187]. The deamidated form of these proteins mimics the activated, GTP-bound state and is important for pathogenicity [188].

Pasteurella multocida toxin (PMT) belongs to the AB superfamily of bacterial toxins and act as a strong mitogen [189, 190]. It is a large protein of approximately 1000 residues which are organized in two main domains and multiple subdomains. The N-terminal domain resembles the CNFs N-terminus and this similarity suggests an analogous function probably as a receptor binding and translocation domain. The C-terminus is organized in three subdomains one of which is a papain-like, deamidase domain [191]. PMT arrests heterotrimeric G proteins in their active state by deamidating a conserved Gln at the switch II of the alpha subunit. The modified Gln is essential for GTP-hydrolysis. Besides the large G proteins, PMT also deamidates the RhoA small G protein.

Bacterial Deamidation of Transcription Factors Pauses Host Protein Synthesis

Burkholderia pseudomallei lethal factor 1 (BLF1) is a toxin directly related to melioidosis [192] and able to deactivate the elongation initiation factor 4A by deamidating Gln339 to Glu. BLF1 has no sequence similarity with the CNFs and lacks a N-terminal translocation domain. Nevertheless, their deamidase domain assumes a fold similar to that of CNFs [193]. Interestingly, it was shown that BLF1 selectively induces apoptosis in neuroblastoma cells and it is considered as a potential anticancer target [194].

Bacterial Deamidation Targets the Ubiquitin/Ubiquitin-Like Protein Signaling Pathways

Cycle inhibiting factor (Cif) proteins are deamidases translocated through the T3SS and are implicated in the disruption of host cell cycle progression [195]. Cifs were first discovered in *E. coli* and later, their homologs were found in many other bacteria such as *Y. pseudotuberculosis* and *B. pseudomallei*. Although the Cif homologs share low sequence similarity, they assume very similar structures, which are usually composed by two domains (Fig. **5A**). The C-terminal domain, which exerts the deamidase activity, folds as a cysteine protease of the papain-like superfamily [196]. It is believed that the N-terminal domain carries the translocation signal and it is responsible for substrate recognition. It was shown that Cif proteins target Gln40 mainly of NEDD8 but also of ubiquitin and modify it to Glu [197] (Fig. **5A**). This deamidation was related with accumulation of cullin-RING E3 ligases (CRLs) in their neddylated form and inhibition of their neddylation/deneddylation cycle. CRLs are activated through conjugation of NEDD8 to the cullin subunit. CRLs neddylation induces substrate ubiquitination. Full activity of CRLs is achieved through a continuous neddylation/deneddylation process. Cifs selectively bind neddylated CRLs, modify the NEDD8 molecule, hamper deneddylation and inhibit CRLs activity. Another Cif protein, the *P. aeruginosa* Cif, selectively increases the ubiquitination and proteasome degradation levels of the transporter associated with antigen processing (TAP1). As a consequence, a lower amount of peptide antigen is available to MHC class I molecules and CD8+ cytotoxic T cell pathogen clearance is impaired [198].

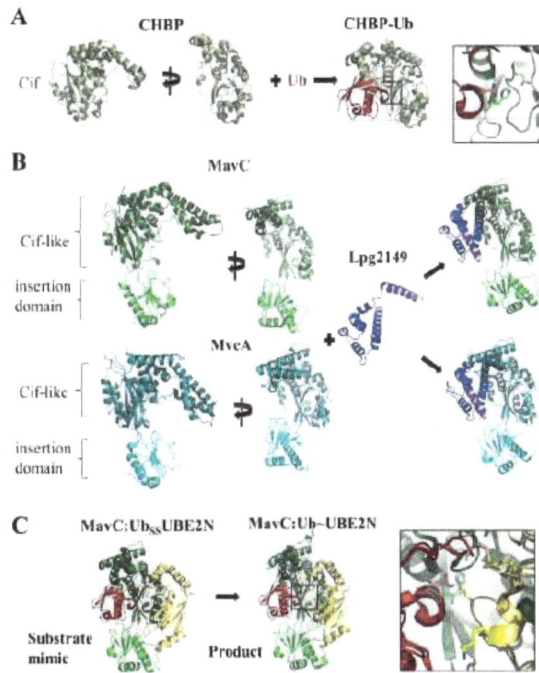

Fig. (5). Crystal structures of Cif deamidases and ubiquitin transglutaminases in ribbon representation. **(A)** The Cif homolog from *B. pseudomallei* (green) is shown in apo (left, PDB 1EIT) and ubiquitin-complexed (right, Ub is colored red, PDB 4HCN) forms. Close up highlights the details of interaction. **(B)** The *Legionella* MavC (green) and MvcA (cyan) Ub transglutaminases (deamidases) are shown in apo forms and in complex with their common inhibitor Lpg2149 (blue). **(C)** The MavC (green) in complex with the substrate mimic Ub$_{ss}$UBE2N and the product is shown. Close up highlights the active site. The figure was prepared using PyMOL [18].

Furthermore, the *S. flexneri,* T3SS translocated, OspI is a deamidase acting on Gln100 of UBE2N, E2-conjucating enzyme [199, 200]. Deamidation inhibits UBE2N which is required for activation of tumor necrosis factor (TNF)-receptor - associated factor 6 (TRAF6). By inhibiting the (TRAF6)-mediated signalling pathway, OspI dampens acute inflammatory responses during bacterial infection.

Bacterial Infection Interferes with the Canonical Ubiquitination

The addition of Ub/Ubl-tags on eukaryotic proteins is of exceptional importance for the precise regulation of cell cycle. This importance renders ubiquitination and Ubl-protein addition networks *i.e.* sumoylation, neddylation *etc*, ideal targets for pathogens to subvert in order to dominate their hosts [201]. Bacterial effectors can interfere with these networks by either modifying their components or be modified by them. A novel mechanism based on engagement of host miRNAs by *Salmonella* to cause an overall alteration of the SUMO proteome of the host has been also described [202]. This mechanism could be supportive of *Salmonella* intracellular lifestyle.

Bacterial Proteins Modify and Disrupt the Host Ubiquitination Network

Bacterial effectors can either mimic enzymatic activities of components of the Ub/Ubl-machinery or directly modify and impair their action. They fall into one of the following groups: bacterial effectors with E3-ligase activity (ubiquitinases), effectors with isopeptidase activity able to remove Ub molecules from the target proteins (deubiquitinases, DUBs) and effectors with Ub/Ubl modifying activity [203 - 205]. The last group includes effectors which target and impair the function of the E1, E2, E3 enzymes and the Ub/Ubl proteins themselves. The Cif/OspI deamidases discussed above belong to this group.

Bacterial E3-ligases can be structural mimics of the known eukaryotic E3-ligase domains such as the HECT and RING domains or they can belong to structurally distinct bacterial families of novel E3 ligases, the so-called NELs [206 - 208]. From the proteins we have already discussed the *P. syringae* AvrPtoB is a RING-like E3 ligase, which ubiquitinates and degradates host kinases and the *Yersinia* YopM is a NEL ligase. *Salmonella* SopA is a T3SS secreted, HECT-like E3 Ub ligase which modulates the innate immune responses [209]. The protein targets members of the TRIM family of host RING-type ligases, namely TRIM56 and TRIM65 [210]. The recent crystal structure of their complex shows that SopA blocks TRIM56 by occluding its E2 ligase interaction interface [211]. Moreover, SopA ubiquitinates TRIM56 and TRIM65 inducing their degradation. NleL is another T3SS secreted HECT-like E3 ligase from the enterohemorrhagic *E. coli* (EHEC). The protein modulates actin pedestral formation [212] with primary target the human JNKs [213]. Ubiquitination of JNKs leads to disruption of JNK-mediated phosphorylation and activation processes. It was recently shown that the NleL also targets multiple proteins including TRAF2, TRAF5, TRAF6, IKKα and IKKβ and disrupts host NF-κB pathway [214]. *Legionella* LubX is a T4SS Ub E3 ligase which targets another T4SS effector, namely SidH as well as the human Clk1 kinase [215]. The protein comprises two U-box domains with distinct functions. The N-terminal U-box is responsible for activation of the E2-conjugated enzymes and ubiquitin ligation while the C-terminal substantially differs from the typical eukaryotic U-box domain and it was proposed to be involved in substrate interactions [216]. *S. flexneri* IpaH9.8 is a NEL E3 ligase translocated into the host cytosol *via* T3SS [217]. The protein is implicated in modulating inflammatory responses during *Shigella* infection. It also plays a role in modulating gene expression since it was shown to ubiquitinate the mammalian splicing factor U2AF35 [218]. IpaH9.8 polyubiquitinates the NEMO protein, a NF-kB pathway activator, and targets it for degradation [219]. The result is a reduction of NF-κB mediated inflammatory response. Moreover, IpaH9.8 is responsible for ubiquitination and proteasome degradation of the human granylate binding protein-1 which is of fundamental importance in antibacterial defence [220, 221].

A well studied example of a canonical, Cys-protease-like, bacterial deubiquitinase (DUB) is the *Salmonella enterica* effector SseL. The protein is translocated into the host cytoplasm through T3SS encoded in SPI-2 and contributes to the systemic virulence of the pathogen [222, 223]. Inactivation of SseL results in bacterial filamentation, unusual localization of *Salmonella* inside the infected cells and a dramatic alteration in host cell lipid metabolism [224]. It is believed that SseL affects host lipid metabolism by modifying the host ubiquitination pattern. Moreove, it is known that infection from *Salmonella* promotes the formation of ubiquitinated protein aggregates around the *Salmonella*-containing vacuole. This is the signal which leads the vacuole to autophagic degradation. However, the pathogen can overcome this recognition mechanism by deubiquitinating the protein aggregates using the bacterial SseL protein [225]. Recently, it was shown that SseL contributes to the phagosome recruitment of the eukaryotic lipid transporter oxysterol binding protein 1, a function which is essential for vacuolar membrane integrity [226]. Legionella RavD is a DUB which inhibits the host NF-κB pathway. The protein is the first identified bacterial DUB specific for hydrolysing linear ubiquitin chains [227]. On the contrary, all the other known bacterial DUBs are active on the isopeptide linkage of polyubiquitin chains. Recently, it was shown that RavD assumes a papain-like fold utilizing a Cys-His-Ser catalytic triad. RavD prevents the accumulation of linear Ub chains on the *Legionella*-containing vacuoles.

Bacterial Proteins Are Modified by the Host Ubiquitination Network

In an alternative strategy, bacteria exploit the host Ub/Ubl machinery to timely modify their own proteins and regulate their catalytic function and cellular location in a manner that promotes virulence, survival or propagation into the host.

We mentioned earlier that YopE is the only Yop which does not catalyse a PTM formation. However, *Y. enterocolitica* YopE undergoes ubiquitination itself and so it is the substrate of post-translational modification [228]. YopE ubiquitination targets the protein for proteasomal degradation. Regulated degradation of YopE is a fine tunning mechanism of bacteria to optimise their virulence since reduced YopE activity has been related with enhanced activity of the remaining Yops [229]. *Salmonella*, T3SS secreted, SopB is a phosphoinositide phosphatase which diversify its function by being localized to different cell loci, at different times during infection [230, 231]. This is achieved in a ubiquitin-dependent manner. During the early stages of infection, SopB is found in the plasma membrane where it modulates actin-mediated bacterial internalization and activates the Akt protein kinase. After establishment of bacterial entry within the host, SopE is found on the *Salmonella*-containing vacuole where it modulates the vesicular traffic and the intracellular bacterial replication.

Ehrlichia chaffeensis TRP120 is the first bacterial protein which was shown to be sumoylated [232]. Sumoylation facilitates bacterial interaction with the host and has a significant impact on intracellular survival. In addition to that activity, TRP120 is a canonical HECT-like E3 Ub ligase. Recently, it was shown that TRP120-mediated ubiquitination and proteasome degradation of host Polycomb Group (PcG) protein family members and the nuclear tumor suppressor F-box and WD domain repeating-containing 7 (FBW7) promotes bacterial survival and infection [233, 234].

Bacteria have Evolved Non-Canonical Ubiquitinases and Deubiquitinases

Besides the canonical bacterial effectors interfereing with the eukaryotic ubiquitination networks, pathogens have evolved enzymes which are able to interact with the host Ub/Ubl systems in a non-typical way. These effectors have been discovered recently and represent non-canonical pathways for disrupting the Ub/Ubl eukaryotic signaling.

Phosphoribosyl Ubiquitinases and Deubiquitinases

Legionella SidE represent a family of four highly conserved effectors which achieve ubiquitination following a catalytic mechanism entirely different from the conventional three-enzyme cascade mechanism followed by eukaryotic ubiquitination systems [235 - 237]. Members of this family are responsible for ubiquitination of endoplasmic reticulum-associated human Rab GTPases, the reticulon 4 protein and proteins involved in membrane recruitment to the *Legionella*-containing vacuole. Ubiquitination of these proteins seems to have a role in endoplasmic reticulum remodeling and fragmentation [236, 238]. Because of the significant contribution to *Legionella*'s pathogenicity, SidE family is considered to be a potential drug target. A recent work has successfully investigated a group of NAD+ mimics as possible inhibitors [239].

SdeA, which is one of the best characterized members of the family, comprises four domains with four distinct functions [238, 240 - 242]. The N-terminal domain is a DUB, which it seems to be dispensable for protein pathogenicity. The second domain is a phosphodiesterase (PDE), the third a mono-ART (mART, mono-ADP-ribosylate) and the C-terminal domain forms a coiled-coil fold. All these three domains are indispensable for pathogenicity and act synergistically achieving ubiquitination in two steps. First, the mART module catalyzes the transfer of an ADP-ribose from a NAD+ to the side chain of Ub-Arg42 to generate an ADP-ribosylated-Ub (ADPR-Ub). Subsequently, the PDE module catalyzes the convertion of the ADP-ribosylated-Ub to a phospho-ribosylated-Ub (PR-Ub) and its ligation to a target-protein Ser residue *via* a phosphodiester bond. In the absence of substrate ADPR-Ub is hydrolyzed to PR-Ub and AMP. The role of the coiled-coil domain is not fully elucidated, even though it has been shown that it is required for optimum activity of mART domain.

Another *Legionella* effector, SidJ pseudokinase, is actually an inhibitor of the ADP-ribosylation activity of SdeA [243]. It was shown that SidJ suppresses SdeA by adding glutamate moieties (polyglutamylation) to a key catalytic residue of SdeA.

In addition, recent evidence demonstrates that phosphoribosyl-Ser-ubiquitination can be reversed [238]. Two *Legionella* proteins, named DupA and DupB, can specifically deubiquitinase phosphoribosyl-Ser-ubiquitinated substrates, while they are inactive on typical, through isopeptide bonds, Lys-ubiquitinated substrates. Dups and SdeA share a highly similar PDE domain, which thus can catalyze two opposite reactions. It is believed that Dups dynamically regulates the endoplasmic reticulum PR-ubiquitination.

Ubiquitin Transglutaminases

MavC and MvcA were originally identified as Ub specific deamidases [244]. Their structure determination demonstrated that both proteins adopt a similar fold which comprises two domains (Fig. **5B**). The main domain resembles a Cif-like fold and the other is actually an insertion domain to the first. Although the Cif-like domain of MavC and MvcA does not exhibit sequence homology with the Cif proteins described above, it does retain the catalytic triad Cys-His-Gln and a helical bundle responsible for substrate binding. Similar to Cifs, MavC and MvcA are able to deamidate Ub-Gln40 to Glu using the same general interface as the one used by Cifs, even though only MavC is able to interact with and deamidate the Ub-UBE2N conjugate [244]. In addition, the proteins are specific for Ub deamidation and unable to deamidate the NEDD8-Gln40 which is the primary target for the canonical Cifs. Very recently, however, new evidence lightened differently some details of the mechanism and demonstrated that the insertion domain of MavC actually induces a more significant functional divergence from the canonical Cifs than it was originally thought. It was confirmed that the MavC substrate is the Ub-UBE2N conjugate and it was shown that the enzyme catalyzes a covalent bond formation between Ub-Gln40 and UBE2N-Lys92, which is a transglutamination [245, 246]. In the absence of an amine donor the reaction results in Ub deamidation which was the activity originally observed. An abundance of crystal structures (Fig. **5C**) explains the functional consequences of this modification and provide details of the catalytic mechanism [246, 247]. The insertion domain is the one which forms most of the interactions with UBE2N and a severe remodelling occurs to accommodate the reaction process. UBE2N-Lys92 is close to the UBE2N active site and its Ub-transglutamination inhibits the E2 conjugating activity. Subsequently, the Lys63 polyubiquitination, which is required for full activation of the NF-κB, is disrupted and the NF-κB signaling is dampened upon infection. MavC is a non-canonical ubiquitinase since it does not require an E1 activated Ub.

Interestingly, MavC and MvcA have also deubiquitinase activity against the non-canonical ubiquitination they induce [248]. A third protein, Lpg2149 which is expressed from a gene adjacent to those expressing for MavC and MvcA was identified as their common bacterial inhibitor [244, 248]. Crystal structure of the complexes shows that Lpg2149 binds both proteins to their Cif-like domain with a manner equivalent to the Ub binding to the same domain (Fig. **5B**).

THE MULTIPLE FACETS OF GLYCOSYLATION IN BACTERIAL PATHOGENICITY

Glycosylation is a common modification present in mammals, bacteria and viruses (Fig. **1C**). Even though the physiological roles of protein glycosylation in bacteria have yet to be thoroughly explored, they are substantially different from those described in eukaryotic cells. In eukaryotes, protein glycosylation plays a vital role in the determination of protein structure, function and stability, subcellular localization, structural stability of the cell, modulation of cell signaling and immune responses. On the contrary, it has been highlighted as a virulence factor, with a significant role in defence mechanisms in bacteria. In this section we describe in detail all facets of glycosylation in bacterial pathogenicity.

Glycosylation is the covalent addition of sugar moieties to proteins, lipids or other organic molecules, in a tightly regulated, reversible manner. It occurs in two common forms: N-linked, when sugars are attached to the nitrogen atom of Asn or Arg residues and O-linked, when sugars are attached to the hydroxyl group of Ser or Thr residues.

O-Glycosylation of Bacterial Flagella

The flagellum is a motility organelle that enables movement and chemotaxis. Bacteria can have one or several flagella which can be either polar or peritrichous. The flagellum is composed of a basal body, anchored to the cell wall that acts as a rotary molecular motor, a hook that connects the basal body to the filament, and a filament that is composed of flagellin proteins and acts as a propeller. Bacterial pathogens utilize flagella-driven motility in order to reach their favorable niche within the host, making flagella essential for infection. Except from its evident role in motility, the flagellum has been shown to be important for adhesion to and invasion of epithelial cells, colonization and biofilm formation [249]. Concerning the host immune defense, flagellin proteins are recognized by the host immune system, triggering innate and adaptive immune responses. Flagellin interacts with cytoplasmic NOD-like receptors, inducing the formation of the inflammasome and it is recognized by TLR5 leading to the activation of NF-κB and members of the MARK family. These signaling pathways activate transcription of pro-inflammatory cytokines like interleukin-1 (IL-1), IL-6, IL-8 and TNF-α in host cells [250].

The process of flagellar glycosylation has been described in a variety of bacterial species from distinct environments. The glycan moieties found on this broad group of bacteria are also very diverse. Glycan diversity suggests potential functional roles which have yet to be revealed. There are several examples of bacteria in which flagellar glycosylation is essential not only for flagellum assembly but also for host-pathogen interactions. These examples are discussed in the following paragraphs.

Campylobacter jejuni, a Gram negative, helical, motile bacterium, is a major human gastrointestinal pathogen that causes infection after consumption of contaminated water or under-cooked poultry. Infected humans typically exhibit mild non-inflammatory diarrhea. However, in some cases, abdominal cramps, bloody diarrhea, vomiting and inflammation are also experienced. Potential severe consequences of this disease are immune-mediated disorders of the peripheral nervous system such as the Guillain-Barré Syndrome and the Miller Fisher Syndrome. *C. jejuni* has the unique ability to modify proteins with either O- or N-linked glycans. The O-glycosylation system of *C. jejuni* decorates flagellar proteins with numerous derivatives of pseudaminic acid (Pse). Flagellar filaments of *C. jejuni* are composed of two flagellin proteins: the major structural protein Flagellin A (FlaA) and a second, slightly larger protein, FlaB. Glycosylation is required for flagellar filament assembly and bacterial motility. FlaA of *C. jejuni* is heavily O-glycosylated, to up to 19 Thr or Ser residues per subunit. Mutation of the Pse biosynthesis A gene (*pseA*) resulted in loss of the acetamidino form of Pse (PseAm) thus changing FlaA glycosylation [251 - 253]. Absence of PseAm glycosylation led to loss of autoagglutination, reduced adherence to and invasion of intestinal epithelial cells *in vitro* as well as reduced virulence in the ferret diarrhea disease model [254]. However, glycosylated flagellin failed to induce TLR5 response. Mutation of five out of 19 O-glycosylation sites in the FlaA subunit resulted in fully motile but autoagglutination defective *C. jejuni* strains. These findings suggest that the five residues are surface exposed and possibly interact with flagellar filaments of other *C. jejuni* cells or with specific ligands on eukaryotic cells [255].

The closely related Gram negative, human gastrointestinal pathogen *Helicobacter pylori* also O-glycosylates its flagellar proteins with Pse. However, *H. pylori* is characterized by glycosylation homogeneity, since flagellins are modified with only a single Pse derivative. FlaA is glycosylated to seven while FlaB to ten Thr or Ser residues in the central region of the molecule. Deletion of any of the Pse biosynthetic pathway genes resulted in nonmotile *H. pylori* that were unable to colonize the stomach in a mouse model. The direct connection of glycosylated flagellar proteins to *H. pylori* pathogenesis highlights the importance of glycoproteins as potential therapeutic targets. Glycan metabolic labelling coupled with mass spectrometry analysis revealed a large number of glycosylated proteins implicated in colonization, persistence and virulence [256]. Even though further characterization of these proteins is necessary, these findings open the door to new vaccination and antibiotic therapies for *H. pylori* elimination.

The Gram negative, opportunistic pathogen *P. aeruginosa* causes fatal infections in immunocompromised human hosts and chronic colonizations in cystic fibrosis patients. Flagellins in *P. aeruginosa* are classified in two types, a- or b-type, depending on their molecular weight and reactivity with specific antisera. Flagellins from two *P. aeruginosa* a-type strains, PAK and JJ692, are O-glycosylated through a rhamnose residue to two sites on their flagellin subunits. *P. aeruginosa* PAK glycan contains up to 11 additional monosaccharides while *P. aeruginosa* JJ692 flagellin is glycosylated with only a single rhamnose residue. Flagellin of *P. aeruginosa* b-type strain PAO1 contains a single deoxyhexose residue attached to two nearby Ser residues and each glycan can be linked to a unique modification of mass 209 Da containing a phosphate moiety. As already mentioned, flagellins from most bacteria are recognized by TLR5, inducing the production of IL-8. However, non-glycosylated flagellin isolated from *P. aeruginosa* PAK mutants stimulated 50% less IL-8 production from A549 human alveolar epithelial cells compared to wild-type flagellin [257 - 259].

An *O*-linked glycosylation system was also identified in members of the Gram positive, spore-forming *Clostridium* species. *Clostridium difficile* is an emerging opportunistic pathogen and the leading cause of antibiotic-associated diarrhea and pseudomembranous colitis in humans. The flagellar proteins of *C. difficile* 630 and clinical isolates are O-glycosylated to up to seven Ser or Thr residues with N-acetylhexoseamine (HexNAc) linked to a methylated Asp through a phosphate bond. Mutation of a glycosyltransferase gene located in the flagellar biosynthesis locus showed that glycosylation is essential for flagellum assembly and motility [260]. On the contrary, the flagellins of *Clostridium botulinum* are O-glycosylated with either a novel derivative of the sialic acid-like nonulosonate sugar legionaminic acid (Leg) or a di-N-acetylhexuronic acid derivative to again up to seven Ser or Thr residues per monomer, depending on the strain. *C. botulinum* produces the potent botulinum neurotoxin, BoNT, which causes botulism, a descending symmetrical paralysis. Infant botulism, the most common form of botulism in the USA, typically occurs in infants under the age of 12 months. Interestingly, the flagellins from strains associated with infant botulism were exclusively modified with Leg derivatives suggesting that identification of the flagellin glycosylation pattern could be utilized as surrogate biomarker of *C. botulinum* infection [261].

The Gram-negative, opportunistic pathogen *Burkholderia cenocepacia*, mainly threatens cystic fibrosis patients by accelerating the decay of lung function. In some cases, this causes lethal necrotizing pneumonia known as the "cepacia syndrome". Nosocomial outbreaks caused by *B. cenocepacia* infection have also been reported. Flagellins from *B. cenocepacia* are classified into two types, type I and II, depending on the pattern resulting from restriction fragment length polymorphism analysis and the molecular weight. *B. cenocepacia* type II strain K56-2 has a single flagellum which induces host immune response through TRL5 activation and contributes to virulence in a mouse infection model. *B. cenocepacia* K56-2 flagellin (FliC) is glycosylated to, at least 10 sites, with a single glycan residue, the viosamine (Qui4N) derivative, D-Qui4N(3OHBut). Qui4N is one of the monosaccharides of the flagellin glycan in *P. aeruginosa* PAK. Flagellins from other *Burkholderia* species are also glycosylated by a single glycan but the molecular masses do not correspond to that of D-Qui4N(3OHBut). One of the genes responsible for the biosynthesis of D-Qui4N(3OHBut) glycan was identified in *B. cenocepacia* K56-2. *rmlB* encodes for a dTDP-D-glucose 4,6-dehydratase and it is one of the dTDP-L-rhamnose biosynthesis genes, located in the O-antigen cluster. RmlB is also implicated in O-antigen synthesis, which contains a rhamnose moiety in its repeating unit. In addition, RmlB has been shown to be essential for *B. cenocepacia* viability even though flagellin glycosylation and O-antigen production are not. In an attempt to study the role of glycosylation in TLR5/flagellin mediated inflammatory responses it was found that non-glycosylated flagellin was more effective in stimulating TLR5-mediated inflammatory response and gene expression in epithelial cells compared to the glycosylated protein [262].

N-Glycosylation of Bacterial Surface Proteins

As already mentioned, *C. jejuni* has the unique ability to modify proteins with either N- or O-linked glycans. The N-linked protein glycosylation (Pgl) pathway was originally described in *C. jejuni* [263] and has been extensively characterized to-date. *C. jejuni* modifies over 100 surface proteins with an heptasaccharide (GalNAc-α1,4-GalNAc-α1,4-[Glcβ1,3]-GalNAc-α1, 4-GalNAc-α1, 4-GalNA--α1, 3-Bac-β1 where Bac is bacillosamine [2,4-diacetamido-2,4,6 trideoxyglucopyranose]) to the Asn residue of the consensus sequence [D/E]XNX[S/T], where X can be any amino acid except Pro. Recently, a proteomics study highlighted *C. jejuni* N-glycosylated proteins as key virulence factors [264]. The seven-residue glycan is synthesized in the cytoplasm, flipped across the membrane and transferred from an undecaprenyl phosphate lipid carrier to target proteins by the PglB oligosaccharyltransferase in the periplasm. PglB can also release the heptasaccharide from the lipid carrier to the periplasm. Once released, the free glycan possibly provides protection of *C. jejuni* against osmotic stress. Deletion of the *pglB* gene or the whole *pgl* gene cluster leads to low adherence of *C. jejuni* to epithelial cells and reduced colonization of the gastrointestinal track in a chicken animal model [265, 266].

Several pathogenic bacterial species, including *Neisseria meningitidis* [265] and *Acinotebacter baumannii* [267], retain a general O-glycosylation system that is able to modify different proteins through the assembly of glycans onto lipid carriers in a process similar to the N-glycosylation system already described in *C. jejuni.*

O-Glycosylation of Host Proteins by Bacterial Toxins

Some pathogenic bacteria contain toxins with glycosyltransferase activities that modify host proteins in order to regulate host innate immune responses and facilitate infection. Two well-studied glycosylating cytotoxins are toxin A (TcdA) and toxin B (TcdB) which constitute the principal pathogenicity factors of *C.*

difficile. TcdA and TcdB are homologous and functionally similar. The glycosyltransferase domain lies in the N-terminus of the protein and it is followed by a protease domain implicated in the auto-proteolytic cleavage of the toxin. Another domain, probably responsible for the translocation and binding of the toxins to host cells, is located at the C-terminus of the protein. Both toxins invade target cells *via* clathrin-mediated endocytosis which is followed by auto-proteolytic cleavage and release of the glycosyltransferase domain into the cytosol. TcdA/B O-glycosylate Rho GTPases, including Rho (RhoA/B/C), Rac (Rac1-3) and Cdc42, to a single highly conserved Thr residue, with either a glucosamine (Glc) or an N-acetylglucosamine (GlcNAc) moiety. This Thr residue is located in the switch I region of Rho proteins and is critical for nucleotide binding. Rho GTPases are involved in many signaling pathways, modulating cell physiology and immune responses. Upon TcdA/B mediated glycosylation, Rho interaction with effectors is inhibited, blocking Rho-dependent signaling. Glycosylation also inhibits Rho activation by GTPase-activating proteins (GAPs) and GEFs leading to host cell bleb formation, rounding and eventually death [266, 268].

C. difficile TcdA and TcdB are the classic examples of the clostridial glycosylating cytotoxin family which also includes *C. perfringens* large toxin (TpeL), *C. novyi* α-toxin (TcnA) and *C. sordellii* lethal (TcsL) and hemorrhagic toxin (TcsH). These toxins also O-glycosylate Rho GTPases on a Thr residue resulting in their inactivation.

Except from *Clostridium*, several *Legionella* species also contain toxins with a glycosyltransferase activity. Such a toxin is Lgt1 which shares high structural homology to the glycosyltransferase domain of the clostridian cytotoxin TcdB. Similarly to other intracellular pathogens, *L. pneumophila* acquires energy for its proliferation from the consumption of nutrients present in the intracellular environment. The life cycle and virulence of *L. pneumophila* are closely related to the levels of nutrient availability in the host. So far, 13 *lgt*1-like genes have been identified in various *L. pneumophila* strains. One of the most studied *L. pneumophila* strains, Philadelphia-1, contains three *lgt* genes, *lgt*1, 2 and 3, whereas other strains only two, *lgt*1 and 3. All 13 Lgt effectors are translocated to host cells *via* the Dot/Icm T4SS in order to modify host proteins by glycosylation. *In vitro* studies have shown that Lgt1 O-glycosylates the eukaryotic elongation factor 1A (eEF1A) to a single Ser residue using UDP-glucose as sugar donor. eEF1A is a conserved, large GTPase, vital for protein synthesis. More specifically, eEF1A is a component of the elongation complex in protein synthesis and it is involved in the delivery of aminoacyl tRNA to the A-site of ribosomes. The Ser residue, which constitutes the target of Lgt1-mediated glycosylation, lies in the GTP-binding domain of eEF1A. The presence of the sugar moiety within the GTPase domain probably prevents conformational changes leading to eEF1A inactivation. When Lgt is delivered to mammalian cells, it mediates glycosylation of eEF1A causing inhibition of host protein synthesis, ultimately leading to cell death [269, 270].

According to a recent study, host protein synthesis inhibition by Lgt effectors activates a master metabolic regulator called mechanistic target of rapamycin complex 1 (mTORC1). mTORC1 is a conserved complex of proteins, including the mTOR kinase and various other regulatory proteins. mTORC1 regulates cell growth in response to amino acid and nutrient availability and when active, it inhibits autophagy and triggers initiation of protein synthesis. In that way, free amino acids are produced, which can be consumed by *L. pneumophila,* in order to obtain energy for intracellular replication [271].

As mentioned earlier, except from Lgt1, most *L. pneumophila* strains produce Lgt3 while some produce Lgt2. The N-terminus of Lgt3 is homologous to that of Lgt1 whereas Lgt2 is significantly similar, but not homologous, to Lgt1. All three Lgt effectors modify eEF1A at the same Ser residue. *lgt*1 and 2 are mainly expressed at stationary phase while *lgt*3 at early phase of growth, highlighting the importance of temporal regulation of gene expression for infection of target cells by *Legionella*. Lastly, recombinant Lgt1, 2 and 3 are able to hinder eukaryotic translation in a cell-free system [268].

L. pneumophila contains another glycosyltransferase effector, named subversion of eukaryotic vesicle trafficking A (SetA). Similarly to Lgt effectors, SetA is translocated to host cells *via* the Dot/Icm T4SS. Sequence analysis of SetA revealed the presence of a glycosyltransferase domain at the N-terminus and a unique phosphatidylinositol-3-phosphate (PI3P)-binding domain at the C-terminus. The PI3P-binding domain is necessary for SetA guidance and localization to vesicular compartments of host cells. SetA has been shown to have glucohydrolase and glucosyltransferase activity *in vitro*. In particular, SetA can specifically hydrolyse UDP-glucose and transfer the sugar moiety to its own Ser and Thr residues but also to a large group of cellular substrates such as actin, histones H3.1 and H4 and the small GTPase Rab1a. Mutations in the glycosyltransferase domain inactivate SetA further blocking histone glycosylation, mammalian cell death and endocytic secretory trafficking [272].

A very recent study demonstrated that when active, SetA glycosylates the transcription factor EB (TFEB) causing its nuclear localization. When amino acids are available, TFEB is phosphorylated by the master regulator mTORC1, triggering its cytoplasmic sequestration through interactions with the regulatory protein 14-3-3. In the absence of amino acids, mTORC1 is inhibited, while phosphatase calcineurin is activated, inducing TFEB dephosphorylation and nuclear translocation. Once in the nucleus, TFEB induces the expression of lysosomal and autophagosomal genes enhancing the activity of degradative organelles. As a result, host macromolecules are hydrolyzed, increasing nutrient availability [273]. Mass spectrometry analysis revealed that SetA O-glycosylates TFEB to three Ser and two Thr residues adjacent to the 14-3-3 binding site, hampering their interaction. SetA also modifies TFEB to a single Ser residue inhibiting GSK3β-mediated phosphorylation on this site, thus promoting retention in the nucleus by hindering export from the nucleus [274]. This is an additional mechanism that *L. pneumophila* has developed in order to acquire host nutrients and ensure its intracellular replication.

N-Glycosylation of Host Proteins by Bacterial Effectors

Enteropathogenic *E. coli* (EPEC) is an extracellular, Gram negative, gastro-intestinal pathogen which constitutes the main cause of infantile diarrhea. Once taken up by the host, EPEC adheres to the apical surface of enterocytes and destroys the brush-border microvilli. The induction of this so-called attaching and effacing (A/E) lesion is crucial for EPEC pathogenesis and it is accompanied by actin redistribution and actin-rich pedestal-like structure formation at the contact site of bacteria. EPEC, similarly to other Gram-negative pathogenic bacteria, utilizes the T3SS in order to inject effector proteins into host intestinal cells. These effectors act to manipulate host cell functions and escape host immune defence. One of these effectors, NleB1, was recently characterized as a glycosyltransferase that irreversibly modifies a conserved Arg residue in death domain (DD) containing adaptor proteins with GlcNAc [275 - 277]. DDs are present in the intracellular region of death receptors such as FAS, TNFR1 and TNF-associated apoptosis-inducing ligand (TRAIL) receptor 1 (TRAIL-R1). Death receptor signaling is vital for apoptosis, inflammatory and immune responses and it is mediated by homotypic/heterotypic interactions between the DDs of the death receptors and the downstream adaptors including FAS-associated death domain protein (FADD), TNFR1-associated death domain protein (TRADD) and receptor-interacting serine/threonine-protein kinase 1 (RIPK1). In particular, once the death receptor is activated by the ligand, FADD and caspase-8 are recruited in order to form the death-inducing signaling complex (DISC) triggering apoptosis. Similarly, TRADD and RIPK1 recruitment induces NF-kB activation for cell survival, inflammation, or differentiation or induces cell death *via* formation of the DISC. The N-glycosylated, by NleB1, DDs of FADD or TRADD adaptor proteins are unable to interact with death receptors and form DISCs thus blocking death receptor signaling, including NF-kB activation and apoptosis, in EPEC infected cells [278].

An NleB1 homologue, called NleB$_{CR}$, is present in *Citrobacter rodentium*, an EPEC-like mucosal pathogen of mice. NleB$_{CR}$, similarly to NleB1, inhibits NF-kB activation and its activity has been recently shown to be necessary for bacterial survival and colonization in a mouse model [279]. *S. enterica* strains also contain NleB1 homologues, named SseK1, SseK2 and SseK3. SseK1 and SseK3, show GlcNAcyltransferase activity and are able to modify the Arg residue of DDs of TRADD and TNFR1. A very recent study showed that SseK3, but not SseK1, targets additional substrates. More specifically, SseK3 transfers GlcNAc to an Arg residue of Rab GTPases, including Rab1, leading to its inactivation. The authors also revealed that "SseK3 blocks the host inflammatory cytokine secretion during *Salmonella* infection and is crucial for bacterial virulence in mice" [280].

VIRAL PATHOGENICITY THOUGH PTMS

Among infectious diseases, the viral infections pose a serious public health threat causing seasonal epidemics, or even pandemics, in humans. It is known that viruses are able to mainly express proteins that help them enter the host cell and proliferate with the help of host cell-machineries. Since PTMs serve as a protein functional switcher of cell, it is not surprising that viruses use PTMs to both make their proteins functional and control host proteins in order to increase virulence. It is observed that in the host cell, viruses are able to mediate PTMs either directly, with some of their proteins that are enzymes or indirectly, implicated with host enzymes. Generally, from influenza virus to human immunodeficiency virus (HIV) and, the newly emerged, Coronavirus (CoV), post-translational modified viral proteins are observed and through PTMs, cell proteins are manipulated by these viruses [281]. The identification of PTMs on viral proteins, the elucidation of how viruses use host cell machineries to induce PTMs or to which host cell proteins they choose to add PTMs will be of great importance in biomedicine and biopharmaceutical sectors in order to understand better virulence and design effective medicine and vaccines. A collection of reviews on "Virus induced and associated post-translational modifications" [282] has been published elsewhere so in this chapter, we will explicitly present how the Coronavirus causative agent of the current pandemic meets PTMs.

Coronavirus (CoV) Family

Coronaviruses are a family of enveloped RNA viruses that are responsible for diseases in humans and animals, as well (Fig. **6**). Impressively, members of the family can cause, except from common colds, more severe diseases with high mortality rates. Such members are the Middle East respiratory syndrome coronavirus (MERS-CoV) and the newly emerged, severe acute respiratory syndrome coronavirus (SARS-CoV) [283, 284].

Coronavirus name is based on the characteristic surface projections of the trimeric S-glycoprotein giving the picture of a corona. Shorter projections can be observed in some coronaviruses, consisting of the homodimeric HE protein. The M-glycoprotein is found embedded into the viral envelope. Its main function is to provide structural support to the virion. Main part of the envelope is the small E protein, as well. It helps virion assembly and release. Finally, the N protein is another important protein that exists in the interior virion, taking part in the helically symmetric nucleocapsid, closely associated with the viral RNA genome [285]. These proteins are the main structural proteins of Coronavirus. Apart from this group, there are also nonstructural proteins (nsps) with diverse functions and accessory proteins with a not well-defined role, so far.

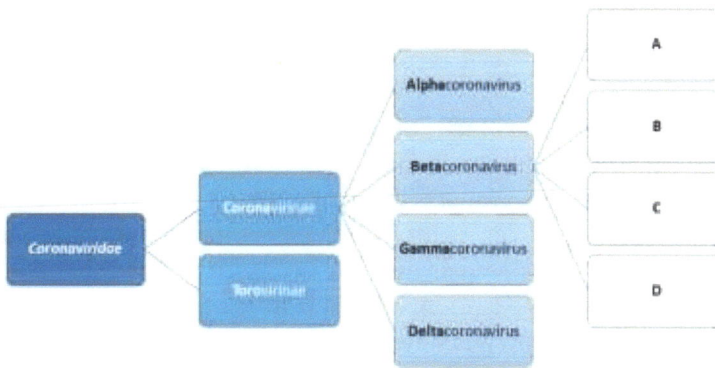

Fig. (6).   Classification of coronaviruses. Coronavidae family is devided into two subfamilies, the *Coronavirinae* and the *Torovirinae*. The subfamily *Coronavirinae* is further divided into four genera, *Alphacoronavirus*, *Betacoronavirus*, *Gammacoronavirus* and *Deltacoronaviruses*. The *Betacoronavirus* genus, is classified in four lineages, A, B, C and D. SARS-CoV is of lineage B.

All of the main structural proteins and most of the nsps are post-translationally modified by glycosylation, phosphorylation, palmitoylation *etc* (Table **1**, Fig. **1**).

Table 1. PTMs of each coronavirus structural protein.

	S Protein	M Protein	E Protein	N Protein
N-glycosylation	√*	√	√	-
O-glycosylation	-	√*	-	-
Palmitoylation	√*	-	√*	-
Phosphorylation	-	-	-	√*
Disulfide Bridge	√	-	-	-
Cleavage	-	-	-	√
ADP-ribosylation	-	-	-	√

(Table 1) cont.....

	S Protein	M Protein	E Protein	N Protein
SUMOylation	-	-	-	√

The PTMs that play a role in pathogenicity are marked with a star (*).

In more detail, the S protein, named by Spike, of SARS-CoV-2 is a glycoprotein and the largest among the four structural proteins [286, 287]. It is a homotrimeric and transmembrane protein and its function is to mediate host-cell entry *via* binding to the angiotensin-converting enzyme 2 (ACE2) receptor [288]. Responsible for the receptor binding is the S1 domain while for the membrane fusion, the S2 domain is responsible, both existed at the N-terminus [289]. For the activation of S protein, a protease cleavage is required, at the boundary between the S1 and S2 domain (S1/S2 boundary) [286, 289, 290]. S protein is post-translationally modified by N-linked glycosylation and disulfide bond formation, while there are cystein residues that are palmitoylated [285].

The E protein, named by Envelope, of SARS-CoV-2 is the smallest (8-12kDa) of the four structural proteins and is found in low amount in the virion [291]. As S protein, E protein is also a transmembrane protein [292] and respectively, the function of E protein is not yet well defined [293]. It is observed that most of the expressed E protein is localized at the endoplasmic reticulum (ER), Golgi and ER-Golgi intermediate compartment where it helps the assembly and budding of the new virions [294] and the remaining, much less amount, is directly incorporated into the formation of newly produced virion envelopes [295]. Studies on CoVs that lack E protein indicate its important role in the virus production and maturation [296, 297]. Moreover, the involvement of E protein to the formation of oligomeric cation-selective ion channels and the consequent of host cell membrane permability, has been studied [298]. Concerning the PTMs, the E protein is reported to be modified by glycosylation and palmitoylation [292] and it has been indicated that through them and several intermediated stages of maturation in the ER and Golgi, the final conformation of the protein can be manipulated according to the physiochemical properties of the membrane [299].

The M protein, named by Membrane, consists of 220-260 amino acids, is transmembrane and the most abundant of the main structural proteins of coronaviruses [300]. The role of M protein is to provide the scaffold for virion assembly and to recruit other structural proteins and virus RNA, by interacting with them in order to mediate incorporation of the nucleocapsid into the newly formed virion [301]. The ectodomain of M protein is glycosylated, O-linked glycosylated in some coronaviruses and N-linked glycosylated in other coronavirues and this is the only PTM reported for M proteins [302].

The N protein is the only among the four structural proteins of coronaviruses that exists entirely in the virion. It is of about 43-50 kDa and is the main protein component of nucleocapsid that also binds the RNA genome [303]. The whole protein interacts with RNA but the C-terminal domain is essential for the N protein dimerization and the interaction with M protein, as well. It is also shown that N protein is involved in the pathway of coronavirus RNA synthesis [304]. The N-terminal domain is phosphorylated and it is also indicated that the whole protein is modified by proteolytic cleavage, SUMOylation and ADP-ribosylation [305, 306] but their role is not yet clarified.

A description of each kind of PTMs that is addressed in each of the CoV and especially the CoV-2 proteins and the role that it may play, is following.

PTMS FOUND IN CORONAVIRUS PROTEINS

Glycosylation

The coronavirus S protein was the first observed to be N-linked glycosylated, for MHV in 1982 [307]. MHV S protein is glycosylated with high mannose oligosaccharides, while the glycans of SARS-CoV S protein were composed of high mannose, hybrid and complex glycans [308]. Notably, even though many glycosylated sites can be noted at the S proteins, they are not all of them functional. The main contribution of N-linked glycosylation is to the final conformation of coronavirus S protein but in this way, it profoundly plays an important role to the receptor binding and antigenicity of the virus. The dependence of the binding of infectious bronchitis virus (IBV) neutralizing antibodies on the glycosylation of the IBV S protein [309] and the reduced antigenicity of both non-glycosylated transmissible gastroenteritis virus (TGEV) S and M proteins [310], showed by early studies on these animal coronaviruses, are examples of the significant roles of N-linked glycosylation. However, there are more recent studies, on SARS-CoV, indicating that the antigenicity of coronavirus S protein does not always depend on its glycosylation status [311 - 313]. Concluding, the glycosylation of coronavirus S protein has a complex effect on the immune response that probably varies according to the specific coronavirus and host system in study. Concerning, though, the SARS-CoV-2, the structure of S protein has demonstrated that the N terminal domain (S1 and S2 domains) is densely decorated with both, host derived, N and unexpected O glycans, helping its folding (by the host cell), the elicitation of humoral immune response and the accessibility to neutralizing antibodies [289, 314, 315]. The S gene encodes 22 N-linked glycan sequons per monomer with S1 domain being slightly more decorated (13 sites) than S2 monomers (9 sites) (Fig. **7**). Hence there are 66 N-linked glycosylation sites, totally, in one S homotrimer [289, 316, 317]. 8 out of the 22 sites contain substantial populations of oligomannose-type glycans while the rest 14 sites are dominated by processed, complex-type glycans [317]. Additionally, from the site-specific glycan analysis by cryo-EM and mass spectrometry that Watanabe *et. al.* have performed, it is revealed that across the 22 N-linked glycosylation sites, 52% are fucosylated and 15% of the glycans contain at least one sialic acid residue. This glycan profile will be an important measure of antigen quality in the manufacture of serological testing kits [317]. Noticeably, the N-linked glycans are conserved among SARS-CoV and SARS-CoV-2 (9 out of 13 glycans in the S1 domain and all 9 glycans in the S2 domain), and the N-linked glycosylation sequons are mostly conserved across glycoproteins of SARS-CoV-related viruses (20 out of 22 concerved sequons) indicating that the recognition and accessibility to Abs is comparable for these two viruses. However, comparison to more human pathogenic coronavirus reveals that the S protein of SARS-CoV-2 is less densely glycosylated [317]. Glycosylation acts as camouflage of immunogenic protein epitopes of virus against host cell. Hence, the sparse glycosylation of S protein of SARS-CoV-2 may limit immune evasion and help the elicitation of humoral immune response. For that reason, S protein would be a key target for drug or vaccine design for COVID-19 disease.

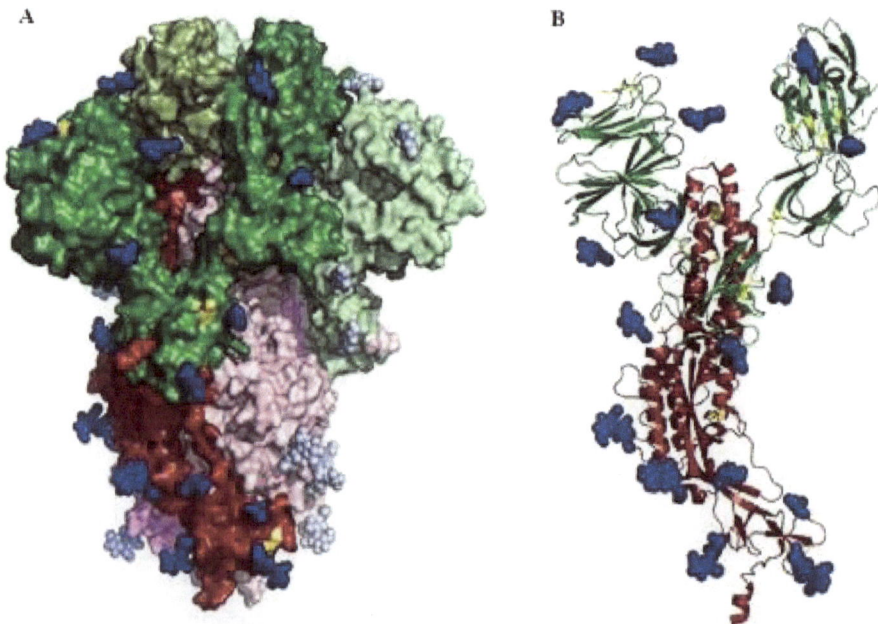

Fig. (7). Crystal structure of SARS-CoV-2 S protein. **(A)** The trimeric S protein with glycans presented as blue spheres. For each monomer the S1 domain is colored green and the S2 domain is colored red. The Cys residues are colored in yellow. **(B)** The S protein monomer in cartoon representation (PDB 6VXX). The figure was prepared using PyMOL [18].

Interestingly, it is observed that host receptors of coronavirus S proteins can be found glycosylated, as well. For example, the N-linked glycosylation of CEACAM1, the cellular receptor protein of MHV, was found essential for the binding to MHV-A59 virions [318]. On the contrary, N-linked glycosylation of human APN, the receptor for HCoV-229E, reduces the binding to HCoV-229E virions [319]. It is profound, that the host tropism of coronavirus infection is affected by the glycosylation modification of receptors but structural characteristics of viral S protein are important, as well and all of them should be taken under consideration for drug or vaccine design [320].

As far as E protein is concerned, it is indicated that its glycosylation may help its trafficking in the cellular production machinery and its final oligomerization and consequently its functional role [293, 299, 315, 321, 322]. IBV E protein contains only one potential N-linked glycosylation sites on N5, whereas SARS-CoV E contains two, N48 and N66 [323]. However, the N5 of IBV E protein and the N48 of SARS-CoV are never glycosylated, whereas the N66 is glycosylated only in one of the two possible membrane topologies that SARS-CoV E protein can adopt. It is suggested that the lack of glycosylation at this position promote oligomerization of the E protein in order, probably, to control its function [293]. Since there is only little information about the glycosylation of CoV E proteins and its role, more research is needed in order to clarify which of the CoV E proteins are glycosylated and when. If only SARS-CoV E protein is indicated to be glycosylated, under specific conditions or viral needs, then it might be a certain pathogenic feature which could be the basis for specific drugs for SARS.

O-linked glycosylation was firstly reported for MHV M protein in early 80's [324]. Although it has not been assumed that it is essential for the virion assembly, the O-linked glycosylation has served as a marker for membrane maturation and localisation of M protein in the cell [325]. Though, there are evidence that the glycosylation of M protein may play a role in the induction of innate immune system [326]. N-linked glycosylation has been reported for SARS-CoV M protein at the Asp4 residue and it seems to help the steady state in the Golgi. More studies on N-glysylated M protein of SARS-CoV has indicated that it does not have any significant affection on protein transport, protein assembly, new virion replication or I-interferon induction or suppression [327, 328].

Finally, most of the nsps and accessory proteins of coronaviruses are found to be glycosylated. In some cases, as for MHV nsp4, glycosylation seems to implicate in viral replication but more studies are required in order to clarify the exact role of glycosylation on these proteins [285].

Disulfide Bond Formation

Structural studies of the SARS-CoV-2 S protein binding to ACE2 have revealed that several Cys residues exist at this area [329 - 331]. It has been, also, indicated that the entry of viral glycoprotein is impacted by thiol–disulfide balance on the cell surface [332]. This happens since, as it is observed, pH change leads to conformational changes and to disulfide-thiol conversion of S protein. However, studies on MHV show that disulfide bond formation is important only for the correct folding of MHV S protein [333] and studies on SARS-CoV show that S1 domain of SARS-CoV S protein is highly insensitivite to redox state [334]. Interestingly, though, molecular dynamics (MD) simulations performed by Hati and Bhattacharyya [335] have indicated that the binding affinity is significantly impaired when all of the disulfide bonds of both ACE2 and SARS-CoV/CoV-2 spike proteins are reduced to thiol groups. The impact on the binding affinity is less severe when the disulfide bridges of only one of the binding partners are reduced to thiols. It is hence, demonstrated that control of oxidative stress may be beneficial since its reduce prevents the viral SARS-CoV-2 S protein binding on the host cell [335].

Concerning the CoV E protein, it is indicated that depending on reducing conditions, there are differences in the oligomerization state of the protein [291]. Site-directed mutagenesis have demonstrated that two Cys residues existed at the transmembrane domain, have a central role at the oligomerization procedure of the CoV protein, forming disulfide bonds that lead to dimers, trimers or pentamers according to the functional need [336]. Additionally, disulfide bond formation has been observed for coronavirus nsp9, whose main role is to act as ssRNA binding protein implicating in the viral genome transcription/replication and it is suggested that disulfind bonds are important for binding affinity to the ssRNA [337]. So, the role of disulfide bond formation must be further analysed since it is significand for specific structure states and binding ability of coronavirus proteins.

Palmitoylation

Biochemical studies based on mutational analysis of Cys residues of S coronavirus proteins have indicated that palmitoylation is essential for the infectivity of MHV [338]. It was found that non palmitoylated cysteins lead the MHV S protein to be trapped in translational folding states almost ten-times longer than the palmitoylated protein with consequent reduced infectivity [339]. Similarly, the lack of palmitoylated cysteins at the SARS-CoV S protein reduces the binding ability to the ACE2 receptor [340]. The only reported difference is that palmitoylation of S protein is essential for the S-M protein interaction of

MHV but not for the SARS-CoV [341]. However, for the SARS-CoV-2, there are no available data concerning the palmitoylation of S protein.

Concerning the E proteins of coronaviruses [145] palmitoylation is broadly reported since the fatty acids, attached to proteins by palmitoylation, increase hydrophobicity which has been indicated to assist in membrane formation and membrane anchoring [342]. Of the coronavirus family, the E protein of IBV, MHV and SARS-CoV, have been found to be palmitoylated [293]. By studies with mutated Cys residues of MHV E protein it has been suggested that palmitoylation plays an important role in E protein structural stability, in VLP formation and consequently to the overall viral assembly [343]. However, similar studies on SARS-CoV E protein shows that palmitoylation might, only affect the interaction with the membrane [343] though, more recent studies indicate that it is not essential for the VLP production [344].

Phosphorylation

Among coronavirus structural proteins, it has been shown, that only the SARS-CoV N protein can be phosphorylated in, at least, four sites by host kinases [345]. Studies on IBV N protein suggest that phosphorylation may play important role in recognition and specific binding of viral RNA [346]. Studies on MHV N protein, have also revealed the role of phosphorylation in regulation of genome replication and transcription [347]. Finally, investigation of the importance of phos-phorylation on SARS-CoV N protein has indicated that they may also be implicated in nucleocytoplasmic shuttling [345], antagonism to host antiviral mechanisms [348] and antigenicity [349].

Ubiquitination

Among coronaviruses, ubiquitination has been reported only for the SARS-CoV E protein and its exact role is not clear yet. It seems that it correlates to the structural stability and half-life of E protein [350, 351].

It is also suggested that nsp16 of SARS-CoV has a ubiquitination site. Though, the main role of nsp16 is to act as a nucleoside-2'O-methyltranferase helping the viral RNA to avoid detection by the host cell, the role of the possible ubiquitination is not clear yet [352].

How Coronaviruses Induce PTMs to Host Proteins

The coronavirus proteins that are involved in the PTMs of host proteins are the nsps. From early 00's, it was known that nsp3 has papain-like protease (PLPro) activity and is responsible for the proteolytic cleavage towards the release of nsp1, nsp2 and nsp3 [353]. Additionally, it has been observed that PLPro of many coronaviruses has deubiquination (DUB) activity and some of them can act as de-ISGylating enzyme, as well [354 - 356]. It is well known that ubiquitination and ISGylation play significant role in immune response by involving in signal transduction of innate immunity. Hence, DUB and deLSGylation are important "tools" of the virus in inhibition of host antiviral response [357]. Several studies have demonstrated that SARS-CoV PLPro can block type I IFN production, inhibit TNFα-induced NF-κB activation and block the production of proinflammatory cytokines and chemokines in activated cells, suppressing the activation of TBK1 and inhibit IRF3 by DUB and dedeISGylation [358 - 361].

Moreover, it has been reported a more indirect way of PTM modulation of host protein by coronaviruses. A characteristic example is that of nsp3, which can enhance a cellular E3 ubiquitin ligase, leading to proteosomal degradation of p53 and consequently help the virulence of SARS-CoV (cellular p53 inhibits virus replication) [362]. Finally, it has been also reported that coronavirus proteins can suppress ubiquitination of host proteins. This is the case of N protein that binds to TRIM25, an E ubiquitin ligase that activates RIG-I and by this binding, inhibit TRIM25 ubiquitination and consequently, RIG-I activation and I IFN production [363]. In the same way, the SARS-CoV accessory protein 6 interacts with a protein of IFN signaling pathway, promoting its ubiquitin degradation and, thus, affect the innate immune response [364].

In conclusion, more research is required in order to be able to elucidate in detail the way that coronaviruses induse PTMs to host proteins in order to recruit them for their virulence.

THE POTENTIAL OF PTMS IN THE NEW ERA OF BIOPHARMACEUTICALS, ANTIBIOTICS AND ANTIVIRALS

The Challenge of Engineering PTMs in Biopharmaceuticals

Biopharmaceuticals is the term for the recombinant therapeutic proteins (*e.g.* recombinant human insulin and antibodies) or nucleic-acid based and cell/tissue-based products. Most of the proteins used as biopharmaceuticals are modified post-translationally, since PTMs affect their biochemical and consequently, therapeutic properties, including stability and binding ability. Here, we will present the most recent advances in the crossroad, where biopharmaceuticals meet PTMs, either as a tool for controlling the main properties (stability, recognition, binding) of the designed protein-based drugs and vaccines or as the main action of the designed drug on the target protein (protein inhibition).

One characteristic example of PTMs in protein-based biopharmaceuticals is disulfide bond formation which is mostly observed in eukaryotic than prokaryotic proteins [365], since prokaryotic cells have limited endogenous mechanisms for this formation. However, prokaryotic expression systems are broadly used for protein pharmaceutical production, since they offer a cost-effective production. It is obvious though, that the choice of the suitable expression system for biopharmaceuticals, concerning the requirements in PTMs, is a critical factor. Hence, research in this field aims to engineer prokaryotic cells in order to improve their capability to produce engineered, intracellular and stable proteins that are post-translationally modified correctly [366].

Another paradigm is glycosylation and the various approaches of glycoengineering. The addition of N-glycosylation sites into recombinant interferon-α provides an interesting example and it is known that the hyperglycosylated interferon shows 20-25 fold increase in plasma half-life [367]. More recently, it has been shown that bacterial engineered glyconjugates can be utilized as vaccine candidates against *B. pseudomallei* [368]. Generally, there are three types of vaccines developed. The first type is vaccines by live attenuated bacteria that are effective but not that easily produced, not very safe nor stable. The second type is by whole-cell-killed bacteria but though they can be produced more easily they are still not that safe nor stable. The third type is vaccines by purified surface carbohydrates but they cannot offer long-term protection or even more effective, vaccines by bacterial surface polysaccharides chemically conjugated to a carrier protein. Garcia-Quintanilla *et al.* have driven this type of vaccines one step further by producing an engineered *E. coli* strain which is able to express the genes of glycosylation machinery and produce the desired glycoconjugates biochemically [368].

Another example of how PTMs can be a significant help for researchers in drug design field is revealed in the design of drug-transporters. These transporters are membrane proteins and their physiological function is to transfer nutrients or other necessary compounds (*e.g.* hormones) into cells. It is observed that these transporters are loose constrained to the molecules that they transport so the researchers have taken advantage of this characteristic and have used the cell transporters as drug-transporters [369]. The control of their physiological function can be occurred for long-term regulation during the steps of transcription and dynamically, for short-term by post-translational modifications. Hence, PTMs are the "tool" for the structural and functional control of drug-transporters. For instance, a glycosylation site (N50) in the peptide transporter 1 (PEPT1) has been identified as the most critical for the efficiency of peptide transport [370]. Additionally, it is indicated that the glycosylation at this point protect PEPT1 form protease degradation [371]. Generally, the implication of PTMs in the control of drug-trasporter function must be fully illuminated since these transporters effect in pharmacokinetics and pharmacodynamics of drugs and in the capacity of drugs to act against off-targets with side-effects [372].

Research in biopharma has also focused on engineered targeted therapy and nowadays, one of the most used types of targeted therapy for several diseases is the small molecules inhibitors. In order to ameliorate the characteristics of the inhibitors and avoid off-target effects or other non-desired effects the PROteolysis-Targeting Chimeras (PROTAC) molecules have been produced to exploit the intracellular ubiquitin-proteasome system to induce selective degradation [373]. PROTAC molecules can be considered as one of the most recent cases where a bio-pharmaceutical use a post-translational modification as the main action of its therapeutic property. These molecules are chimeras of three linkers, the first one is a linker to the inhibition target protein, the second one is a linker to the E3 ubiquitin ligase and the last one is a linker for these two linkers. Pharmaceutical companies have already made efforts for clinical trials of specific PROTACs against prostate and estrogen cancer [374]. The research about PROTAC is in progress for more proteins that could be targeted and for more E3 ligases that could be recruited, as well.

Finally, in the field of biopharmaceuticals, it is approved that the most protein-based biocharmaceuticals use PTMs in order to fulfill their therapeutic effect since the drug-target interaction (protein-protein interaction and drug-protein binding) occurs through PTMs. Su *et al.* have recently developed CruxTPM a novel, integrative web platform for structural characterization and 3D visualization of PTM sites, as well as the investigation of their relationship with drug-target binding and PPI. This tool will implicate in the understanding of the biological mechanisms associated with PTMs and improve the efficiency of drug design [375].

A review about the post-translation modifications of protein biopharmaceuticals in general, is recently written by Walsh *et al.* [376]. Here we will focus on anti-viral and anti-microbial drug design used for infectious diseases emphasizing on the significance of PTMs.

Potential Anti-Viral Drugs

It has been described in detail above that viruses exploits host cell machinery to their advantaged by extensively manipulating the physiological network of protein PTMs which usually regulate cellular processes. Proteins and pathways involved in this process are all possible drug targets, since if they are blocked, the virulence will be blocked. The research in this field is not yet very advanced and here we will present briefly only two recent paradigms of how anti-viral drug design meets PTMs.

The first paradigm, as it is reviewed recently, is the Lysine-specific modifications [9] that affect main cellular mechanisms such as regulation of gene expression [377], immune response [378] and cell cycle [379]. The understanding of these procedures can be extremely useful for antiviral drug design. For instance, inhibitors of deubiquitinases of the MERS-CoV and the Crimean-Congo hemorrhagic fever virus [380] and several inhibitors of lysine-deacetylases (HDAC) for treatment against Epstain-Barr virus-derived cancers have been produced [381].

The second example of research target for drug design and therapy development against viruses, relative to PTMs, is the 14-3-3 family of eukaryotic proteins because of the very important role they play in several diseases and their implication in viral infection that is recently revealed [382]. The 14-3-3 proteins consists of seven isoforms in mammalians (β, γ, ε, ζ, η, σ και τ) and regulate intracellular signaling pathways by binding to protein-targets [383]. In order to act, they bind to phosphorylated Ser and Thr residues (rarely to non-phosphorylated targets) of protein-targets and lead to conformational changes, to masking the phosphorylated region or help the binding to other proteins [384]. It was indicated that their function and specificity is regulated by post-translational modifications. Their function is recently reviewed [385] but it is worth mentioned as paradigms the association of 14-3-3 proteins with hepatitis C virus (HCV) core protein in order to activate the RAF-1 kinase pathway and consequently control the hepatocyte growth or to induce Bax-mediated apoptosis [386, 387]. Moreover, the association of 14-3-3 ε and η proteins with the NS3 protein of Zika virus that lead to the inhibition of melanoma differentiation-associated protein 5 (MDA5) signaling pathway [388]. More interestingly, the association of 14-3-3 proteins with phosphorylated N protein of SARS virus, through phosphorylation-dependent protein-protein interactions, in order to interfere with cellular machinery [389]. It is obvious that the elucidation of 14-3-3 protein function and protein-protein interaction could be a potential drug target in antiviral strategy.

Promising Antimicrobial Targets

Common pathogenic bacteria have developed increasing antibiotic resistance, threatening the future of global human health. Conventional antibiotics, *i.e.* bactericidal and bacteriostatic, are considered to be broadly effective drugs since they target conserved bacterial structures or processes essential for growth [390]. However, this feature makes them non-selective, as they have the ability to kill or inhibit not only pathogenic bacteria but also commensal microbiota. Alteration of the microbiota composition induced by antibiotic therapy has detrimental side effects in human health including asthma, infectious and metabolic diseases [391]. In addition, antibiotic treatment induces resistance to commensal gut flora which can be obtained by pathogens *via* horizontal gene transfer [392]. The development of new antibiotic agents is significantly slower compared to the rapid increase in antibiotic resistance. If our inability to control bacterial infections continues, antibiotic- resistant pathogens are predicted to cause 10 million deaths per year globally by 2050 [393].

In the past two decades, antibiotic research has shifted from traditional antibiotics to antibacterial drugs that attempt to solely attack pathogenic bacteria without affecting normal microflora. These antibiotic alternatives are also known as virulence blockers or pathoblockers and they target virulence factors which are present only in a small group of bacteria [390]. Their selectivity should apply pressure only on specific bacteria thus reducing the evolution and spread of antibiotic resistant genes [394].

Specialized secretion systems are an obvious target for virulence blockers as they are crucial for host infection [393, 394]. As previously mentioned in this chapter, many pathogenic bacteria express secretion systems in order to inject and translocate bacterial effector proteins into target host cells. Several of those effectors are able to modify host proteins using PTMs resulting in host immune defense disruption, pathogen replication and disease progression.

Over the years, numerous natural and synthetic molecules have been screened for their ability to inhibit secretion systems in one or multiple pathogens. For example, thiazolidinone, a small molecule, which was originally screened for its potential inhibition of the *Salmonella* T3SS. Thiazolidinone was shown to reduce the secretion of a *S. typhimurium* effector protein while it could also inhibit the assembly of the needle complex, blocking T3-dependent secretion by *Y. enterocolitica* [395].

Eight more small molecules from a natural/synthetic compound library were discovered and characterized when screening for blockers of translocation of *Y. pseudotuberculosis* effectors into mammalian cells. The compounds blocked Yop effector translocation *in vitro*, inducing their release into the cell environment. The compounds function without affecting T3SS needle formation and structure but possibly by modifying pore formation on host cells or by disrupting the interaction between the *Yersinia* T3SS and the host cell [396].

RWJ-60475 is another small molecule which was selected from a library of more than 2500 molecules in an attempt to identify specific inhibitors of effector translocation by *L. pneumophila* 1 cm/Dot T4SS. RWJ-60475 inhibits bacterial uptake by blocking the host receptor protein tyrosine phosphate phosphatase CD45 which was found to be essential for *L. pneumophila* phagocytocis and effector translocation [397].

Antitoxins are the most established class of virulence blockers [394] and are able to inhibit the secreted toxins of pathogens including TcdA and TcdB toxins from *C. difficile*. One such example is the binding agent X-aptamer. X-aptamers are small nucleic acid molecules which have the ability to bind to specific targets such as small molecules, proteins, cells and tissues [398, 399]. Their function is similar to that of antibodies with the difference that they exhibit no immunogenicity in the host since they are generated *in vitro*. In addition, X-aptamers are extremely stable and can be easily modified for increased specificity. *C. difficile* TcdA and TcdB toxins were used as targets for the design and generation of X-aptamers that bind with high affinity to their N-terminal glycosyltransferase domain leading to their sequestration and inactivation [400]. Bile salts such as taurocholate [401], tolevamer, cholestyramines and colestipol can also be used as potential toxin-binding agents [400]. Tolevamar, in particular, is an anion polymer which was designed to bind and sequester TcdA and TcdB toxins. Patients treated with tolevamar exhibited milder *C. difficile* infection. Despite their advantages, toxin-binding agents could potentialy interact with antibiotics, like vancomycin, when administered at the same time [402].

Several studies have attempted to identify promising small molecules that target bacterial effectors which perform PTMs on host proteins, setting the stage for the discovery of new and more potent derivatives. Histidine kinases, especially those which are part of bacterial two-component systems (TCS), are the focus of the majority of these studies [403, 404]. Histidine kinases are considered promising drug targets because they contain a highly conserved ATP-binding site which plays an essential role in TCS signaling [403]. TCS are also considered attractive drug targets as they are present in pathogenic bacteria and absent in mammals, while several of them have been shown to be essential for bacterial viability. TCS signal transduction occurs in response to changes in the environment, altering expression of genes implicated, among others, in virulence, antibiotic resistance and regulation of secretion systems [405]. So far, many small molecule inhibitors have been designed or identified from compound libraries with the most recent targeting histidine kinase from *S. pneumoniae* [406] and *Bacillus subtilis* [407].

Only one study has so far identified inhibitors against a *V. parahaemolyticus* AMPylator which is delivered into host cells by T3SS. A screen of a 1280 compound library led to the discovery of three molecules (GW7646, MK886 and calmidazolium) which were selective for the *V. parahaemolyticus* VopS. VopS mediates the transfer of the AMP moiety of ATP to Thr residues present in the host GTPases, Cdc42 and Rac1, leading to cell rounding and ultimately cell death. AMPylation has also been demonstrated to be an indispensable mechanism for *L. pneumophila* and *H. somni* infections. All three compounds could decrease protein AMPylation in VopS transfected cells but they were unable to prevent the cell rounding phenotype. Calmidazolium in particular, displayed cellular toxicity which limits its potential application as a VopS inhibitor. However, the imidazoline core of calmidazolium and GW7646 both bind to the N-terminal region of VopS causing conformational changes and destabilizing the whole protein [408].

Bacterial E3 ubiquitin ligases are considered to be another attractive but challenging target for the development of antimicrobial drugs. The limited availability of high-throughput screening assays against E3 ubiquitin ligases makes them a difficult-to-target group of enzymes [409]. Furthermore, the absence of ATP-binding domains from the HECT- and RING-containing types poses additional challenges for the design of novel inhibitors [409]. Despite the limitations, two high-throughput screening assays for inhibitors against eukaryotic Ub ligases have been developed [410, 411]. Similar approaches could be applied for the generation of small molecule inhibitors against bacterial Ub ligase-like enzymes.

Even though small molecules dominate the field of antimicrobial drug development, several studies have turned their focus on humanized monoclonal antibodies (Hu-mAbs). Hu-mAbs have advantages over small molecules such as reduced toxicity, longevity, enhanced specificity, rapid and sustained killing of target pathogenic bacteria through several different processes including "direct killing, anti-virulence, neutralization, complement deposition, and opsonization by phagocytes". The involvement of these processes results in bacterial elimination from different sites of the body, limiting toxic shock [412]. Small molecules alone are unable to completely clear bacteria from the host, rendering the contribution of the immune system absolutely indispensable. Hu-mAbs can be used as a prophylactic treatment to prevent bacterial infection or as a therapeutic treatment. mAbs have the ability to disrupt bacterial infection displaying anti-toxin [413, 414] or bactericidal action [415, 416] or by interfering with a variety of mechanism including biofilm formation [417, 418], attachment and adhesion to host cells [419, 420].

PTMS IN NATURAL ANTIMICROBIAL PEPTIDES AID SEARCH FOR NOVEL THERAPEUTICS

Single cell organisms have developed their own shield against other pathogens. These natural products have long been the focus point for the development of novel therapeutics due to their antimicrobial activity [421, 422]. This activity comes from ribosomally synthesized and post-translationally modified peptides (RiPPs). A comprehensive database is available to help with the ever-growing list of identified and characterized antimicrobial peptides [423]. Although strides in genome mining have revealed a plethora of unknown RiPPs [424], their use in a clinical setting is not yet possible due to solubility issues. The biochemical and functional characterization of these anti-microbial peptides is crucial in the development of therapeutics against drug-resistant microbes [425, 426]. Their complex topology and unusual post-translational modifications, along with poor solubility issues, are also hindering factors for the efficient large-scale production of these molecules [427].

All proteins affiliated with the formation and maturation of a RiPP are encoded from dedicated Biosynthesis Gene Clusters (BGCs). The biosynthesis of these peptides relies heavily on the ribosomal expression of a precursor peptide that consists of a C-terminal core peptide and a N-terminal leader peptide (LP). Proteins part of the biosynthetic pathway bind to a conserved amino acid sequence of the leader peptide and modify the core peptide in order to create the mature RiPP molecule [428]. The maturation of the precursor molecule is complete when the core peptide is released from the leader. Here, we will discuss lasso peptides, thiopeptides and lanthipeptides, the main RiPP categories that have been shown to exhibit prominent antimicrobial activity (Fig. **8**). Understanding their biosynthetic pathway and the PTMs that govern their maturation process can help in the pursuit of new antibiotic drugs.

Lasso Peptides

Lasso peptides take their name from their distinct topology, as the C-terminal region of the core peptide is practically threaded through a N-terminal macrolactam ring. The molecule is kept in place by bisulfide bonds and/or steric interactions from the side chains of the macrolactam ring [429]. The way lasso peptides prevent unthreading of the C-tail also distinguishes them into three categories (Class I-III). Class I members, like Siamycin-I, Sviceucin and Specialicin from *Streptomyces sp.*, bear two disulfide bonds each connecting the loop and the tail of the peptide to the macrocycle ring (Fig. **8B**) [430, 431]. Class II, the most populated category with almost 35 members, lack disulfide bonds and the unravelling of the tail is prevented *via* steric restrains. The most notable and well characterized Class II lasso peptide is microcin J25 (MccJ25) from *E. coli* (Fig. **8A**) [432], although most members derive from *Streptomyces sp.* and *Rhodococcus sp.* BI-32169, the sole member of Class III, exhibits a single disulfide bond between the tail and the ring part of the peptide structure [433].

This intricate folding of the lasso peptides provides thermostability and protects them against proteolysis.

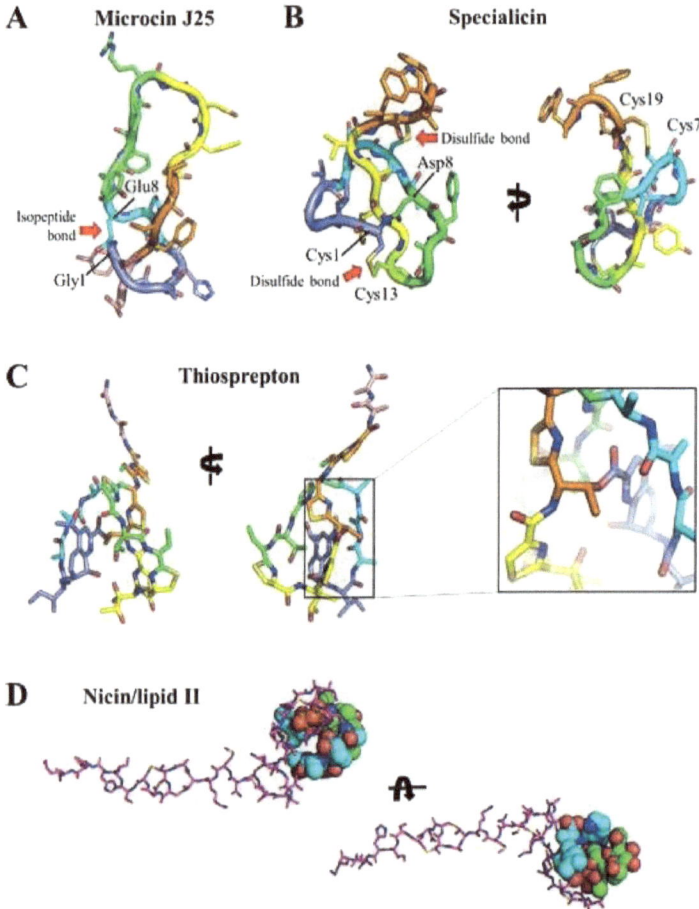

Fig. (8). Ribosomally synthesised and post-translationally modified peptides (RiPPs) with proven antibiotic activity. **(A)** Microcin J25 is a Class II lasso peptide from *E. coli*. An isopeptide bond is formed between Gly1 and Glu8. The tail that passes through the macrocycle is prevented from unthreading due to steric inhibition from the adjacent phenyl rings. **(B)** Specialicin is a Class I lasso peptide from *Streptomyces specialis*. An isopeptide bond between Cys1 and Asp8 create a macrocycle. The unravelling of the tail is prevented by two disulfide bonds, one between Cys1 and Cys13 and one between Cys19 and Cys7. **(C)** Thiostrepton is a thiopeptide for *Streptomyces sp*. Thiopeptides are heavily decorated with post-translational modifications including dehydrated Ser (Dha) and dehydrated Thr (Dhb) residues, enzymatic cycloaddition between two Dha residues and secondary macrocycles (zoom). **(D)** Nisin (stick representation) is a Class I lantibiotic from *Lactococcus lactis*. Nisin binds to lipid II (spacefill model) and creates pores that cause instability to the cell membrane. Unlike other lantibiotics, nisin is not heavily decorated with PTMs. It bears five lanthionine thioester rings created enzymatically during biosynthesis. The figure was prepared using PyMOL [18].

Despite their diverse nature in regard to size and amino acid composition the biosynthetic pathway for all lasso peptides is quite straight-forward and rather universal. All lasso biosynthesis affiliated genes are part of an ABCD type gene cluster. Lasso peptide synthase protein B1 binds to the conserved L12, P14 and Y17 amino acids of the LP in the precursor peptide A and the B2 protein cleaves it revealing a Cys or Gly residue at the N-terminus [434]. B1 and B2 can also be expressed as a merged protein B, as is the case for microcin J25 that exhibits the full cysteine protease activity. The newly formed N-terminus of the released core peptide is linked with an isopeptide bond to the side chain of a conserved Asp or Glu residue, present between positions 7 and 9, by the ATP-dependent lactam synthase known as protein C.

Cys/Gly and Asp/Glu residues necessary for the formation of the macrolactam are highly conserved [435]. Most lasso BGCs also encode a D protein (an ABC-transporter) or other enzymes that aid lasso biosynthesis [436]. Through studies on lasso peptide biosynthesis in heterologous expression studies [437, 438], the biosynthetic enzymes show unprecedented tolerance for alternative peptide substrates, as long as the substitution is not a residue critical for RiPP modification and maturation [439]. These properties make lasso peptides a favourable target for drug design with biomedical and clinical applications [440].

Lasso peptides characteristically function as antimicrobial agents against other microorganisms and enzymatic inhibitory activity. RP71955 and siamycins, Class I lasso peptides produced in *Streptomyces sp.*, showcase potent antibiotic activity against *B. subtilis*, *Staphylococcus aureus* and *E. coli* Juhl [441]. They are also known for their anti-HIV activity, with RP71955 inhibiting HIV-1 aspartyl protease and halting the production of the viral reverse transcriptase [441 - 443]. Siamycin-I was recently revealed to bind lipid II, prevent peptidoglycan formation and cell wall biosynthesis [444]. The newly characterized specialicin bears high conformational similarity to siamycin-I and exhibits antibacterial activity against *Micrococcus luteus* and anti-viral-activity against HIV [445]. The most well studied, structurally and functionally characterized lasso peptide is microcin J25 from *E. coli* and it has been shown to target RNA polymerases in Gram negative bacteria, like other *E. coli* and *Salmonella* strains [432]. MccJ25 highjacks the iron receptor FhuA and proteins from the TonB pathway to enter the cell walls of "enemy" strains [446]. Once inside, MccJ25 binds to pathogen RNA polymerase (RNAP) and blocks the active site [447]. MccJ25 derivatives are also tested for their antimicrobial activity but further research is required [448]. Produced from a single precursor peptide in *Rhodococcus sp.*, lariatin A and B have been shown to provide antibiotic activity against *Mycobacterium tuberculosis* but there is no further elucidation into their molecular function, mechanism and target [449]. Another lasso peptide that targets *M. tuberculosis* is lassomycin from *Lentzea kentuckyensis sp.* Lassomycin specifically targets the ClpC1 ATPase domain of the *M. tuberculosis* caseinolytic protease causing its disassociation from ATP and inhibiting its proteolytic activity [450].

Thiopeptides

Thiopeptides (or thiazolyl peptides) are one of the most structurally and chemically diverse groups of NPs, with an array of post-translational modifications necessary for their biosynthesis and maturation. The main structural feature that is observed in a thiopeptide is a six-membered macrocycle which usually contains azole heterocycles and dehydroamino acids [451]. Further modifications that are usually involved in a thiopeptide structure include a secondary heterocycle, glycosylation, hydroxylation, and methylation (Fig. **8C**). Thiopeptides are known for their strong antimicrobial activity against Gram-positive bacteria, as protein synthase inhibitors, by targeting elongation factor Tu (EF-Tu) and the interface between ribosomal proteins S23 and L11 [451 - 454].

The majority of thiopeptide compounds, like thiostrepton, berninamycins, thiocillin and noheptide-like molecules, target bacterial ribosomal subunit interface belonging to a conserved GTPase-associated centre (GAC) that binds translational GTPases EF4 and EF-G [455 - 457]. These two proteins are responsible for the translocation of tRNA and mRNA promoting the newly synthesised amino acid chain. Binding of thiostrepton and nosiheptides to the GAC site inhibits protein synthesis by sterically interfering with the association of translation factors to the bacterial ribosome [454, 458]. Additionally, it can prevent binding of IF-2 (initiation factor 2) to the ribosome [458]. IF-2 is considered responsible for the delivery and binding of fMet-tRNA^{fMet}, and hence the initiation of translation, has been shown to utilise the same GAC site during ribosomal assembly. Thiomuracine-like compound GE2270A, exhibit a similar inhibitory function towards protein synthesis by targeting bacterial elongation factor Tu (EF-Tu) [459]. GE2270A fits in an almost-perfect way to the 3'-tRNA site of the EF-Tu/GDP conformation, locked in place by a salt bridge created between two Arg residues. This prevents the conformational change that will allow the release of GDP and the association with a new GTP molecule. Thus, EF-Tu can no longer bind new aminoacyl-tRNAs.

Similar to other RiPPs and secondary metabolites, all genes involved in thiopeptide biosynthesis are positioned within the same BGC. Most of the data available on thiopeptide biosynthesis and maturation are from studies on thiomuracin, lactazole and GE2270A biosynthesis [460]. It is evident that the starting point in the biosynthetic pathway of thiomuracins and thiocillins is the formation of thi- and ox-azoles from Ser/Thr/Cys residues [461]. Oxazole formation in thiopeptides is rather scarce due to being energetically demanding compared to thiazoles but it can be found in berninamycins like sulfomycin. Initially, a Thif-Ocin-like protein binds to the LP and brings it closer to an enzyme of the YcaO superfamily to allow association. YcaO uses ATP to create azolines by performing a cyclodehydration reaction between the residue side chain and the backbone amide [462]. The second step would be to convert the azolines to azoles *via* FMN-dependent oxidation catalysed by dehydrogenases encoded from the BGC [463].

The other essential PTM is the formation of dehydroamino acids. Specifically, the formation of dehydroalanine (Dha) and dehydrobutyrine (Dhb) from Ser and Thr residues, respectively. This process occurs in two stages by two enzymes with distinct functions. The first one catalyses the glutamylation of a Ser or Thr residue by transferring glutamic acid from a charged glutamyl-tRNA to the side chain of the substrate [464]. The second enzyme performs a retro-Michael reaction, upon recognition of the O-glutamylated residues. Subsequent eliminylation of the glutamate molecule leads to the formation of the dehydroamino acids. While most biosynthetic glutamylation enzymes carry a RiPP recognition element (RRE) that binds to LP; this is not the case for TbtB, the glutamylase from thiomuracin biosynthetic pathway. TbtB specifically binds the thiazoles formed in the core peptide, as mentioned earlier, practically mandating the dehydration of Ser/Thr [465]. In GE2270A biosynthesis, this is catalysed by PbtH which exhibits a C-terminal amidase activity [466]. The aforementioned PTMs also occur in lactazole maturation, though not in such an ordered manner as in thiomuracins.

The formation of thiazoles and dehydroamino acids Dha/Dhb is fundamental for the macrocyclization reaction. TbtD catalyses the aza-Diels-Alder (aza-DA) [4+2]-cycloaddition reaction between two Dha residues, creating a dehydropiperidine in the macrocyclization junction [467]. This process signals the end of the lactazole precursor peptide maturation, but additional secondary macrocycles and modifications of the C-terminus are a rather prominent feature in thiopeptide structures of thiostrepton, nosiheptides, berninamycins and GE2270A [460, 468].

Thiazomycin has been proven very effective against *Mycobacterium tuberculosis* and various cocci strains [469], thiostrepton is only used as a topical ointment for veterinary practices [470], while nosiheptide is commonly used as a food additive in livestock feeding [471]. The newly characterized semi-synthetic molecule LFF571, deriving from GE2270A, has been proposed as a new drug against *C. difficile* infection [472]. NAI003, another GE2270A derivative, is used as a topical antibiotic in acne treatment due to its potent activity against *Propionibacterium acnes* [453]. Despite their potent antimicrobial activity, thiopeptides are characterized by poor aqueous solubility and metabolic stability. They are known to lose antibiotic activity in serum and are mostly effective when administered locally at the site of infection [473]. Deciphering steps and characteristics of RiPP biosynthesis will increase their bioengineering potential and this, in turn, will allow the design of novel and more efficient antibiotic drugs [438, 466, 469, 474, 475].

Lanthipeptides/lantibiotics

Another RiPP group with prominent structural and chemical diversity, as well as potent antimicrobial activity, is the lanthipeptides or lanthibiotics. Lanthibiotics are named after the lanthionine/Lan (or methyllanthionine/MeLan) thioester cross-links that are formed during biosynthesis, with the hetero-conjugate addition of Cys to dehydrated Ser (or Thr) residues [476]. The mechanism employed for the Ser/Thr dehydration reaction is the distinguishing factor in lanthipeptide classification into four classes (Class I-IV). The potent antibiotic activity of these compounds lays heavily on the PTMs installed during biosynthesis but, like other RiPPs, they also face difficulties in large scale production. In a recent study, the accumulation of epidermin and gallidermin in *Staphylococcus sp.* cells has been proven toxic for the producing strains [477].

Class I lantibiotics

The first and best characterized Class I lantibiotic is nisin from *Lactococcus lactis* which will be used here as an example of Class I lantibiotic biosynthesis [478]. Nisin has been shown to inhibit the growth of many Gram-positive bacteria, like *Lactobacillus bulgaricus*, and it has been used as a food preservative for over 40 years. It binds to lipid II and uses it to dock itself at the cell membrane where it forms pores (Fig. **8C**) [479]. The first PTM for the formation of the Lan and MeLan cross-links is the dehydration of Ser/Thr *via* polyglutamylation. A single enzyme, NisB, uses free glutamyl-tRNA^{Glu} to transfer multiple Glu onto target residues of the precursor peptide and then eliminates the glutamate to produce the dehydroamino acids [464, 480 - 482]. Nisin is host to five thioester rings created *via* 1,4-conjugate addition of Cys to the newly formed Dha/Dhb residues. Though this reaction can occur spontaneously in basic pH, enzymatic catalysis of peptide cyclization is mandatory for the creation of the correct ring topology in the active compound [483]. The cyclization reaction that yields the Lan (and/or MeLan) thioester rings is catalysed by a metalloenzyme, NisC [484, 485]. Similar to every RiPP biosynthetic pathway, the removal of the leader peptide and release of the mature nisin compound is catalysed by the NisP protease [486].

Additional PTMs that can be found in individual lanthibiotics usually come from enzymes outside the lanthibiotic BGC and most of them are LP-independent.

Epilancin 15X from *Staphylococcus sp.*, bears a N-terminal lactyl group (Lac) that requires the dehydration of Ser1 and a nonenzymatic hydrolysis before a oxidoreductase yields the lactyl cap [487]. In paenibacillin, a PaeN enzyme from *Paenibacillus polymyxa* has been proved to cause N-acetylation of the end Ala residue after leader peptide removal [488]. Potential therapeutic lanthipeptides epidermin and gallidermin, from *Staphylococcus epidermis* and *Staphylococcus gallinarum* respectively, have a C-terminal AviCys (S-[(Z)-2-aminovynil]-$_D$-cystein) installed by a flavin-decarboxylase [489]. Interestingly, a lanthibiotic from *Microspora sp.* 107891 known as NAI-107 contains two novel modifications, the first is the halogenation of Trp4 catalysed by two FMN dependent proteins, a halogenase and a reductase [490]. Bromination of NAI-107, catalysed by the same enzymes, actually increases its antimicrobial activity [491]. The second modification is the hydroxylation of Pro14 by MibO, which is similar to cytochrome P450, but further biochemical characterization is required [492].

Class II Lantibiotics

The major difference in Class II lantibiotics is the presence of the LanM biosynthetic protein in place of LanBs and LanCs [493]. The N-terminal domain is responsible for the dehydration of Ser/Thr residues with an enzymatic reaction that is novel to lanthipeptide biosynthesis. Instead of glutamylation, the Ser/Thr residues get phosphorylated by LanM before the same enzyme eliminates the phosphorylated residues [494, 495]. A group of class II lantibiotics appear to act in a two-component system, where the α-peptide binds the lipid II and the β-peptide putatively binds this complex to form pores on the cell membrane [496, 497]. In most cases the two peptide factors are dehydrated by two different LanMs but only the precursor peptides for Cytolysin are processed by the same CylM [498].

In lacticin 3147 of *Lactobacillus lactis* both peptide components are host of $_D$-Ala residues that provide proteolytic stability and bioactivity to the peptides that carry them [499]. The installation of $_D$-Ala is catalysed by an enzyme that performs diasteroselevtive hydrogenation on the LanM-produced Dha to form the $_D$-Ala residue but it does not seem able to act on Dhb residues [499]. Dehydrated Ser can also take part in the formation of Lysoalanine, where the attack of Lys to Dha is catalysed by Cinorf7, as it was elucidated in cinnamycin from *Streptomyces cinnamoneus* [500]. Another PTM present in cinnamycin is a hydroxylated Asp15 that is installed by an α-ketoglutarate/iron (II)-dependent hydroxylase [500, 501]. Lastly, in a few Class II lanthipeptides, like actagardine from *Actinoplanes garbadinensis*, a sulfoxide is formed *via* oxidation of a thioester MeLan cross-link by a flavo-monoxygenase with homology to luciferase-like proteins [502].

Class III and IV Lantibiotics

The last two Classes of lanthipeptides are distinct from the rest due to their Lan synthases. In Class III and IV the reactions of phosphorylation, phosphate elimination and cyclisation are catalysed by a single enzyme with distinct active sites [503, 504]. Their lyase domain has homology with Type 3 effectors from *Salmonella sp.*, *Shingella sp* [505]. The distinction between Class III and IV lanthipeptide synthases lies in their cyclase domain, where zinc-binding ligands are present in Class IV but absent in Class III [506]. As the most newly characterized lantibiotic Classes, there is a lot that remains to be discovered in the characterisation of biochemistry, structure and activity of LanKCs and LanLs. Surprisingly, many Class III lanthipeptides do not possess antibiotic activity when tested against other bacteria [507].

In Class III lanthipeptides the formation of another type of thioester cross-linkage called labionin (or Lab) is formed when an enolate of a Lan (or MeLan) thioester is then attacked by Cys to form the second thioester bond [508, 509]. The presence of labionin structures is a distinguishing factor, as they are rather prevalent in Class III lantibiotics and can rarely be found across other Classes [510]. Variety of tailoring PTMs in Class III/IV lanthipeptides, compared to other classes, is scarce to say the least. A disulfide bond was discovered in Class III labyrinthopeptins [511] and a novel glycosylation of Trp4, with a 6-deoxyhexose attached to the indole nitrogen, in NAI-112 [512]. As these Classes were recently established not much is known for the biochemical and physiological properties of their compounds and further research would produce promising results.

CONCLUSION AND FUTURE PERSPECTIVES

PTMs constitute a flexible mechanism for quick, on-demand responses of biological systems to intracellular and extracellular stimuli [172]. Since it largely relies on fine-tuned chemistry, rather than genetical regulation, it has unique, advantageous characteristics such as high versatility and adaptability [3]. An ever-growing number of studies has discovered numerous biochemical pathways where PTMs are implicated, including cell homeostasis, adaptation to environmental and intracellular changes, stress response, defence and virulence.

Eukaryotes have developed an elaborate network of interactions, namely innate and adaptive immunity, in order to timely recognize and eliminate invaders. PTMs play an important role to these defence mechanisms, taking part in pathogen recognition, protein activation and translocation [21 - 23]. PAMP receptors depend on interferon and NF-κB signaling pathways that require cascades of phosphorylation and ubiquitination, among other PTMs, in order to achieve a generalised immunity response against invaders. The host can also respond to a threat through adaptive immunity, with the production of antibodies. Antibodies are decorated with a variety of PTMs throughout their structure, from disulfide bonds, which provide structural stability, to modifications in the variable domains, which aid the sensing of distinct pathogens.

On the other side, pathogenic bacteria have evolved sophisticated mechanisms to subvert eukaryotic defence and dominate against them [6, 14]. Similar to eukaryotes, bacteria take advantage of the unique PTM properties and widely use them to design effective attacking strategies, which enable pathogens to disrupt host physiological processes or exploit them for their own advantage. Bacteria have evolved three main strategies to promote their survival and propagation at the expense of their host. First, they express a large class of diverse enzymatic activities whose substrates are eukaryotic proteins [206]. A nice example here, comes from the *Yersinia* Yop effectors. Five out of six Yops directly induce PTMs on eukaryotic proteins, having protease, kinase, phosphatase, acetyltransferase and ubiquitinase activities [85, 95, 108]. Second, another class of bacterial proteins are effectively modified by eukaryotic factors resulting in their activation or localization within the host cell. For example, the sixth Yop mentioned above, undergoes ubiquitination from the host machinery. Another typical example is the bacterial protein lipidation at a specific motif from eukaryotic transferases. Lipidations usually target the bacterial protein to plasma, cell-organelle or pathogen-containing vacuole membranes where their targets are accumulated [143 - 145]. A third class of bacterial proteins are modified inside the bacterial cell in order to be more efficient during host invasion. A characteristic example is bacterial flagellar proteins which are usually decorated with a variety of sugar moieties depending on the bacterial species. Despite their small genomes, bacteria contain a large number of putative glycosyl-transferases which they use to modify target proteins. Glycosylation catalyzed by bacterial pathogens displays high divergence in both glycosidic linkage and glycan structure [268]. An interesting question that occurs is how different glycan structures are selected to serve different functional purposes in bacterial pathogens. Bacterial glycosylation can be identified by host immune response but it also be exploited as a putative target of novel antimicrobial agents [266].

Similar to bacteria, viruses use PTMs to facilitate their entry inside the host cell, avoid immune response and control the activity of the host proteins to the advantage of viral survival and propagation. Here, the coronavirus, the causative agent of the new pandemic, is used to exemplify the details of how viruses use PTMs. It has been observed that most of coronavirus proteins are post-translationally modified *via* glycosylation, palmitoylation, phosphorylation or disulfide bond formation [285]. Glycosylation seems to play an important role in host cell receptor binding of the virus [289, 315], disulfide bond formation is probably significant for the entry of viral proteins to the host cell [335], palmitoylation is indicated to help the membrane formation and anchoring to the host cell membrane [145] while phosphorylation, as well as glycosylation, are crucial for the antigenicity of the virus [349]. Moreover, ubiquitination is used to control the host cell machineries [362, 363]. Although the exact functional implication and biological significance requires further investigation, it is believed that elucidation of PTM mechanisms in coronavirus proteins will boost the development of effective vaccines and novel antiviral drugs.

The extensive implication of PTMs in almost every aspect of infectious pathogenicity makes them promising drug targets for developing new therapeutics for a wide range of diseases. The last decade, significant progress has been made on our understanding of the mechanisms that control PTMs and the mechanisms through which PTMs regulate protein structure and function. This makes now the identification of relevant molecular targets, the design of specific drugs and the discovery of medicine based on PTMs more feasible than ever [176, 194, 393, 513]. For example, the natural membrane transporters can be used for drug delivery and engineering PTMs on them could help to improve their stability and target specificity [371, 372]. Moreover, small inhibitors can be used as drugs to inhibit, *via* ubiquitination, targeted pathways [373]. Another challenge would be the design of antiviral drugs utilizing the machineries that normally add PTMs to viral proteins in order to render them invisible to host immune system [385, 388]. PTMs are significantly helpful with biopharmaceutics in order to induce stability and avoid off-target effects. Biopharmaceutical research has also been focused on engineering expression systems able to produce protein-based therapeutics decorated with the desired PTMs.

Furthermore, it has been shown that natural antimicrobial compounds are dominated by the presence of PTMs. These are mostly ribosomally synthesized and post-translationally modified peptides called RiPPs. They all share a similar biosynthetic pathway, where a precursor peptide, containing a leader and a core sequence, is expressed and various enzymes get attached to the leader peptide in order to dock PTMs to the core peptide [514]. In all cases, the removal of the leader sequence by a protease is mandatory for the maturation of the compound. While the same principle for the main biosynthetic pathway is shared, more often than not individual compounds bear distinct modifications. There is a vast list of RiPPs and their respective categories, though lasso peptides, thiopeptides and lanthipeptides are the most abundant and well characterized [429, 451, 504]. PTMs are involved in the biosynthesis and maturation of these compounds so intrinsically that without them, RiPPs would not be able to achieve their characteristic structure and antimicrobial activity, in respect to the group they belong to. Their antibiotic properties include disruption of the integrity of the bacterial cell wall and inhibition of protein synthesis in bacteria [440, 454, 515]. Continuous progress on elucidating the biochemistry and biology of PTMs renders them a promising field for investigation and discovery of new therapeutics for many infectious diseases.

Efforts in genome mining have unveiled a plethora of compounds unknown until now [424]. The ever-growing list of RiPPs has provided and almost equal amount of potential antibiotics that await characterization. Additionally, bioengineering of the RiPPs is required to solve issues that deter their mass production and use in clinical trials. They are plagued by solubility issues and toxicity for the producing strains, which limit their commercial use, as many studies on the heterologous production of RiPPs have pointed [438, 477, 507, 516]. Among other approaches, many efforts target the leader sequence where biosynthetic enzymes dock in order to modify the core peptide [474, 507, 517, 518]. As a result, these derivatives are now decorated with different PTMs than the original enzyme and most likely hold different properties that need to be studied. There is no doubt that the bioengineering of natural products for the production of novel pharmaceuticals is a promising field of research.

CONSENT FOR PUBLICATION

Not applicable.

CONFLICT OF INTEREST

The author declares no conflict of interest, financial or otherwise.

ACKNOWLEDGEMENTS

We apologize to all authors whose work in the field was practically unfeasible to be cited here.

REFERENCES

[1]   Millar AH, Heazlewood JL, Giglione C, Holdsworth MJ, Bachmair A, Schulze WX. The scope, functions, and dynamics of posttranslational protein modifications. Annu Rev Plant Biol 2019; 70: 119-51.
        [http://dx.doi.org/10.1146/annurev-arplant-050718-100211] [PMID: 30786234]

[2]   Fadouloglou VE, Kapanidou M, Agiomirgianaki A, *et al.* Structure determination through homology modelling and torsion-angle simulated annealing: application to a polysaccharide deacetylase from *Bacillus cereus.* Acta Crystallogr D Biol Crystallogr 2013; 69(Pt 2): 276-83.
        [http://dx.doi.org/10.1107/S0907444912045829] [PMID: 23385463]

[3]   Fadouloglou VE, Balomenou S, Aivaliotis M, *et al.* Unusual α-carbon hydroxylation of proline promotes active-site maturation. J Am Chem Soc 2017; 139(15): 5330-7.
        [http://dx.doi.org/10.1021/jacs.6b12209] [PMID: 28333455]

[4]   Prejanò M, Romeo I, Sgrizzi L, Russo N, Marino T. Why hydroxy-proline improves the catalytic

power of the peptidoglycan N-deacetylase enzyme: insight from theory. Phys Chem Chem Phys 2019; 21(42): 23338-45.
[http://dx.doi.org/10.1039/C9CP03804C] [PMID: 31617504]

[5]   Suprun EV. Protein post-translational modifications – A challenge for bioelectrochemistry. TrAC -. Trends Analyt Chem 2019; 116: 44-60.
[http://dx.doi.org/10.1016/j.trac.2019.04.019]

[6]   Macek B, Forchhammer K, Hardouin J, Weber-Ban E, Grangeasse C, Mijakovic I. Protein post-translational modifications in bacteria. Nat Rev Microbiol 2019; 17(11): 651-64. [Internet].
[http://dx.doi.org/10.1038/s41579-019-0243-0] [PMID: 31485032]

[7]   Ravikumar V, Jers C, Mijakovic I. Elucidating host-pathogen interactions based on post-translational modifications using proteomics approaches. Front Microbiol 2015; 6(NOV): 1313.
[http://dx.doi.org/10.3389/fmicb.2015.01312] [PMID: 26635773]

[8]   Michard C, Doublet P. Post-translational modifications are key players of the *Legionella pneumophila* infection strategy. Front Microbiol 2015; 6(FEB): 87.
[http://dx.doi.org/10.3389/fmicb.2015.00087] [PMID: 25713573]

[9]   Loboda AP, Soond SM, Piacentini M, Barlev NA. Lysine-specific post-translational modifications of proteins in the life cycle of viruses. Cell Cycle 2019; 18(17): 1995-2005.
[http://dx.doi.org/10.1080/15384101.2019.1639305] [PMID: 31291816]

[10]   Chiang C, Gack MU. Post-translational Control of Intracellular Pathogen Sensing Pathways. 2017.
[http://dx.doi.org/10.1016/j.it.2016.10.008]

[11]   Nally JE, Grassmann AA, Planchon S, *et al.* Pathogenic leptospires modulate protein expression and post-translational modifications in response to mammalian host signals. Front Cell Infect Microbiol 2017; 7(AUG): 362.
[http://dx.doi.org/10.3389/fcimb.2017.00362] [PMID: 28848720]

[12]   Malet JK, Impens F, Carvalho F, Hamon MA, Cossart P, Ribet D. Rapid remodeling of the host epithelial cell proteome by the listeriolysin O (LLO) pore-forming toxin. Mol Cell Proteomics 2018; 17(8): 1627-36.
[http://dx.doi.org/10.1074/mcp.RA118.000767] [PMID: 29752379]

[13]   Marcelino I, Colomé-Calls N, Holzmuller P, *et al.* Sweet and sour Ehrlichia: Glycoproteomics and phosphoproteomics reveal new players in Ehrlichia ruminantium physiology and pathogenesis. Front Microbiol 2019; 10(MAR): 450.
[http://dx.doi.org/10.3389/fmicb.2019.00450] [PMID: 30930869]

[14]   El Qaidi S, Wu M, Zhu C, Hardwidge PR. *Salmonella, E. coli,* and Citrobacter Type III Secretion System Effector Proteins that Alter Host Innate Immunity. Adv Exp Med Biol 2019; 1111: 205-18.
[http://dx.doi.org/10.1007/5584_2018_289] [PMID: 30411307]

[15]   Wang M, Qazi IH, Wang L, Zhou G, Han H. Salmonella virulence and immune escape. Microorganisms 2020; 8(3): 1-25.
[http://dx.doi.org/10.3390/microorganisms8030407] [PMID: 32183199]

[16]   Schroeder GN. The toolbox for uncovering the functions of legionella Dot/Icm Type IVb secretion system effectors: Current state and future directions. Front Cell Infect Microbiol 2018; 7(JAN): 528.
[http://dx.doi.org/10.3389/fcimb.2017.00528] [PMID: 29354599]

[17]   Ribet D, Cossart P. Pathogen-mediated posttranslational modifications: A re-emerging field. Cell 2010; 143(5): 694-702.
[http://dx.doi.org/10.1016/j.cell.2010.11.019] [PMID: 21111231]

[18]   DeLano WL. The PyMOL Molecular Graphics System 2002. https://www.scirp.org/ (S(vtj3fa45qm1ean45vvffcz55))/reference/ReferencesPapers.aspx? ReferenceID=1958992

[19]   Notredame C, Higgins DG, Heringa J. T-Coffee: A novel method for fast and accurate multiple sequence alignment. J Mol Biol 2000; 302(1): 205-17.

[http://dx.doi.org/10.1006/jmbi.2000.4042] [PMID: 10964570]

[20]   Robert X, Gouet P. Deciphering key features in protein structures with the new ENDscript server. Nucleic Acids Res 2014; 42(W1): W320-4.http://espript.ibcp.fr
[http://dx.doi.org/10.1093/nar/gku316]

[21]   Liu J, Qian C, Cao X. Post-translational modification control of innate immunity. Immunity 2016; 45: 15-30.
[http://dx.doi.org/10.1016/j.immuni.2016.06.020]

[22]   Panda S, Ding JL, Alerts E. Natural antibodies bridge innate and adaptive immunity. J Immunol 2015; 194(1): 13-20.
[http://dx.doi.org/10.4049/jimmunol.1400844] [PMID: 25527792]

[23]   Akira S, Uematsu S, Takeuchi O. Pathogen recognition and innate immunity. Cell 2006; 124(4): 783-801.
[http://dx.doi.org/10.1016/j.cell.2006.02.015] [PMID: 16497588]

[24]   Cai X, Chiu YH, Chen ZJ. The cGAS-cGAMP-STING pathway of cytosolic DNA sensing and signaling. Mol Cell 2014; 54(2): 289-96.
[http://dx.doi.org/10.1016/j.molcel.2014.03.040] [PMID: 24766893]

[25]   Vallabhapurapu S, Karin M. Regulation and function of NF-kappaB transcription factors in the immune system. Annu Rev Immunol 2009; 27: 693-733.
[http://dx.doi.org/10.1146/annurev.immunol.021908.132641] [PMID: 19302050]

[26]   Lamkanfi M, Dixit VM. Mechanisms and functions of inflammasomes. Cell 2014; 157(5): 1013-22.
[http://dx.doi.org/10.1016/j.cell.2014.04.007] [PMID: 24855941]

[27]   Thaiss CA, Levy M, Itav S, Elinav E. Integration of innate immune signaling. Trends in Immunology. Elsevier Ltd 2016; 37: pp. 84-101.
[http://dx.doi.org/10.1016/j.it.2015.12.003]

[28]   Yang J, Liu Z, Xiao TS. Post-translational regulation of inflammasomes. Cell Mol Immunol 2017; 14(1): 65-79.
[http://dx.doi.org/10.1038/cmi.2016.29] [PMID: 27345727]

[29]   Rahman AH, Taylor DK, Turka LA. The contribution of direct TLR signaling to T cell responses. Immunol Res 2009; 45(1): 25-36.
[http://dx.doi.org/10.1007/s12026-009-8113-x] [PMID: 19597998]

[30]   Kaparakis-Liaskos M. The intracellular location, mechanisms and outcomes of NOD1 signaling. Cytokine 2015; 74(2): 207-12.
[http://dx.doi.org/10.1016/j.cyto.2015.02.018] [PMID: 25801093]

[31]   Kawasaki T, Kawai T. Toll-like receptor signaling pathways. Front Immunol 2014; 5(SEP): 461.
[PMID: 25309543]

[32]   Deguine J, Barton GM. MyD88: a central player in innate immune signaling. F1000Prime Rep 2014; 6(November): 97.
[http://dx.doi.org/10.12703/P6-97] [PMID: 25580251]

[33]   Arthur JSC, Ley SC. Mitogen-activated protein kinases in innate immunity. Nat Rev Immunol 2013; 13(9): 679-92.
[http://dx.doi.org/10.1038/nri3495] [PMID: 23954936]

[34]   Kanarek N, London N, Schueler-Furman O, Ben-Neriah Y. Ubiquitination and degradation of the inhibitors of NF-kappaB. Cold Spring Harb Perspect Biol 2010; 2(2): a000166.
[http://dx.doi.org/10.1101/cshperspect.a000166] [PMID: 20182612]

[35]   Sato S, Sugiyama M, Yamamoto M, *et al.* Toll/IL-1 receptor domain-containing adaptor inducing IFN-β (TRIF) associates with TNF receptor-associated factor 6 and TANK-binding kinase 1, and activates two distinct transcription factors, NF-κ B and IFN-regulatory factor-3, in the Toll-like

receptor signaling. J Immunol 2003; 171(8): 4304-10.
[http://dx.doi.org/10.4049/jimmunol.171.8.4304] [PMID: 14530355]

[36]   Yamamoto M, Sato S, Hemmi H, *et al.* Role of adaptor TRIF in the MyD88-independent toll-like receptor signaling pathway. Science 2003; 301(5633): 640-3.
[http://dx.doi.org/10.1126/science.1087262] [PMID: 12855817]

[37]   Liu S, Cai X, Wu J. Phosphorylation of innate immune adaptor proteins MAVS, STING, and TRIF induces IRF3 activation. Science (80-) 2015; 347(6227)

[38]   Botos I, Liu L, Wang Y, Segal DM, Davies DR. The toll-like receptor 3:dsRNA signaling complex. Biochim Biophys Acta 2009; 1789(9-10): 667-74.
[http://dx.doi.org/10.1016/j.bbagrm.2009.06.005] [PMID: 19595807]

[39]   Sun J, Duffy KE, Ranjith-Kumar CT, *et al.* Structural and functional analyses of the human Toll-like receptor 3. Role of glycosylation. J Biol Chem 2006; 281(16): 11144-51.
[http://dx.doi.org/10.1074/jbc.M510442200] [PMID: 16533755]

[40]   Geng PL, Song LX, An H, Huang JY, Li S, Zeng XT. Toll-like receptor 3 is associated with the risk of HCV infection and HBV-related diseases. Medicine (Baltimore) 2016; 95(21): e2302.
[http://dx.doi.org/10.1097/MD.0000000000002302] [PMID: 27227908]

[41]   Philpott DJ, Sorbara MT, Robertson SJ, Croitoru K, Girardin SE. NOD proteins: regulators of inflammation in health and disease. Nat Rev Immunol 2014; 14(1): 9-23.
[http://dx.doi.org/10.1038/nri3565] [PMID: 24336102]

[42]   Takeuchi O, Akira S. Pattern recognition receptors and inflammation. Cell 2010; 140(6): 805-20.
[http://dx.doi.org/10.1016/j.cell.2010.01.022] [PMID: 20303872]

[43]   Franchi L, Eigenbrod T, Muñoz-Planillo R, Nuñez G. The inflammasome: a caspase-1-activation platform that regulates immune responses and disease pathogenesis. Nat Immunol 2009; 10(3): 241-7.
[http://dx.doi.org/10.1038/ni.1703] [PMID: 19221555]

[44]   Zamaraev AV, Kopeina GS, Prokhorova EA, Zhivotovsky B, Lavrik IN. Post-translational Modification of Caspases: The other side of apoptosis regulation. Trends Cell Biol 2017; 27(5): 322-39.
[http://dx.doi.org/10.1016/j.tcb.2017.01.003] [PMID: 28188028]

[45]   Vladimer GI, Weng D, Paquette SWM, *et al.* The NLRP12 inflammasome recognizes *Yersinia pestis.* Immunity 2012; 37(1): 96-107.
[http://dx.doi.org/10.1016/j.immuni.2012.07.006] [PMID: 22840842]

[46]   Nathan C, Ding A. Nonresolving inflammation. Cell 2010; 140(6): 871-82.
[http://dx.doi.org/10.1016/j.cell.2010.02.029] [PMID: 20303877]

[47]   Saxena M, Yeretssian G. NOD-like receptors: Master regulators of inflammation and cancer. Front Immunol 2014; 5(JUL): 327.
[http://dx.doi.org/10.3389/fimmu.2014.00327] [PMID: 25071785]

[48]   Chen L, Deng H, Cui H, *et al.* Inflammatory responses and inflammation-associated diseases in organs. Oncotarget 2017; 9(6): 7204-18.
[http://dx.doi.org/10.18632/oncotarget.23208] [PMID: 29467962]

[49]   Rehwinkel J, Gack MU. RIG-I-like receptors: their regulation and roles in RNA sensing. Nat Rev Immunol 2020; 20(9): 537-51.
[http://dx.doi.org/10.1038/s41577-020-0288-3] [PMID: 32203325]

[50]   Reikine S, Nguyen JB, Modis Y. Pattern recognition and signaling mechanisms of RIG-I and MDA5. Front Immunol 2014; 5(JUL): 342.
[http://dx.doi.org/10.3389/fimmu.2014.00342] [PMID: 25101084]

[51]   Brisse M, Ly H. Comparative structure and function analysis of the RIG-I-like receptors: RIG-I and MDA5. Front Immunol 2019; 10(JULY): 1586.

[http://dx.doi.org/10.3389/fimmu.2019.01586] [PMID: 31379819]

[52]   Tan X, Sun L, Chen J, Chen ZJ. Detection of microbial infections through innate immune sensing of nucleic acids. Annu Rev Microbiol 2018; 72: 447-78.
[http://dx.doi.org/10.1146/annurev-micro-102215-095605] [PMID: 30200854]

[53]   Gupta S, Ylä-Anttila P, Sandalova T, Achour A, Masucci MG. Interaction with 14-3-3 correlates with inactivation of the rig-i signalosome by herpesvirus ubiquitin deconjugases. Front Immunol 2020; 11(March): 437.
[http://dx.doi.org/10.3389/fimmu.2020.00437] [PMID: 32226432]

[54]   Chan YK, Gack MU. Viral evasion of intracellular DNA and RNA sensing. Nat Rev Microbiol 2016; 14(6): 360-73.
[http://dx.doi.org/10.1038/nrmicro.2016.45] [PMID: 27174148]

[55]   Soderstrom K. Viral replication. xPharm Compr Pharmacol Ref 2007; 1-5.

[56]   Sun L, Wu J, Du F, Chen X, Chen ZJ. Cyclic GMP-AMP synthase is a cytosolic dna sensor that activates the type-I interferon pathway. Science (80-) 2013; 339(6121)
[http://dx.doi.org/10.1126/science.1232458]

[57]   Wu J, Sun L, Chen X, Du F, Shi H, Chen C, *et al.* Cyclic-GMP-AMP is an endogenous second messenger in innate immune signaling by cytosolic DNA. Science (80-) 2013; 339(6121)
[http://dx.doi.org/10.1126/science.1229963]

[58]   Ablasser A, Schmid-Burgk JL, Hemmerling I, *et al.* Cell intrinsic immunity spreads to bystander cells *via* the intercellular transfer of cGAMP. Nature 2013; 503(7477): 530-4.
[http://dx.doi.org/10.1038/nature12640] [PMID: 24077100]

[59]   Song B, Greco TM, Lum KK, Taber CE, Cristea IM. The DNA sensor cGAS is decorated by acetylation and phosphorylation modifications in the context of immune signaling. Mol Cell Proteomics 2020; 19(7): 1193-208.
[http://dx.doi.org/10.1074/mcp.RA120.001981] [PMID: 32345711]

[60]   Wakabayashi C, Adachi T, Wienands J, Tsubata T. A distinct signaling pathway used by the IgG-containing B cell antigen receptor. Science (80-) 2002; 298(5602): 2392-5.

[61]   Bournazos S, Wang TT, Dahan R, Maamary J, Ravetch JV. Signaling by antibodies: recent progress. Annu Rev Immunol 2017; 35: 285-311.
[http://dx.doi.org/10.1146/annurev-immunol-051116-052433] [PMID: 28446061]

[62]   Wang LD, Clark MR. B-cell antigen-receptor signalling in lymphocyte development. Immunology 2003; 110(4): 411-20.
[http://dx.doi.org/10.1111/j.1365-2567.2003.01756.x] [PMID: 14632637]

[63]   Tanaka S, Baba Y. B cell receptor signaling. Adv Exp Med Biol 2020; 1254: 23-36.
[http://dx.doi.org/10.1007/978-981-15-3532-1_2] [PMID: 32323266]

[64]   Kwak K, Akkaya M, Pierce SK. B cell signaling in context. Nat Immunol 2019; 20(8): 963-9.
[http://dx.doi.org/10.1038/s41590-019-0427-9] [PMID: 31285625]

[65]   Janeway CA, Travers P, Walport M, Shlomchik MJ. The structure of a typical antibody molecule. Immunobiology 5th editio. New York: Garland Science 2001.

[66]   Schroeder HW Jr, Cavacini L. Structure and function of immunoglobulins. J Allergy Clin Immunol 2010; 125(2) (Suppl. 2): S41-52.
[http://dx.doi.org/10.1016/j.jaci.2009.09.046] [PMID: 20176268]

[67]   Liu H, May K. Disulfide bond structures of IgG molecules: structural variations, chemical modifications and possible impacts to stability and biological function. MAbs 2012; 4(1): 17-23.
[http://dx.doi.org/10.4161/mabs.4.1.18347] [PMID: 22327427]

[68]   Hmiel LK, Brorson KA, Boyne MT II. Post-translational structural modifications of immunoglobulin G and their effect on biological activity. Anal Bioanal Chem 2015; 407(1): 79-94.

[http://dx.doi.org/10.1007/s00216-014-8108-x] [PMID: 25200070]

[69]   Wacker C, Berger CN, Girard P, Meier R. Glycosylation profiles of therapeutic antibody pharmaceuticals. Eur J Pharm Biopharm 2011; 79(3): 503-7.
       [http://dx.doi.org/10.1016/j.ejpb.2011.06.010] [PMID: 21745568]

[70]   Costa AR, Rodrigues ME, Henriques M, Oliveira R, Azeredo J. Glycosylation: impact, control and improvement during therapeutic protein production. Crit Rev Biotechnol 2014; 34(4): 281-99.
       [http://dx.doi.org/10.3109/07388551.2013.793649] [PMID: 23919242]

[71]   Asrat S, de Jesús DA, Hempstead AD, Ramabhadran V, Isberg RR. Bacterial pathogen manipulation of host membrane trafficking. Annu Rev Cell Dev Biol 2014; 30(1): 79-109. [Internet].
       [http://dx.doi.org/10.1146/annurev-cellbio-100913-013439] [PMID: 25103867]

[72]   Mattock E, Blocker AJ. How do the virulence factors of shigella work together to cause disease? Front Cell Infect Microbiol 2017; 7(MAR): 64.
       [http://dx.doi.org/10.3389/fcimb.2017.00064] [PMID: 28393050]

[73]   Hervé JC, Bourmeyster N. Rho GTPases at the crossroad of signaling networks in mammals. Small GTPases 2015; 6(2): 43-8.https://pubmed.ncbi.nlm.nih.gov/26110743
       [http://dx.doi.org/10.1080/21541248.2015.1044811]

[74]   Phuyal S, Farhan H. Multifaceted Rho GTPase signaling at the endomembranes. Front Cell Dev Biol 2019; 7: 127.https://www.frontiersin.org/article/10.3389/fcell.2019.00127 [Internet].
       [http://dx.doi.org/10.3389/fcell.2019.00127] [PMID: 31380367]

[75]   Ribet D, Cossart P. Ubiquitin, SUMO, and NEDD8: key targets of bacterial pathogens. Trends in Cell Biology. Elsevier Ltd 2018; 28: pp. 926-40.

[76]   Song L, Luo ZQ. Post-translational regulation of ubiquitin signaling. J Cell Biol 2019; 218(6): 1776-86.
       [http://dx.doi.org/10.1083/jcb.201902074] [PMID: 31000580]

[77]   Kerscher O, Felberbaum R, Hochstrasser M. Modification of proteins by ubiquitin and ubiquitin-like proteins. Annu Rev Cell Dev Biol 2006; 22(1): 159-80. [Internet].
       [http://dx.doi.org/10.1146/annurev.cellbio.22.010605.093503] [PMID: 16753028]

[78]   Hochstrasser M. Origin and function of ubiquitin-like proteins. Nature 2009; 458(7237): 422-9. [Internet].
       [http://dx.doi.org/10.1038/nature07958] [PMID: 19325621]

[79]   Cappadocia L, Lima CD. Ubiquitin-like protein conjugation: structures, chemistry, and mechanism. Chem Rev 2018; 118(3): 889-918. [Internet].
       [http://dx.doi.org/10.1021/acs.chemrev.6b00737] [PMID: 28234446]

[80]   Pickart CM, Eddins MJ. Ubiquitin: structures, functions, mechanisms. Biochim Biophys Acta 2004; 1695(1-3): 55-72.
       [http://dx.doi.org/10.1016/j.bbamcr.2004.09.019] [PMID: 15571809]

[81]   Deol KK, Lorenz S, Strieter ER. Enzymatic logic of ubiquitin chain assembly. Front Physiol 2019; 10(July): 835.
       [http://dx.doi.org/10.3389/fphys.2019.00835] [PMID: 31333493]

[82]   Buetow L, Huang DT. Structural insights into the catalysis and regulation of E3 ubiquitin ligases. Nat Rev Mol Cell Biol 2016; 17(10): 626-42.
       [http://dx.doi.org/10.1038/nrm.2016.91] [PMID: 27485899]

[83]   Pickart CM. Mechanisms underlying ubiquitination. Annu Rev Biochem 2001; 70: 503-33.
       [http://dx.doi.org/10.1146/annurev.biochem.70.1.503] [PMID: 11395416]

[84]   Cornelis GR. Yersinia type III secretion: send in the effectors. J Cell Biol 2002; 158: 401-8.https://pubmed.ncbi.nlm.nih.gov/12163464/

[85]   Grabowski B, Schmidt MA, Rüter C. Immunomodulatory Yersinia outer proteins (Yops)-useful tools

for bacteria and humans alike. Virulence 2017; 8(7): 1124-47. [Internet].
[http://dx.doi.org/10.1080/21505594.2017.1303588] [PMID: 28296562]

[86] Zhu M, Shao F, Innes RW, Dixon JE, Xu Z. The crystal structure of Pseudomonas avirulence protein AvrPphB: A papain-like fold with a distinct substrate-binding site. Proc Natl Acad Sci U S A 2004; 101(1): 302-7.
[http://dx.doi.org/10.1073/pnas.2036536100]

[87] Bogdanovic X, Schneider S, Levanova N, Wirth C, Trillhaase C, Steinemann M, *et al.* A cysteine protease–like domain enhances the cytotoxic effects of the Photorhabdus asymbiotica toxin PaTox. J Biol Chem 2019; 294(3): 1035-44. http://www.jbc.org/lookup/doi/10.1074/jbc.RA118.005043

[88] Prehna G, Ivanov MI, Bliska JB, Stebbins CE. Yersinia virulence depends on mimicry of host rho-family nucleotide dissociation inhibitors. Cell 2006; 126(5): 869-0.
[PMID: 16959567] [http://dx.doi.org/10.1016/j.cell.2006.06.056]

[89] Galyov EE, Håkansson S, Forsberg Å, Wolf-Watz H. A secreted protein kinase of *Yersinia pseudotuberculosis* is an indispensable virulence determinant. Nature 1993; 361(6414): 730-2.
[PMID: 8441468] [http://dx.doi.org/10.1038/361730a0]

[90] Juris SJ, Rudolph AE, Huddler D, Orth K, Dixon JE. A distinctive role for the Yersinia protein kinase: Actin binding, kinase activation, and cytoskeleton disruption. Proc Natl Acad Sci U S A 2000; 97(17): 9431-6.https://pubmed.ncbi.nlm.nih.gov/10920208/

[91] Barz C, Abahji TN, Trülzsch K, Heesemann J. The Yersinia Ser/Thr protein kinase YpkA/YopO directly interacts with the small GTPases RhoA and Rac-1. FEBS Lett 2000; 482(1-2): 139-43.
[http://dx.doi.org/10.1016/S0014-5793(00)02045-7] [PMID: 11018537]

[92] Peter MF, Tuukkanen AT, Heubach CA, *et al.* Studying conformational changes of the yersinia type-III-secretion effector YopO in solution by integrative structural biology. Structure 2019; 27(9): 1416-1426.e3.
[http://dx.doi.org/10.1016/j.str.2019.06.007] [PMID: 31303480]

[93] Trasak C, Zenner G, Vogel A, Yüksekdag G, Rost R, Haase I, *et al.* Yersinia protein kinase YopO is activated by a novel G-actin binding process. J Biol Chem 2007; 282(4): 2268-77.
[PMID: 17121817]

[94] Lee WL, Grimes JM, Robinson RC. Yersinia effector YopO uses actin as bait to phosphorylate proteins that regulate actin polymerization. Nat Struct Mol Biol 2015; 22(3): 248-55.
[PMID: 25664724] [http://dx.doi.org/10.1038/nsmb.2964]

[95] Lee WL, Singaravelu P, Wee S, Xue B, Ang KC, Gunaratne J, *et al.* Mechanisms of Yersinia YopO kinase substrate specificity. Sci Rep 2016; 2017(7): 1-12.
[http://dx.doi.org/10.1038/srep39998] [PMID: 28051168]

[96] Singaravelu P, Lee WL, Wee S, Ghoshdastider U, Ding K, Gunaratne J, *et al.* Yersinia effector protein (YopO)-mediated phosphorylation of host gelsolin causes calcium-independent activation leading to disruption of actin dynamics. J Biol Chem 2017; 292(19): 8092-100.

[97] Navarro L, Koller A, Nordfelth R, Wolf-Watz H, Taylor S, Dixon JE. Identification of a molecular target for the Yersinia protein kinase A. Mol Cell 2007; 26(4): 465-77. [Internet].
[http://dx.doi.org/10.1016/j.molcel.2007.04.025] [PMID: 17531806]

[98] de la Puerta ML, Trinidad AG, Rodríguez M del C, Bogetz J. Characterization of new substrates targeted by Yersinia tyrosine phosphatase yopH. In: Bozza P, Ed. PLoS One 2009; 4(2): e4431.
[http://dx.doi.org/10.1371/journal.pone.0004431]

[99] Malik HS, Bliska JB. The pyrin inflammasome and the Yersinia effector interaction. Immunological Reviews 2020; 297: 96-107.
[PMID: 32721043]

[100] Medici NP, Rashid M, Bliska JB. Characterization of pyrin dephosphorylation and inflammasome activation in macrophages as triggered by the Yersinia effectors YopE and YopT. Infect Immun 2019;

87(3).
[http://dx.doi.org/10.1128/IAI.00822-18]

[101] Chung LK, Park YH, Zheng Y, Brodsky IE, Hearing P, Kastner DL, *et al.* The yersinia virulence factor YopM hijacks host kinases to inhibit type III effector-triggered activation of the pyrin inflammasome. Cell Host Microbe 2016; 20(3): 296-306.
[http://dx.doi.org/10.1016/j.chom.2016.07.018]

[102] Ratner D, Orning MPA, Proulx MK, Wang D, Gavrilin MA, Wewers MD, *et al.* The *Yersinia pestis* effector YopM inhibits pyrin inflammasome activation. In: Brodsky IE, Ed. PLOS Pathog 2016; 12(12): e1006035.
[http://dx.doi.org/10.1371/journal.ppat.1006035]

[103] Wei C, Wang Y, Du Z, Guan K, Cao Y, Yang H, *et al.* The yersinia type III secretion effector YopM is an E3 ubiquitin ligase that induced necrotic cell death by targeting NLRP3. Cell Death Dis 2016; 7(12>): e2519-9.www.nature.com/cddis
[http://dx.doi.org/10.1038/cddis.2016.413]

[104] Spinner JL, Hasenkrug AM, Shannon JG, Kobayashi SD, Hinnebusch BJ. Role of the Yersinia YopJ protein in suppressing interleukin-8 secretion by human polymorphonuclear leukocytes. Microbes Infect 2016; 18(1): 21-9. [Internet].
[http://dx.doi.org/10.1016/j.micinf.2015.08.015] [PMID: 26361732]

[105] Mukherjee S, Keitany G, Li Y, Wang Y, Ball HL, Goldsmith EJ, *et al.* Yersinia YopJ acetylates and inhibits kinase activation by blocking phosphorylation. Science (80-) 2006; 312(5777): 1211-4.
https://science.sciencemag.org/content/312/5777/1211
[http://dx.doi.org/10.1126/science.1126867]

[106] Paquette N, Conlon J, Sweet C, Rus F, Wilson L, Pereira A, *et al.* Serine/threonine acetylation of TGFβ-activated kinase (TAK1) by *Yersinia pestis* YopJ inhibits innate immune signaling. Proc Natl Acad Sci U S A 2012; 109(31): 12710-5.
[http://dx.doi.org/10.1073/pnas.1008203109]

[107] Ma K-W, Ma W. YopJ family effectors promote bacterial infection through a unique acetyltransferase activity. Microbiol Mol Biol Rev 2016; 80(4): 1011-27.http://mmbr.asm.org/
[http://dx.doi.org/10.1128/MMBR.00032-16]

[108] Zhang ZM, Ma KW, Gao L, Hu Z, Schwizer S, Ma W, *et al.* Mechanism of host substrate acetylation by a YopJ family effector. Nat Plants 2017; 3(8): 1-10.https://www.nature.com/articles/nplants2017115
[http://dx.doi.org/10.1038/nplants.2017.115]

[109] Popa CM, Tabuchi M, Valls M. Modification of bacterial effector proteins inside Eukaryotic host cells. Front Cell Infect Microbiol 2016; 6(JUL): 73.
[http://dx.doi.org/10.3389/fcimb.2016.00073] [PMID: 27489796]

[110] Belyy A, Raoux-Barbot D, Saveanu C, Namane A, Ogryzko V, Worpenberg L, *et al.* Actin activates *Pseudomonas aeruginosa* ExoY nucleotidyl cyclase toxin and ExoY-like effector domains from MARTX toxins. Nat Commun 2016; 7(1): 1-14.www.nature.com/naturecommunications
[http://dx.doi.org/10.1038/ncomms13582]

[111] Kloth C, Schirmer B, Munder A, Stelzer T, Rothschuh J, Seifert R. The role of *Pseudomonas aeruginosa* exoy in an acute mouse lung infection model. Toxins (Basel) 2018; 10
[http://dx.doi.org/10.3390/toxins10050185]

[112] Mancl JM, Suarez C, Liang WG, Kovar DR, Tang WJ. *Pseudomonas aeruginosa* exoenzyme Y directly bundles actin filaments. J Biol Chem 2020; 295(11): 3506-17. http://www.jbc.org/content/295/11/3506.full

[113] Sato H, Frank DW. ExoU is a potent intracellular phospholipase. Mol Microbiol 2004; 53(5): 1279-90.
[http://dx.doi.org/10.1111/j.1365-2958.2004.04194.x] [PMID: 15387809]

[114] Gendrin C, Contreras-Martel C, Bouillot S, Elsen S, Lemaire D, Skoufias DA, *et al.* Structural basis of cytotoxicity mediated by the type III secretion toxin ExoU from *Pseudomonas aeruginosa*. PLoS Pathog 2012; 8(4): 0-11.

[115] Halavaty AS, Borek D, Tyson GH, Veesenmeyer JL, Shuvalova L, Minasov G, *et al.* Structure of the type III secretion effector protein ExoU in complex with its chaperone SpcU. In: Kaufmann GF, Ed. PLoS One 2012; 7(11): e49388.
[http://dx.doi.org/10.1371/journal.pone.0049388]

[116] Stirling FR, Cuzick A, Kelly SM, Oxley D, Evans TJ. Eukaryotic localization, activation and ubiquitinylation of a bacterial type III secreted toxin. Cell Microbiol 2006; 8(8): 1294-309.
[http://dx.doi.org/10.1111/j.1462-5822.2006.00710.x] [PMID: 16882033]

[117] Anderson DM, Feix JB, Monroe AL, Peterson FC, Volkman BF, Haas AL, *et al.* dentification of the major ubiquitin-binding domain of the *Pseudomonas aeruginosa* ExoU A2 Phospholipase. J Biol Chem 2013; 288(37): 26741-52.

[118] Tessmer MH, Anderson DM, Pickrum AM, Riegert MO, Moretti R, Meiler J, *et al.* Identification of a ubiquitin-binding interface using Rosetta and DEER. Proc Natl Acad Sci U S A 2018; 115(3): 525-30.www.pnas.org/cgi/doi/10.1073/pnas.1716861115
[http://dx.doi.org/10.1073/pnas.1716861115]

[119] Tessmer MH, Anderson DM, Pickrum AM, Riegert MO, Frank DW. Identification and verification of ubiquitin-activated bacterial phospholipases. J Bacteriol 2019; 201(4)

[120] Tessmer MH, Anderson DM, Buchaklian A, Frank DW, Feix JB. Cooperative substrate-cofactor interactions and membrane localization of the bacterial phospholipase A2 (PLA2) enzyme, ExoU. J Biol Chem 2017; 292(8): 3411-9.https://pubmed.ncbi.nlm.nih.gov/28069812/

[121] Wang W, Liu N, Gao C, Rui L, Tang D. The pseudomonas syringae effector avrptob associates with and ubiquitinates arabidopsis exocyst subunit EXO70B1. Front Plant Sci 2019; 10: 1027.https://www.frontiersin.org/article/10.3389/fpls.2019.01027/full
[http://dx.doi.org/10.3389/fpls.2019.01027]

[122] Lei L, Stevens DM, Coaker G. Phosphorylation of the pseudomonas effector avrptob by arabidopsis snrk2.8 is required for bacterial virulence. Mol Plant 2020; 13(10): 1513-22.
[http://dx.doi.org/10.1016/j.molp.2020.08.018] [PMID: 32889173]

[123] Oh CS, Martin GB. Effector-triggered immunity mediated by the Pto kinase. Trends Plant Sci 2011; 16(3): 132-40. [Internet].
[http://dx.doi.org/10.1016/j.tplants.2010.11.001] [PMID: 21112235]

[124] Xing W, Zou Y, Liu Q, Liu J, Luo X, Huang Q, *et al.* The structural basis for activation of plant immunity by bacterial effector protein AvrPto. Nature 2007; 449(7159): 243-7. https://www.nat ure.com/articles/nature06109
[http://dx.doi.org/10.1038/nature06109]

[125] Dong J, Xiao F, Fan F, Gu L, Cang H, Martin GB, *et al.* Crystal structure of the complex between pseudomonas effector avrptob and the tomato pto kinase reveals both a shared and a unique interface compared with avrpto-pto. Plant Cell 2009; 21(6): 1846-59.
[http://dx.doi.org/10.1105/tpc.109.066878]

[126] Yeam I, Nguyen HP, Martin GB. Phosphorylation of the Pseudomonas syringae effector AvrPto is required for FLS2/BAK1-independent virulence activity and recognition by tobacco. Plant J 2010; 61: 1-24.: 16-24.
[PMID: 19793077]

[127] Mathieu J, Schwizer S, Martin GB. Pto kinase binds two domains of avrptob and its proximity to the effector e3 ligase determines if it evades degradation and activates plant immunity. In: He S, Ed. PLoS Pathog 2014; 10(7): e1004227.
[http://dx.doi.org/10.1371/journal.ppat.1004227]

[128]   Lan KH, Lee WP, Wang YS, Liao SX, Lan KH. *Helicobacter pylori* CagA protein activates Akt and attenuates chemotherapeutics-induced apoptosis in gastric cancer cells. Oncotarget 2017; 8(69): 113460-71.
        [http://dx.doi.org/10.18632/oncotarget.23050]

[129]   Chen SY, Zhang RG, Duan GC. Pathogenic mechanisms of the oncoprotein CagA in H. pylori-induced gastric cancer (Review). Oncology Reports 2016; 36: 3087-94.
        http://www.spandidos-publications.com/10.3892/or.2016.5145/abstract

[130]   Hatakeyama M. Structure and function of *Helicobacter pylori* caga, the first-identified bacterial protein involved in human cancer. Proceedings of the Japan Academy Series B: Physical and Biological Sciences. 93: 196-219.

[131]   Hayashi T, Senda M, Suzuki N, Nishikawa H, Ben C, Tang C, *et al.* Differential mechanisms for shp2 binding and activation are exploited by geographically distinct *Helicobacter pylori* CagA oncoproteins. Cell Rep 2017; 20(12): 2876-90.
        [http://dx.doi.org/10.1016/j.celrep.2017.08.080]

[132]   Wong K, Perpich JD, Kozlov G, Cygler M, Abu Kwaik Y, Gehring K. Structural mimicry by a bacterial f box effector hijacks the host ubiquitin-proteasome system. Structure 2017; 25(2): 376-83.
        [http://dx.doi.org/10.1016/j.str.2016.12.015] [PMID: 28111017]

[133]   Price C, Merchant M, Jones S, *et al.* Host FIH-mediated asparaginyl hydroxylation of translocated *Legionella pneumophila* effectors. Front Cell Infect Microbiol 2017; 7(MAR): 54.
        [http://dx.doi.org/10.3389/fcimb.2017.00054] [PMID: 28321389]

[134]   Lando D, Peet DJ, Gorman JJ, Whelan DA, Whitelaw ML, Bruick RK. FIH-1 is an asparaginyl hydroxylase enzyme that regulates the transcriptional activity of hypoxia-inducible factor. Genes Dev 2002; 16(12): 1466-71.

[135]   Huszczynski SM, Lam JS, Khursigara CM. The role of *Pseudomonas aeruginosa* lipopolysaccharide in bacterial pathogenesis and physiology. Pathogens 2019; 9(1): E6.
        [http://dx.doi.org/10.3390/pathogens9010006] [PMID: 31861540]

[136]   Weigele BA, Orchard RC, Jimenez A, Cox GW, Alto NM. A systematic exploration of the interactions between bacterial effector proteins and host cell membranes. Nat Commun 2017; 8(1): 532. [Internet].
        [http://dx.doi.org/10.1038/s41467-017-00700-7] [PMID: 28912547]

[137]   Swart AL, Hilbi H. Phosphoinositides and the fate of legionella in phagocytes Frontiers in Immunology 2020; 11.
        [PMID: 32117224]

[138]   Hsu FS, Luo X, Qiu J, Teng Y. The legionella effector SidC defines a unique family of ubiquitin ligases important for bacterial phagosomal remodeling. Proc Natl Acad Sci USA 2014; 111(29): 10538-43.
        [http://dx.doi.org/10.1073/pnas.1402605111]

[139]   Luo X, Wasilko DJ, Liu Y, Sun J, Wu X, Luo Z-Q, *et al.* Structure of the legionella virulence factor, sidc reveals a unique PI(4)P-specific binding domain essential for its targeting to the bacterial phagosome. In: Roy CR, Ed. PLOS Pathog 2015; 11(6): e1004965.
        [http://dx.doi.org/10.1371/journal.ppat.1004965]

[140]   Geissler B. Bacterial toxin effector-membrane targeting: outside in, then back again. Front Cell Infect Microbiol 2012; 2(May): 75.
        [http://dx.doi.org/10.3389/fcimb.2012.00075] [PMID: 22919666]

[141]   Turnbull D, Hemsley PA. Fats and function: protein lipid modifications in plant cell signalling. Curr Opin Plant Biol 2017; 40: 63-70.
        [http://dx.doi.org/10.1016/j.pbi.2017.07.007] [PMID: 28772175]

[142]   Brown RW, Sharma AI, Engman DM. Dynamic protein S-palmitoylation mediates parasite life cycle progression and diverse mechanisms of virulence. Crit Rev Biochem Mol Biol 2017; 52(2):

145-62.https://www.ncbi.nlm.nih.gov/pmc/articles/PMC5560270/pdf/nihms887669.pdf [Internet].
[http://dx.doi.org/10.1080/10409238.2017.1287161] [PMID: 28228066]

[143] Udenwobele DI, Su RC, Good SV, Ball TB, Shrivastav SV, Shrivastav A. Myristoylation: An important protein modification in the immune response. Frontiers in Immunology. Frontiers Media S.A. 2017; 8: p. 1.www.frontiersin.org [cited 2020 Oct 24]

[144] Yuan M, Song Z han, Ying M dan, *et al.* N-myristoylation: from cell biology to translational medicine. Acta Pharmacologica Sinica. Springer Nature 2020; 41: pp. 1005-15. https://www.nature.com/articles/s41401-020-0388-4 [cited 2020 Oct 24]

[145] Sobocińska J, Roszczenko-Jasińska P, Ciesielska A, Kwiatkowska K. Protein palmitoylation and its role in bacterial and viral infections. Front Immunol 2018; 8: 2003.
[http://dx.doi.org/10.3389/fimmu.2017.02003] [PMID: 29403483]

[146] Ohlson MB, Huang Z, Alto NM, *et al.* Structure and function of Salmonella SifA indicate that its interactions with SKIP, SseJ, and RhoA family GTPases induce endosomal tubulation. Cell Host Microbe 2008; 4(5): 434-46.
[http://dx.doi.org/10.1016/j.chom.2008.08.012] [PMID: 18996344]

[147] Reinicke AT, Hutchinson JL, Magee AI, Mastroeni P, Trowsdale J, Kelly AP. A *Salmonella typhimurium* effector protein SifA is modified by host cell prenylation and S-acylation machinery. J Biol Chem 2005; 280(15): 14620-7.
[http://dx.doi.org/10.1074/jbc.M500076200] [PMID: 15710609]

[148] Zhao W, Moest T, Zhao Y, *et al.* The Salmonella effector protein SifA plays a dual role in virulence. Sci Rep 2015; 5: 12979.
[http://dx.doi.org/10.1038/srep12979] [PMID: 26268777]

[149] Patel S, Wall DM, Castillo A, McCormick BA. Caspase-3 cleavage of salmonella type III secreted effector protein SifA is required for localization of functional domains and bacterial dissemination. Gut Microbes 2019; 10(2): 172-87.
[http://dx.doi.org/10.1080/19490976.2018.1506668] [PMID: 30727836]

[150] Hicks SW, Charron G, Hang HC, Galán JE. Subcellular targeting of salmonella virulence proteins by host-mediated S-palmitoylation. Cell Host Microbe 2011; 10(1): 9-20.

[151] Bhaskaran SS, Stebbins CE. Structure of the catalytic domain of the Salmonella virulence factor SseI. Acta Crystallogr D Biol Crystallogr 2012; 68(Pt 12): 1613-21.
[http://dx.doi.org/10.1107/S0907444912039042] [PMID: 23151626]

[152] Brink T, Leiss V, Siegert P, *et al. Salmonella typhimurium* effector SseI inhibits chemotaxis and increases host cell survival by deamidation of heterotrimeric Gi proteins. PLoS Pathog 2018; 14(8): e1007248-.
[http://dx.doi.org/10.1371/journal.ppat.1007248] [PMID: 30102745]

[153] Spera JM, Comerci DJ, Ugalde JE. Brucella alters the immune response in a prpA-dependent manner. Microb Pathog 2014; 67-68(1): 8-13.
[http://dx.doi.org/10.1016/j.micpath.2014.01.003]

[154] Spera JM, Guaimas F, Corvi MM, Ugalde JE. Brucella hijacks host-mediated palmitoylation to stabilize and localize PrpA to the plasma membrane. Infect Immun 2018; 86: 11.
[http://dx.doi.org/10.1128/IAI.00402-18]

[155] Burnaevskiy N, Peng T, Reddick LE, Hang HC, Alto NM. Myristoylome profiling reveals a concerted mechanism of ARF GTPase deacylation by the bacterial protease IpaJ. Mol Cell 2015; 58(1): 110-22.
[PMID: 25773595] [http://dx.doi.org/10.1016/j.molcel.2015.01.040]

[156] Burnaevskiy N, Fox TG, Plymire DA, Ertelt JM, Weigele BA, Selyunin AS, *et al.* Proteolytic elimination of N-myristoyl modifications by the Shigella virulence factor IpaJ. Nature 2013; 496(7443): 106-9.
[PMID: 23535599]

[157] Ke Z, Smith GK, Zhang Y, Guo H. Molecular mechanism for eliminylation, a newly discovered post-translational modification. J Am Chem Soc 2011; 133(29): 11103-5.
[http://dx.doi.org/10.1021/ja204378q] [PMID: 21710993]

[158] Zhu Y, Li H, Long C, *et al.* Structural insights into the enzymatic mechanism of the pathogenic MAPK phosphothreonine lyase. Mol Cell 2007; 28(5): 899-913.
[http://dx.doi.org/10.1016/j.molcel.2007.11.011] [PMID: 18060821]

[159] Mazurkiewicz P, Thomas J, Thompson JA, *et al.* SpvC is a Salmonella effector with phosphothreonine lyase activity on host mitogen-activated protein kinases. Mol Microbiol 2008; 67(6): 1371-83.
[http://dx.doi.org/10.1111/j.1365-2958.2008.06134.x] [PMID: 18284579]

[160] Meijer BM, Jang SM, Guerrera IC, Chhuon C, Lipecka J, Reisacher C, *et al.* Threonine eliminylation by bacterial phosphothreonine lyases rapidly causes cross-linking of mitogen-activated protein kinase (MAPK) in live cells. J Biol Chem 2017; 292(19): 7784-94.
[PMID: 28325837]

[161] Haneda T, Ishii Y, Shimizu H, *et al.* Salmonella type III effector SpvC, a phosphothreonine lyase, contributes to reduction in inflammatory response during intestinal phase of infection. Cell Microbiol 2012; 14(4): 485-99. [Internet].
[http://dx.doi.org/10.1111/j.1462-5822.2011.01733.x] [PMID: 22188134]

[162] Gulig PA, Chiodo VA. Genetic and DNA sequence analysis of the *Salmonella typhimurium* virulence plasmid gene encoding the 28,000-molecular-weight protein. Infect Immun 1990; 58(8): 2651-8. [Internet].
[http://dx.doi.org/10.1128/IAI.58.8.2651-2658.1990] [PMID: 2164511]

[163] Matsui H, Bacot CM, Garlington WA, Doyle TJ, Roberts S, Gulig PA. Virulence Plasmid-Borne spvB and spvC Genes Can Replace the 90-Kilobase Plasmid in Conferring Virulence to Salmonella enterica Serovar Typhimurium in Subcutaneously Inoculated Mice. J Bacteriol 2001; 183(15): 4652-8.http://jb.asm.org/content/183/15/4652

[164] Li H, Xu H, Zhou Y, Zhang J, Long C, Li S, *et al.* The phosphothreonine lyase activity of a bacterial type III effector family. Science (80-) 2007; 315(5814): 1000-3. https://science.sciencemag.org/content/315/5814/1000
[http://dx.doi.org/10.1126/science.1138960]

[165] Brennan DF, Barford D. Eliminylation: a post-translational modification catalyzed by phosphothreonine lyases. Trends Biochem Sci 2009; 34(3): 108-14. [Internet].
[http://dx.doi.org/10.1016/j.tibs.2008.11.005] [PMID: 19233656]

[166] Arbibe L, Kim DW, Batsche E, *et al.* An injected bacterial effector targets chromatin access for transcription factor NF-kappaB to alter transcription of host genes involved in immune responses. Nat Immunol 2007; 8(1): 47-56. [Internet].
[http://dx.doi.org/10.1038/ni1423] [PMID: 17159983]

[167] Woolery A. AMPylation: something old is new again. Front Microbiol 2010; 1(OCT): 113.http://journal.frontiersin.org/article/10.3389/fmicb.2010.00113/abstract
[http://dx.doi.org/10.3389/fmicb.2010.00113]

[168] Yarbrough ML, Li Y, Kinch LN, Grishin NV, Ball HL, Orth K. AMPylation of Rho GTPases by Vibrio VopS disrupts effector binding and downstream signaling. Science (80-) 2009; 323(5911): 269-72.https://pubmed.ncbi.nlm.nih.gov/19039103/
[http://dx.doi.org/10.1126/science.1166382]

[169] Zekarias B, Mattoo S, Worby C, Lehmann J, Rosenbusch RF, Corbeil LB. Histophilus somni IbpA DR2/Fic in virulence and immunoprotection at the natural host alveolar epithelial barrier. Infect Immun 2010; 78(5): 1850-8.http://iai.asm.org/

[170] Barthelmes K, Ramcke E, Kang HS, Sattler M, Itzen A. Conformational control of small GTPases by AMPylation. Proc Natl Acad Sci USA 2020; 117(11): 5772-81.

[http://dx.doi.org/10.1073/pnas.1917549117] [PMID: 32123090]

[171] Casey AK, Orth K. Enzymes Involved in AMPylation and deAMPylation. Chemical Reviews 2018; 118: 1199-215. https://pubmed.ncbi.nlm.nih.gov/28819965/

[172] Kokkinidis M, Glykos NM, Fadouloglou VE. Catalytic activity regulation through post-translational modification: the expanding universe of protein diversity. Adv Protein Chem Struct Biol 2020; 122 https://pubmed.ncbi.nlm.nih.gov/32951817/ [http://dx.doi.org/10.1016/bs.apcsb.2020.05.001]

[173] Chambers KA, Scheck RA. Bacterial virulence mediated by orthogonal post-translational modification. Nature Chemical Biology. Nature Research 2020; 16: pp. 1043-51. https://pubmed.ncbi.nlm.nih.gov/32943788/ [cited 2020 Oct 24]

[174] O'Sullivan J, Tedim Ferreira M, Gagné JP, Sharma AK, Hendzel MJ, Masson JY, *et al.* Emerging roles of eraser enzymes in the dynamic control of protein ADP-ribosylation. Nature Communications. Nature Publishing Group 2019; 10: pp. 1-14. [cited 2020 Oct 25]

[175] Palazzo L, Mikoč A, Ahel I. ADP-ribosylation: new facets of an ancient modification. FEBS J 2017; 284(18): 2932-46.http://doi.wiley.com/10.1111/febs.14078

[176] Catara G, Corteggio A, Valente C, Grimaldi G, Palazzo L. Targeting ADP-ribosylation as an antimicrobial strategy. Biochem Pharmacol 2019; 167: 13-26.

[177] Rocha CL, Coburn J, Rucks EA, Olson JC. Characterization of *Pseudomonas aeruginosa* exoenzyme S as a bifunctional enzyme in J774A.1 macrophages. Infect Immun 2003; 71(9): 5296-305. [http://dx.doi.org/10.1128/IAI.71.9.5296-5305.2003] [PMID: 12933877]

[178] Barbieri JT, Sun J. *Pseudomonas aeruginosa* ExoS and ExoT. Rev Physiol Biochem Pharmacol 2004; 152: 79-92. [PMID: 15375697]

[179] Rangel SM, Diaz MH, Knoten CA, Zhang A, Hauser AR. The role of exos in dissemination of *Pseudomonas aeruginosa* during pneumonia. PLoS Pathog 2015; 11(6): e1004945. [http://dx.doi.org/10.1371/journal.ppat.1004945] [PMID: 26090668]

[180] Sun Y, Karmakar M, Taylor PR, Rietsch A, Pearlman E. ExoS and ExoT ADP ribosyltransferase activities mediate *Pseudomonas aeruginosa* keratitis by promoting neutrophil apoptosis and bacterial survival . J Immunol 2012; 188(4): 1884-95. http://www.jimmunol.org/content/188/4/1884

[181] Robinson NE, Robinson AB. Molecular clocks. Proc Natl Acad Sci U S A 2001; 98(3): 944-.www.pnas.org [http://dx.doi.org/10.1073/pnas.98.3.944]

[182] Washington EJ, Banfield MJ, Dangl JL. What a difference a Dalton makes: bacterial virulence factors modulate eukaryotic host cell signaling systems *via* deamidation. Microbiol Mol Biol Rev 2013; 77(3): 527-39. [http://dx.doi.org/10.1128/MMBR.00013-13] [PMID: 24006474]

[183] Zhao J, Li J, Xu S, Feng P. Emerging roles of protein deamidation in innate immune signaling. J Virol 2016; 90(9): 4262-8. http://jvi.asm.org/

[184] Schweer J, Kulkarni D, Kochut A, Pezoldt J, Pisano F, Pils MC, *et al.* The cytotoxic necrotizing factor of *Yersinia pseudotuberculosis* (CNFY) enhances inflammation and yop delivery during infection by activation of Rho GTPases. PLoS Pathog 2013; 9(11): 1003746.

[185] Twittenhoff C, Heroven AK, Mühlen S, Dersch P, Narberhaus F. An RNA thermometer dictates production of a secreted bacterial toxin. PLoS Pathog 2020; 16: 1.

[186] Zhang L, Krachler AM, Broberg CA, *et al.* Type III effector VopC mediates invasion for Vibrio species. Cell Rep 2012; 1(5): 453-60. [http://dx.doi.org/10.1016/j.celrep.2012.04.004] [PMID: 22787576]

[187] Okada R, Zhou X, Hiyoshi H, *et al.* The Vibrio parahaemolyticus effector VopC mediates Cdc42-

dependent invasion of cultured cells but is not required for pathogenicity in an animal model of infection. Cell Microbiol 2014; 16(6): 938-47.
[http://dx.doi.org/10.1111/cmi.12252] [PMID: 24345190]

[188] Yang H, Santos M de S, Lee J, Law HT, Chimalapati S, Verdu EF, *et al.* A novel mouse model of enteric vibrio parahaemolyticus infection reveals that the type iii secretion system 2 effector vopc plays a key role in tissue invasion and gastroenteritis. MBio 2019; 10: 6. http://mbio.asm.org/

[189] Orth JHC, Aktories K. Pasteurella multocida toxin activates various heterotrimeric G proteins by deamidation. Toxins (Basel) 2010; 2(2): 205-14.
[http://dx.doi.org/10.3390/toxins2020205] [PMID: 22069582]

[190] Wilson BA, Ho M. Pasteurella multocida toxin interaction with host cells: entry and cellular effects. Curr Top Microbiol Immunol 2012; 361: 93-111.
[http://dx.doi.org/10.1007/82_2012_219] [PMID: 22552700]

[191] Kitadokoro K, Kamitani S, Miyazawa M, *et al.* Crystal structures reveal a thiol protease-like catalytic triad in the C-terminal region of Pasteurella multocida toxin. Proc Natl Acad Sci USA 2007; 104(12): 5139-44.
[http://dx.doi.org/10.1073/pnas.0608197104] [PMID: 17360394]

[192] Hautbergue GM, Wilson SA. BLF1, the first *Burkholderia pseudomallei* toxin, connects inhibition of host protein synthesis with melioidosis. In: Biochemical Society Transactions 2012; 842-5.
[http://dx.doi.org/10.1042/BST20120057]

[193] Cruz-Migoni A, Hautbergue GM, Artymiuk PJ, Baker PJ, Bokori-Brown M, Te Chang C, *et al.* A *Burkholderia pseudomallei* toxin inhibits helicase activity of translation factor eIF4A. Science (80-) 2011; 334(6057): 821-4. https://science.sciencemag.org/content/334/6057/821

[194] Rust A, Shah S, Hautbergue GM, Davletov B. Burkholderia lethal factor 1, a novel anti-cancer toxin, demonstrates selective cytotoxicity in MYCN-amplified neuroblastoma cells. Toxins (Basel) 2018; 10(7): 1-13.
[http://dx.doi.org/10.3390/toxins10070261] [PMID: 29954071]

[195] Taieb F, Nougayrède J-P, Oswald E. Cycle inhibiting factors (Cifs): cyclomodulins that usurp the ubiquitin-dependent degradation pathway of host cells. Toxins (Basel) 2011; 3(4): 356-68.
http://www.mdpi.com/2072-6651/3/4/356

[196] Crow A, Hughes RK, Taieb F, Oswald E, Banfield MJ. The molecular basis of ubiquitin-like protein NEDD8 deamidation by the bacterial effector protein Cif. Proc Natl Acad Sci USA 2012; 109(27): E1830-8.
[http://dx.doi.org/10.1073/pnas.1112107109]

[197] Jubelin G, Taieb F, Duda DM, Hsu Y, Samba-Louaka A. Pathogenic bacteria target NEDD8-conjugated cullins to hijack host-cell signaling pathways 2010. https://hal.inrae.fr/hal-02662283
[http://dx.doi.org/10.1371/journal.ppat.1001128]

[198] Bomberger JM, Ely KH, Bangia N, Ye S, Green KA, Green WR, *et al. Pseudomonas aeruginosa* Cif protein enhances the ubiquitination and proteasomal degradation of the transporter associated with antigen processing (TAP) and reduces major histocompatibility complex (MHC) class I antigen presentation. J Biol Chem 2014; 289(1): 152-62.

[199] Sanada T, Kim M, Mimuro H, *et al.* The *Shigella flexneri* effector OspI deamidates UBC13 to dampen the inflammatory response. Nature 2012; 483(7391): 623-6.
[http://dx.doi.org/10.1038/nature10894] [PMID: 22407319]

[200] Nishide A, Kim M, Takagi K, Himeno A, Sanada T, Sasakawa C, *et al.* Structural basis for the recognition of Ubc13 by the *Shigella flexneri* effector ospi. J Mol Biol 2013; 425(15): 2623-31.
[PMID: 23542009]

[201] Narayanan LA, Edelmann MJ. Ubiquitination as an efficient molecular strategy employed in Salmonella infection. Frontiers in Immunology 2014; 5.

[202] Verma S, Mohapatra G, Ahmad SM, *et al.* Salmonella engages host micrornas to modulate sumoylation: a new arsenal for intracellular survival. Mol Cell Biol 2015; 35(17): 2932-46. [http://dx.doi.org/10.1128/MCB.00397-15] [PMID: 26100020]

[203] Kim M, Otsubo R, Morikawa H, *et al.* Bacterial effectors and their functions in the ubiquitin-proteasome system: insight from the modes of substrate recognition. Cells 2014; 3(3): 848-64. [http://dx.doi.org/10.3390/cells3030848] [PMID: 25257025]

[204] Kubori T, Kitao T, Nagai H. Emerging insights into bacterial deubiquitinases. Curr Opin Microbiol. Elsevier Ltd 2019; 47: pp. 14-9. [http://dx.doi.org/10.1016/j.mib.2018.10.001]

[205] Hermanns T, Hofmann K. Bacterial DUBs: deubiquitination beyond the seven classes. Biochem Soc Trans 2019; 47(6): 1857-66. [Internet]. [http://dx.doi.org/10.1042/BST20190526] [PMID: 31845741]

[206] Ashida H, Sasakawa C. Bacterial E3 ligase effectors exploit host ubiquitin systems. Current Opinion in Microbiology. Elsevier Ltd 2017; 35: pp. 16-22. [http://dx.doi.org/10.1016/j.mib.2016.11.001]

[207] Maculins T, Fiskin E, Bhogaraju S, Dikic I. Bacteria-host relationship: Ubiquitin ligases as weapons of invasion. Cell Research. Nature Publishing Group 2016; 26: pp. 499-510.www.nature.com/cr [cited 2020 Oct 24]

[208] Pisano A, Albano F, Vecchio E, Renna M, Scala G, Quinto I, *et al.* Revisiting bacterial ubiquitin ligase effectors: Weapons for host exploitation. Int J Mol Sci 2018; 19

[209] Zhang Y, Higashide WM, McCormick BA, Chen J, Zhou D. The inflammation-associated Salmonella SopA is a HECT-like E3 ubiquitin ligase. Mol Microbiol 2006; 62(3): 786-93.https://pubmed.ncbi.nlm.nih.gov/17076670/

[210] Kamanova J, Sun H, Lara-Tejero M, Galán JE. The salmonella effector protein SopA modulates innate immune responses by targeting TRIM E3 ligase family members. In: Baumler AJ, Ed. PLOS Pathog 2016; 12(4): e1005552. [http://dx.doi.org/10.1371/journal.ppat.1005552]

[211] Fiskin E, Bhogaraju S, Herhaus L, Kalayil S, Hahn M, Dikic I. Structural basis for the recognition and degradation of host TRIM proteins by Salmonella effector SopA. Nat Commun 2017; 8(1): 1-14.www.nature.com/naturecommunications [http://dx.doi.org/10.1038/ncomms14004]

[212] Piscatelli H, Kotkar SA, McBee ME, Muthupalani S, Schauer DB, Mandrell RE, *et al.* The EHEC Type III Effector NleL Is an E3 Ubiquitin Ligase That Modulates Pedestal Formation. In: van der Goot FG, Ed. PLoS One 2011; 6(4): e19331. [http://dx.doi.org/10.1371/journal.pone.0019331]

[213] Sheng X, You Q, Zhu H, Chang Z, Li Q, Wang H, *et al.* Bacterial effector NleL promotes enterohemorrhagic *E. coli*-induced attaching and effacing lesions by ubiquitylating and inactivating JNK. In: Mulvey MA, Ed. PLOS Pathog 2017; 13(7): e1006534. [http://dx.doi.org/10.1371/journal.ppat.1006534]

[214] Sheng X, You Q, Zhu H, Li Q, Gao H, Wang H, *et al.* Enterohemorrhagic *E. coli* effector NleL disrupts host NF-κB signaling by targeting multiple host proteins. J Mol Cell Biol 2020; 12(4): 318-21.

[215] Kubori T, Hyakutake A, Nagai H. Legionella translocates an E3 ubiquitin ligase that has multiple U-boxes with distinct functions. Mol Microbiol 2008; 67(6): 1307-9. [PMID: 18284575]

[216] Quaile AT, Urbanus ML, Stogios PJ, Nocek B, Skarina T, Ensminger AW, *et al.* Molecular characterization of LubX: functional divergence of the u-box fold by *Legionella pneumophila*. Structure 2015; 23(8): 1459-69.

[217]   Keszei AFA, Sicheri F. Mechanism of catalysis, E2 recognition,& autoinhibition for the IpaH family of bacterial E3 ubiquitin ligases. Proc Natl Acad Sci USA 2017; 114(6): 1311-6.
[http://dx.doi.org/10.1073/pnas.1611595114]

[218]   Okuda J, Toyotome T, Kataoka N, *et al.* Shigella effector IpaH9.8 binds to a splicing factor U2AF(35) to modulate host immune responses. Biochem Biophys Res Commun 2005; 333(2): 531-9.
[http://dx.doi.org/10.1016/j.bbrc.2005.05.145] [PMID: 15950937]

[219]   Ashida H, Kim M, Schmidt-Supprian M, Ma A, Ogawa M, Sasakawa C. A bacterial E3 ubiquitin ligase IpaH9.8 targets NEMO/IKKγ to dampen the host NF-κB-mediated inflammatory response. Nature Cell Biology. Nature Publishing Group 2010; Vol. 12: pp. 66-73. [cited 2020 Oct 24]
[PMID: 20010814]

[220]   Li P, Jiang W, Yu Q, Liu W, Zhou P, Li J, *et al.* Ubiquitination and degradation of GBPs by a Shigella effector to suppress host defence. Nature 2017; 551(7680): 378-83.
[http://dx.doi.org/10.1038/nature24467] [PMID: 29144452]

[221]   Ji C, Du S, Li P, Zhu Q, Yang X, Long C, *et al.* Structural mechanism for guanylate-binding proteins (GBPs) targeting by the Shigella E3 ligase IpaH9.8. In: Ghosh P, Ed. PLOS Pathog 2019; 15(6): e1007876.
[http://dx.doi.org/10.1371/journal.ppat.1007876]

[222]   Coombes BK, Lowden MJ, Bishop JL, Wickham ME, Brown NF, Duong N, *et al.* SseL is a Salmonella-specific translocated effector integrated into the SsrB-controlled Salmonella pathogenicity island 2 type III secretion system. Infect Immun 2007; 75(2): 574-80.http://iai.asm.org/
[http://dx.doi.org/10.1128/IAI.00985-06]

[223]   Rytkönen A, Poh J, Garmendia J, Boyle C, Thompson A, Liu M, *et al.* SseL, a Salmonella deubiquitinase required for macrophage killing and virulence. Proc Natl Acad Sci U S A 2007; 104(9): 3502-7.
[http://dx.doi.org/10.1073/pnas.0610095104]

[224]   Arena ET, Auweter SD, Antunes LCM, Vogl AW, Han J, Guttman JA, *et al.* The deubiquitinase activity of the salmonella pathogenicity island 2 effector, ssel, prevents accumulation of cellular lipid droplets. Infect Immun 2011; 79(11): 4392-00.http://iai.asm.org/

[225]   Mesquita FS, Thomas M, Sachse M, Santos AJM, Figueira R, Holden DW. The salmonella deubiquitinase ssel inhibits selective autophagy of cytosolic aggregates. In: Roy CR, Ed. PLoS Pathog 2012; 8(6): e1002743.
[http://dx.doi.org/10.1371/journal.ppat.1002743]

[226]   Kolodziejek AM, Altura MA, Fan J, Petersen EM, Cook M, Brzovic PS, *et al.* Salmonella translocated effectors recruit OSBP1 to the phagosome to promote vacuolar membrane integrity. Cell Rep 2019; 27(7): 2147-56.
[http://dx.doi.org/10.1016/j.celrep.2019.04.021] [PMID: 31091452]

[227]   Wan M, Wang X, Huang C, Xu D, Wang Z, Zhou Y, *et al.* A bacterial effector deubiquitinase specifically hydrolyses linear ubiquitin chains to inhibit host inflammatory signalling. Nat Microbiol 2019; 4(8): 1282-93.https://www.nature.com/articles/s41564-019-0454-1
[http://dx.doi.org/10.1038/s41564-019-0454-1]

[228]   Aepfelbacher M, Roppenser B, Hentschke M, Ruckdeschel K. Activity modulation of the bacterial Rho GAP YopE: An inspiration for the investigation of mammalian Rho GAPs. Eur J Cell Biol. Urban & Fischer 2011; 90: pp. 951-4.

[229]   Gaus K, Hentschke M, Czymmeck N, Novikova L, Trülzsch K, Valentin-Weigand P, *et al.* Destabilization of YopE by the ubiquitin-proteasome pathway fine-tunes yop delivery into host cells and facilitates systemic spread of *Yersinia enterocolitica* in host lymphoid tissue. Infect Immun 2011; 79(3): 1166-75.
[PMID: 21149597] [http://dx.doi.org/10.1128/IAI.00694-10]

[230]   Knodler LA, Winfree S, Drecktrah D, Ireland R, Steele-Mortimer O. Ubiquitination of the bacterial inositol phosphatase, SopB, regulates its biological activity at the plasma membrane. Cell Microbiol 2009; 11(11): 1652-70.https://pubmed.ncbi.nlm.nih.gov/19614667/

[231]   Patel JC, Hueffer K, Lam TT, Galán JE. Diversification of a salmonella virulence protein function by ubiquitin-dependent differential localization. Cell 2009; 137(2): 283-94.
[http://dx.doi.org/10.1016/j.cell.2009.01.056]

[232]   Dunphy PS, Luo T, McBride JW. Ehrlichia chaffeensis exploits host SUMOylation pathways to mediate effector-host interactions and promote intracellular survival. Infect Immun 2014; 82(10): 4154-68.
[http://dx.doi.org/10.1128/IAI.01984-14] [PMID: 25047847]

[233]   Mitra S, Dunphy PS, Das S, Zhu B, Luo T, McBride JW. Ehrlichia chaffeensis TRP120 effector targets and recruits host polycomb group proteins for degradation to promote intracellular infection. Infect Immun 2018; 86(4)

[234]   Wang JY, Zhu B, Patterson LL, Rogan MR, Kibler CE, McBride JW. Ehrlichia chaffeensis TRP120-mediated ubiquitination and proteasomal degradation of tumor suppressor FBW7 increases oncoprotein stability and promotes infection. In: Voth DE, Ed. PLOS Pathog 2020; 16(4): e1008541.
[http://dx.doi.org/10.1371/journal.ppat.1008541]

[235]   Bhogaraju S, Kalayil S, Liu Y, *et al.* Phosphoribosylation of ubiquitin promotes serine ubiquitination and impairs conventional ubiquitination. Cell 2016; 167(6): 1636-1649.e13.
[http://dx.doi.org/10.1016/j.cell.2016.11.019] [PMID: 27912065]

[236]   Qiu J, Sheedlo MJ, Yu K, Tan Y, Nakayasu ES, Das C, *et al.* Ubiquitination independent of E1 and E2 enzymes by bacterial effectors. Nature 2016; 533(7601): 120-4.
[http://dx.doi.org/10.1038/nature17657]

[237]   Wang Y, Shi M, Feng H, Zhu Y, Liu S, Gao A, *et al.* Structural Insights into Non-canonical Ubiquitination Catalyzed by SidE. Cell 2018; 173(5): 1231-43.
[PMID: 29731171] [http://dx.doi.org/10.1016/j.cell.2018.04.023]

[238]   Puvar K, Luo ZQ, Das C. Uncovering the structural basis of a new twist in protein ubiquitination. Trends Biochem Sci 2019; 44(5): 467-77.
[http://dx.doi.org/10.1016/j.tibs.2018.11.006] [PMID: 30583962]

[239]   Madern JM, Kim RQ, Misra M, *et al.* Synthesis of stable NAD$^+$ mimics as inhibitors for the *Legionella pneumophila* phosphoribosyl ubiquitylating enzyme SdeC. Chem Bio Chem 2020; 21(20): 2903-7.
[http://dx.doi.org/10.1002/cbic.202000230] [PMID: 32421893]

[240]   Akturk A, Wasilko DJ, Wu X, *et al.* Mechanism of phosphoribosyl-ubiquitination mediated by a single Legionella effector. Nature 2018; 557(7707): 729-33.
[http://dx.doi.org/10.1038/s41586-018-0147-6] [PMID: 29795346]

[241]   Dong Y, Mu Y, Xie Y, *et al.* Structural basis of ubiquitin modification by the Legionella effector SdeA. Nature 2018; 557(7707): 674-8. [Internet].
[http://dx.doi.org/10.1038/s41586-018-0146-7] [PMID: 29795342]

[242]   Kim L, Kwon DH, Kim BH, *et al.* Structural and biochemical study of the mono-ad--ribosyltransferase domain of sdea, a ubiquitylating/deubiquitylating enzyme from *Legionella pneumophila*. J Mol Biol 2018; 430(17): 2843-56.
[http://dx.doi.org/10.1016/j.jmb.2018.05.043] [PMID: 29870726]

[243]   Sulpizio A, Minelli ME, Wan M, *et al.* Protein polyglutamylation catalyzed by the bacterial calmodulin-dependent pseudokinase SidJ. eLife 2019; 8: e51162.
[http://dx.doi.org/10.7554/eLife.51162] [PMID: 31682223]

[244]   Valleau D, Quaile AT, Cui H, *et al.* Discovery of ubiquitin deamidases in the pathogenic arsenal of *Legionella pneumophila*. Cell Rep 2018; 23(2): 568-83.
[http://dx.doi.org/10.1016/j.celrep.2018.03.060] [PMID: 29642013]

[245] Gan N, Nakayasu ES, Hollenbeck PJ, Luo ZQ. *Legionella pneumophila* inhibits immune signalling *via* MavC-mediated transglutaminase-induced ubiquitination of UBE2N. Nat Microbiol 2019; 4(1): 134-43.
[http://dx.doi.org/10.1038/s41564-018-0282-8] [PMID: 30420781]

[246] Puvar K, Iyer S, Fu J, *et al.* Legionella effector MavC targets the Ube2N~Ub conjugate for noncanonical ubiquitination. Nat Commun 2020; 11(1): 2365.
[http://dx.doi.org/10.1038/s41467-020-16211-x] [PMID: 32398758]

[247] Mu Y, Wang Y, Huang Y, *et al.* Structural insights into the mechanism and inhibition of transglutaminase-induced ubiquitination by the Legionella effector MavC. Nat Commun 2020; 11(1): 1774.
[http://dx.doi.org/10.1038/s41467-020-15645-7] [PMID: 32286321]

[248] Wang Y, Zhan Q, Wang X, *et al.* Insights into catalysis and regulation of non-canonical ubiquitination and deubiquitination by bacterial deamidase effectors. Nat Commun 2020; 11(1): 2751.
[http://dx.doi.org/10.1038/s41467-020-16587-w] [PMID: 32488130]

[249] Nakamura S, Minamino T. Flagella-driven motility of bacteria. Biomolecules 2019; 9(7): 279.
[http://dx.doi.org/10.3390/biom9070279] [PMID: 31337100]

[250] Hajam IA, Dar PA, Shahnawaz I, Jaume JC, Lee JH. Bacterial flagellin-a potent immunomodulatory agent. Exp Mol Med 2017; 49(9): e373-3.
[http://dx.doi.org/10.1038/emm.2017.172] [PMID: 28860663]

[251] Thibault P, Logan SM, Kelly JF, *et al.* Identification of the carbohydrate moieties and glycosylation motifs in Campylobacter jejuni flagellin. J Biol Chem 2001; 276(37): 34862-70. http://www.jbc.org/content/276/37/34862 [Internet].
[http://dx.doi.org/10.1074/jbc.M104529200] [PMID: 11461915]

[252] McNally DJ, Hui JPM, Aubry AJ, *et al.* Functional characterization of the flagellar glycosylation locus in Campylobacter jejuni 81-176 using a focused metabolomics approach. J Biol Chem 2006; 281(27): 18489-98.http://www.jbc.org/content/281/27/18489 [Internet].
[http://dx.doi.org/10.1074/jbc.M603777200] [PMID: 16684771]

[253] Schirm M, Schoenhofen IC, Logan SM, Waldron KC, Thibault P. Identification of unusual bacterial glycosylation by tandem mass spectrometry analyses of intact proteins. Anal Chem 2005; 77(23): 7774-82. [Internet].
[http://dx.doi.org/10.1021/ac051316y] [PMID: 16316188]

[254] Guerry P, Ewing CP, Schirm M, *et al.* Changes in flagellin glycosylation affect Campylobacter autoagglutination and virulence. Mol Microbiol 2006; 60(2): 299-311.
[http://dx.doi.org/10.1111/j.1365-2958.2006.05100.x] [PMID: 16573682]

[255] Ewing CP, Andreishcheva E, Guerry P. Functional characterization of flagellin glycosylation in campylobacter jejuni 81-176. J Bacteriol 2009; 191(22): 7086-93.
http://jb.asm.org/cont-ent/191/22/7086

[256] Champasa K, Longwell SA, Eldridge AM, Stemmler EA, Dube DH. Targeted identification of glycosylated proteins in the gastric pathogen *Helicobacter pylori* (Hp). Mol Cell Proteomics 2013; 12(9): 2568-86.
[PMID: 23754784]

[257] Verma A, Arora SK, Kuravi SK, Ramphal R. Roles of specific amino acids in the N terminus of *Pseudomonas aeruginosa* flagellin and of flagellin glycosylation in the innate immune response. Infect Immun 2005; 73(12): 8237-46.
[http://dx.doi.org/10.1128/IAI.73.12.8237-8246.2005] [PMID: 16299320]

[258] Verma A, Schirm M, Arora SK, Thibault P, Logan SM, Ramphal R. Glycosylation of b-Type flagellin of *Pseudomonas aeruginosa*: structural and genetic basis. J Bacteriol 2006; 188(12): 4395-403.
[http://dx.doi.org/10.1128/JB.01642-05] [PMID: 16740946]

[259] Schirm M, Arora SK, Verma A, Vinogradov E, Thibault P, Ramphal R, *et al.* Structural and genetic characterization of glycosylation of type a flagellin in *Pseudomonas aeruginosa.* J Bacteriol 2004; 186(9): 2523-31.http://jb.asm.org/content/186/9/2523

[260] Twine SM, Reid CW, Aubry A, McMullin DR, Fulton KM, Austin J, *et al.* Motility and flagellar glycosylation in *Clostridium difficile.* J Bacteriol 2009; 191(22): 7050-62. http://jb.asm.org/content/191/22/7050

[261] Twine SM, Paul CJ, Vinogradov E, *et al.* Flagellar glycosylation in clostridium botulinum. FEBS J 2008; 275(17): 4428-44.
[http://dx.doi.org/10.1111/j.1742-4658.2008.06589.x] [PMID: 18671733]

[262] Hanuszkiewicz A, Pittock P, Humphries F, Moll H, Rosales AR, Molinaro A, *et al.* Identification of the flagellin glycosylation system in Burkholderia cenocepacia and the contribution of glycosylated flagellin to evasion of human innate immune responses. J Biol Chem 2014; 289(27): 19231-44.
[PMID: 24841205]

[263] Wacker M, Linton D, Hitchen PG, Nita-Lazar M, Haslam SM, North SJ, *et al.* N-Linked glycosylation in *Campylobacter jejuni* and its functional transfer into *E. coli.* Science 2002; 298(5599): 1790-3. http://science.sciencemag.org/content/298/5599/1790

[264] Cain JA, Dale AL, Niewold P, Klare WP, Man L, White MY, *et al.* Proteomics reveals multiple phenotypes associated with N-linked Glycosylation in Campylobacter jejuni. Mol Cell Proteomics 2019; 18(4): 715-34. http://www.mcponline.org/content/18/4/715

[265] Nothaft H, Szymanski CM. Protein glycosylation in bacteria: sweeter than ever. Nat Rev Microbiol 2010; 8(11): 765-78.
[http://dx.doi.org/10.1038/nrmicro2383] [PMID: 20948550]

[266] Lu Q, Li S, Shao F. Sweet talk: protein glycosylation in bacterial interaction with the host. Trends Microbiol 2015; 23(10): 630-41. http://www.sciencedirect.com/science/article/pii/S096684 2X15001523 [Internet].
[http://dx.doi.org/10.1016/j.tim.2015.07.003] [PMID: 26433695]

[267] Iwashkiw JA, Seper A, Weber BS, Scott NE, Vinogradov E, Stratilo C, *et al.* Identification of a general O-linked protein glycosylation system in Acinetobacter baumannii and its role in virulence and biofilm formation. PLoS Pathog 2012; 8(6): e1002758-.
[PMID: 22685409]

[268] Jank T, Belyi Y, Aktories K. Bacterial glycosyltransferase toxins. Cell Microbiol 2015; 17(12): 1752-65.
[http://dx.doi.org/10.1111/cmi.12533] [PMID: 26445410]

[269] Belyi Y, Tabakova I, Stahl M, Aktories K. Lgt: a family of cytotoxic glucosyltransferases produced by *Legionella pneumophila.* J Bacteriol 2008; 190(8): 3026-35.
[http://dx.doi.org/10.1128/JB.01798-07] [PMID: 18281405]

[270] Belyi Y, Jank T, Aktories K. Effector glycosyltransferases in legionella. Front Microbiol 2011; 2: 76.
[http://dx.doi.org/10.3389/fmicb.2011.00076] [PMID: 21833323]

[271] De Leon JA, Qiu J, Nicolai CJ, *et al.* Positive and negative regulation of the master metabolic regulator MTORC1 by two families of *Legionella pneumophila* effectors. Cell Rep 2017; 21(8): 2031-8.http://www.sciencedirect.com/science/article/pii/S2211124717315516 [Internet].
[http://dx.doi.org/10.1016/j.celrep.2017.10.088] [PMID: 29166595]

[272] Wang Z, McCloskey A, Cheng S, *et al.* Regulation of the small GTPase Rab1 function by a bacterial glucosyl transferase. Cell Discov 2018; 4: 53. [Internet].
[http://dx.doi.org/10.1038/s41421-018-0055-9] [PMID: 30323948]

[273] Beck WHJ, Kim D, Das J, Yu H, Smolka MB, Mao Y. glucosylation by the legionella effector seta promotes the nuclear localization of the transcription factor TFEB. iScience 2020; 23(7): 101300.
[PMID: 32622269]

[274]   Levanova N, Steinemann M, Böhmer KE, *et al.* Characterization of the glucosyltransferase activity of *Legionella pneumophila* effector SetA. Naunyn Schmiedebergs Arch Pharmacol 2019; 392(1): 69-79.
[http://dx.doi.org/10.1007/s00210-018-1562-9] [PMID: 30225797]

[275]   Pearson JS, Giogha C, Ong SY, *et al.* A type III effector antagonizes death receptor signalling during bacterial gut infection. Nature 2013; 501(7466): 247-51. [Internet].
[http://dx.doi.org/10.1038/nature12524] [PMID: 24025841]

[276]   Li S, Zhang L, Yao Q, *et al.* Pathogen blocks host death receptor signalling by arginine GlcNAcylation of death domains. Nature 2013; 501(7466): 242-6. [Internet].
[http://dx.doi.org/10.1038/nature12436] [PMID: 23955153]

[277]   Scott NE, Giogha C, Pollock GL, Kennedy CL, Webb AI, Williamson NA, *et al.* The bacterial arginine glycosyltransferase effector NleB preferentially modifies Fas-associated death domain protein (FADD). J Biol Chem 2017; 292(42): 17337-50.
[PMID: 28860194]

[278]   Ding J, Pan X, Du L, *et al.* Structural and functional insights into host death domains inactivation by the bacterial arginine glcnacyltransferase effector. Mol Cell 2019; 74(5): 922-935.e6.
http://www.sciencedirect.com/science/article/pii/S1097276519302321 [Internet].
[http://dx.doi.org/10.1016/j.molcel.2019.03.028] [PMID: 30979585]

[279]   Wong Fok Lung T, Giogha C, Creuzburg K, *et al.* Mutagenesis and functional analysis of the bacterial arginine glycosyltransferase effector nleb1 from enteropathogenic *Escherichia coli*. Infect Immun 2016; 84(5): 1346-60.
[http://dx.doi.org/10.1128/IAI.01523-15] [PMID: 26883593]

[280]   Meng K, Zhuang X, Peng T, *et al.* Arginine GlcNAcylation of Rab small GTPases by the pathogen *Salmonella typhimurium*. Commun Biol 2020; 3(1): 287. [Internet].
[http://dx.doi.org/10.1038/s42003-020-1005-2] [PMID: 32504010]

[281]   Salomon D, Orth K. What pathogens have taught us about posttranslational modifications. Cell Host and Microbe. Cell Press 2013; 14: pp. 269-79.
[http://dx.doi.org/10.1016/j.chom.2013.07.008]

[282]   Salinas S, Kremer EJ. Virus induced and associated post-translational modifications. Biol Cell 2012; 104(3): 119-20.
[http://dx.doi.org/10.1111/boc.201290008] [PMID: 22380478]

[283]   Ksiazek TG, Erdman D, Goldsmith CS, *et al.* SARS Working Group. A novel coronavirus associated with severe acute respiratory syndrome. N Engl J Med 2003; 348(20): 1953-66.
[http://dx.doi.org/10.1056/NEJMoa030781] [PMID: 12690092]

[284]   de Groot RJ, Baker SC, Baric RS, *et al.* Middle East respiratory syndrome coronavirus (MERS-CoV): announcement of the Coronavirus Study Group. J Virol 2013; 87(14): 7790-2.
[http://dx.doi.org/10.1128/JVI.01244-13] [PMID: 23678167]

[285]   Fung TS, Liu DX. Post-translational modifications of coronavirus proteins: Roles and function. Future Virology. Future Medicine Ltd. 2018; 13: pp. 405-30.

[286]   Wrapp D, Wang N, Corbett KS, Goldsmith JA, Hsieh CL, Abiona O, *et al.* Cryo-EM structure of the 2019-nCoV spike in the prefusion conformation. Science 2020; 367(6483): 1260-3.

[287]   Mittal A, Manjunath K, Ranjan RK, Kaushik S, Kumar S, Verma V. COVID-19 pandemic: Insights into structure, function, and hACE2 receptor recognition by SARS-CoV-2. PLoS Pathog 2020; 16(8): e1008762.
[http://dx.doi.org/10.1371/journal.ppat.1008762] [PMID: 32822426]

[288]   Letko M, Marzi A, Munster V. Functional assessment of cell entry and receptor usage for SARS-Co-2 and other lineage B betacoronaviruses. Nat Microbiol 2020; 5(4): 562-9.
[http://dx.doi.org/10.1038/s41564-020-0688-y] [PMID: 32094589]

[289] Walls AC, Park YJ, Tortorici MA, Wall A, McGuire AT, Veesler D. Structure, Function, and antigenicity of the SARS-CoV-2 spike glycoprotein. Cell 2020; 181(2): 281-292.e6.
[http://dx.doi.org/10.1016/j.cell.2020.02.058]

[290] Hoffmann M, Kleine-Weber H, Pöhlmann S. A multibasic cleavage site in the spike protein of SARS-CoV-2 is essential for infection of human lung cells. Mol Cell 2020; 78(4): 779-784.e5.
[http://dx.doi.org/10.1016/j.molcel.2020.04.022] [PMID: 32362314]

[291] Liao Y, Yuan Q, Torres J, Tam JP, Liu DX. Biochemical and functional characterization of the membrane association and membrane permeabilizing activity of the severe acute respiratory syndrome coronavirus envelope protein. Virology 2006; 349(2): 264-75.
[http://dx.doi.org/10.1016/j.virol.2006.01.028] [PMID: 16507314]

[292] Yuan Q, Liao Y, Torres J, Tam JP, Liu DX. Biochemical evidence for the presence of mixed membrane topologies of the severe acute respiratory syndrome coronavirus envelope protein expressed in mammalian cells. FEBS Lett 2006; 580(13): 3192-200.
[http://dx.doi.org/10.1016/j.febslet.2006.04.076] [PMID: 16684538]

[293] Schoeman D, Fielding BC. Coronavirus envelope protein: current knowledge. Virol J 2019; 16(1): 69.
[http://dx.doi.org/10.1186/s12985-019-1182-0] [PMID: 31133031]

[294] Nieto-Torres JL, Dediego ML, Álvarez E, *et al.* Subcellular location and topology of severe acute respiratory syndrome coronavirus envelope protein. Virology 2011; 415(2): 69-82.
[http://dx.doi.org/10.1016/j.virol.2011.03.029] [PMID: 21524776]

[295] Venkatagopalan P, Daskalova SM, Lopez LA, Dolezal KA, Hogue BG. Coronavirus envelope (E) protein remains at the site of assembly. Virology 2015; 478: 75-85.
[http://dx.doi.org/10.1016/j.virol.2015.02.005] [PMID: 25726972]

[296] Ortego J, Ceriani JE, Patiño C, Plana J, Enjuanes L. Absence of E protein arrests transmissible gastroenteritis coronavirus maturation in the secretory pathway. Virology 2007; 368(2): 296-308.
[http://dx.doi.org/10.1016/j.virol.2007.05.032] [PMID: 17692883]

[297] DeDiego ML, Álvarez E, Almazán F, *et al.* A severe acute respiratory syndrome coronavirus that lacks the E gene is attenuated in vitro and in vivo. J Virol 2007; 81(4): 1701-13.
[http://dx.doi.org/10.1128/JVI.01467-06] [PMID: 17108030]

[298] Wilson L, McKinlay C, Gage P, Ewart G. SARS coronavirus E protein forms cation-selective ion channels. Virology 2004; 330(1): 322-31.
[http://dx.doi.org/10.1016/j.virol.2004.09.033] [PMID: 15527857]

[299] Mukherjee S, Bhattacharyya D, Bhunia A. Host-membrane interacting interface of the SARS coronavirus envelope protein: Immense functional potential of C-terminal domain. Biophys Chem 2020; 266: 106452.
[http://dx.doi.org/10.1016/j.bpc.2020.106452] [PMID: 32818817]

[300] Masters PS. The molecular biology of coronaviruses. Adv Virus Res 2006; 66: 193-292.
[http://dx.doi.org/10.1016/S0065-3527(06)66005-3] [PMID: 16877062]

[301] Hogue BG, Machamer CE. Coronavirus structural proteins and virus assembly. In: Nidoviruse. 2014.

[302] Voss D, Kern A, Traggiai E, *et al.* Characterization of severe acute respiratory syndrome coronavirus membrane protein. FEBS Lett 2006; 580(3): 968-73.
[http://dx.doi.org/10.1016/j.febslet.2006.01.026] [PMID: 16442106]

[303] Chang CK, Sue SC, Yu TH, *et al.* Modular organization of SARS coronavirus nucleocapsid protein. J Biomed Sci 2006; 13(1): 59-72.
[http://dx.doi.org/10.1007/s11373-005-9035-9] [PMID: 16228284]

[304] Hurst KR, Koetzner CA, Masters PS. Characterization of a critical interaction between the coronavirus nucleocapsid protein and nonstructural protein 3 of the viral replicase-transcriptase complex. J Virol 2013; 87(16): 9159-72.

[http://dx.doi.org/10.1128/JVI.01275-13] [PMID: 23760243]

[305] Fang S, Xu L, Huang M, Qisheng Li F, Liu DX. Identification of two ATR-dependent phosphorylation sites on coronavirus nucleocapsid protein with nonessential functions in viral replication and infectivity in cultured cells. Virology 2013; 444(1-2): 225-32.
[http://dx.doi.org/10.1016/j.virol.2013.06.014] [PMID: 23849791]

[306] Li FQ, Xiao H, Tam JP, Liu DX. Sumoylation of the nucleocapsid protein of severe acute respiratory syndrome coronavirus. FEBS Lett 2005; 579(11): 2387-96.
[http://dx.doi.org/10.1016/j.febslet.2005.03.039] [PMID: 15848177]

[307] Niemann H, Boschek B, Evans D, Rosing M, Tamura T, Klenk HD. Post-translational glycosylation of coronavirus glycoprotein E1: inhibition by monensin. EMBO J 1982; 1(12): 1499-504.
[http://dx.doi.org/10.1002/j.1460-2075.1982.tb01346.x] [PMID: 6327272]

[308] Ritchie G, Harvey DJ, Feldmann F, et al. Identification of N-linked carbohydrates from severe acute respiratory syndrome (SARS) spike glycoprotein. Virology 2010; 399(2): 257-69.
[http://dx.doi.org/10.1016/j.virol.2009.12.020] [PMID: 20129637]

[309] Koch G, Kant A. Binding of antibodies that strongly neutralise infectious bronchitis virus is dependent on the glycosylation of the viral peplomer protein. Advances in Experimental Medicine and Biology 1990.
[http://dx.doi.org/10.1007/978-1-4684-5823-7_21]

[310] Delmas B, Laude H. Carbohydrate-induced conformational changes strongly modulate the antigenicity of coronavirus TGEV glycoproteins S and M. Virus Res 1991; 20(2): 107-20.
[http://dx.doi.org/10.1016/0168-1702(91)90103-3] [PMID: 1950169]

[311] Chen WH, Du L, Chag SM, Ma C, Tricoche N, Tao X, et al. Yeast-expressed recombinant protein of the receptor-binding domain in SARS-CoV spike protein with deglycosylated forms as a SARS vaccine candidate. Hum Vaccines Immunother 2014; 10(3): 648-58.
[http://dx.doi.org/10.4161/hv.27464]

[312] Chakraborti S, Prabakaran P, Xiao X, Dimitrov DS. The SARS coronavirus S glycoprotein receptor binding domain: fine mapping and functional characterization. Virol J 2005; 2: 73.
[http://dx.doi.org/10.1186/1743-422X-2-73] [PMID: 16122388]

[313] Li F, Li W, Farzan M, Harrison SC. Structural biology: Structure of SARS coronavirus spike receptor-binding domain complexed with receptor. Science 2005; 309(5742): 1864-8.

[314] Shajahan A, Supekar NT, Gleinich AS, Azadi P. Deducing the N- and O-glycosylation profile of the spike protein of novel coronavirus SARS-CoV-2. Glycobiology 2020; 30(12): 981-8.
[http://dx.doi.org/10.1093/glycob/cwaa042] [PMID: 32363391]

[315] Vigerust DJ, Shepherd VL. Virus glycosylation: role in virulence and immune interactions. Trends Microbiol 2007; 15(5): 211-8.
[http://dx.doi.org/10.1016/j.tim.2007.03.003] [PMID: 17398101]

[316] Millet JK, Whittaker GR. Physiological and molecular triggers for SARS-CoV membrane fusion and entry into host cells. Virology 2018; 517: 3-8.
[http://dx.doi.org/10.1016/j.virol.2017.12.015] [PMID: 29275820]

[317] Watanabe Y, Allen JD, Wrapp D, McLellan JS, Crispin M. Site-specific glycan analysis of the SARS-CoV-2 spike. Science 2020; 369(6501): 330-3.

[318] Pensiero MN, Dveksler GS, Cardellichio CB, et al. Binding of the coronavirus mouse hepatitis virus A59 to its receptor expressed from a recombinant vaccinia virus depends on posttranslational processing of the receptor glycoprotein. J Virol 1992; 66(7): 4028-39.
[http://dx.doi.org/10.1128/JVI.66.7.4028-4039.1992] [PMID: 1318394]

[319] Wentworth DE, Holmes KV. Molecular determinants of species specificity in the coronavirus receptor aminopeptidase N (CD13): influence of N-linked glycosylation. J Virol 2001; 75(20): 9741-52.
[http://dx.doi.org/10.1128/JVI.75.20.9741-9752.2001] [PMID: 11559807]

[320] Peck KM, Scobey T, Swanstrom J, *et al.* Permissivity of dipeptidyl peptidase 4 orthologs to middle East respiratory syndrome coronavirus is governed by glycosylation and other complex determinants. J Virol 2017; 91(19): e00534-17.
[http://dx.doi.org/10.1128/JVI.00534-17] [PMID: 28747502]

[321] Zhou Y, Lu K, Pfefferle S, *et al.* A single asparagine-linked glycosylation site of the severe acute respiratory syndrome coronavirus spike glycoprotein facilitates inhibition by mannose-binding lectin through multiple mechanisms. J Virol 2010; 84(17): 8753-64.
[http://dx.doi.org/10.1128/JVI.00554-10] [PMID: 20573835]

[322] Westerbeck JW, Machamer CE. A coronavirus e protein is present in two distinct pools with different effects on assembly and the secretory pathway. J Virol 2015; 89(18): 9313-23.
[http://dx.doi.org/10.1128/JVI.01237-15] [PMID: 26136577]

[323] Wu Q, Zhang Y, Lü H, Wang J, He X, Liu Y, *et al.* The E protein is a multifunctional membrane protein of SARS-CoV. Genomics, proteomics Bioinforma / Beijing Genomics Inst 2003.

[324] Holmes KV, Doller EW, Sturman LS. Tunicamycin resistant glycosylation of coronavirus glycoprotein: demonstration of a novel type of viral glycoprotein. Virology 1981; 115(2): 334-44.
[http://dx.doi.org/10.1016/0042-6822(81)90115-X] [PMID: 7314449]

[325] de Haan CAM, Kuo L, Masters PS, Vennema H, Rottier PJM. Coronavirus particle assembly: primary structure requirements of the membrane protein. J Virol 1998; 72(8): 6838-50.
[http://dx.doi.org/10.1128/JVI.72.8.6838-6850.1998] [PMID: 9658133]

[326] de Haan CAM, de Wit M, Kuo L, *et al.* The glycosylation status of the murine hepatitis coronavirus M protein affects the interferogenic capacity of the virus *in vitro* and its ability to replicate in the liver but not the brain. Virology 2003; 312(2): 395-406.
[http://dx.doi.org/10.1016/S0042-6822(03)00235-6] [PMID: 12919744]

[327] Voss D, Pfefferle S, Drosten C, *et al.* Studies on membrane topology, N-glycosylation and functionality of SARS-CoV membrane protein. Virol J 2009; 6: 79.
[http://dx.doi.org/10.1186/1743-422X-6-79] [PMID: 19534833]

[328] Siu KL, Chan CP, Kok KH, Chiu-Yat Woo P, Jin DY. Suppression of innate antiviral response by severe acute respiratory syndrome coronavirus M protein is mediated through the first transmembrane domain. Cell Mol Immunol 2014; 11(2): 141-9.
[http://dx.doi.org/10.1038/cmi.2013.61] [PMID: 24509444]

[329] Chen Y, Guo Y, Pan Y, Zhao ZJ. Structure analysis of the receptor binding of 2019-nCoV. Biochem Biophys Res Commun 2020; S0006-291X(20)30339-9.
[http://dx.doi.org/10.1016/j.bbrc.2020.02.071] [PMID: 32081428]

[330] Yan R, Zhang Y, Li Y, Xia L, Guo Y, Zhou Q. Structural basis for the recognition of SARS-CoV-2 by full-length human ACE2. Science 2020; 367(6485): 1444-8.

[331] Wang Q, Zhang Y, Wu L, *et al.* Structural and functional basis of SARS-CoV-2 entry by using human ACE2. Cell 2020; 181(4): 894-904.e9.
[http://dx.doi.org/10.1016/j.cell.2020.03.045] [PMID: 32275855]

[332] Mathys L, Balzarini J. The role of cellular oxidoreductases in viral entry and virus infection-associated oxidative stress: potential therapeutic applications. Expert Opin Ther Targets 2016; 20(1): 123-43.
[http://dx.doi.org/10.1517/14728222.2015.1068760] [PMID: 26178644]

[333] Opstelten DJ, de Groote P, Horzinek MC, Vennema H, Rottier PJ. Disulfide bonds in folding and transport of mouse hepatitis coronavirus glycoproteins. J Virol 1993; 67(12): 7394-401.
[http://dx.doi.org/10.1128/JVI.67.12.7394-7401.1993] [PMID: 8230460]

[334] Lavillette D, Barbouche R, Yao Y, *et al.* Significant redox insensitivity of the functions of the SARS-CoV spike glycoprotein: comparison with HIV envelope. J Biol Chem 2006; 281(14): 9200-4.
[http://dx.doi.org/10.1074/jbc.M512529200] [PMID: 16418166]

[335] Hati S, Bhattacharyya S. Impact of thiol-disulfide balance on the binding of covid-19 spike protein with angiotensin-converting enzyme 2 receptor. ACS Omega 2020; 5(26): 16292-8.
[http://dx.doi.org/10.1021/acsomega.0c02125] [PMID: 32656452]

[336] Li PP, Nakanishi A, Clark SW, Kasamatsu H. Formation of transitory intrachain and interchain disulfide bonds accompanies the folding and oligomerization of simian virus 40 Vp1 in the cytoplasm. Proc Natl Acad Sci USA 2002; 99(3): 1353-8.
[http://dx.doi.org/10.1073/pnas.032668699] [PMID: 11805304]

[337] Ponnusamy R, Moll R, Weimar T, Mesters JR, Hilgenfeld R. Variable oligomerization modes in coronavirus non-structural protein 9. J Mol Biol 2008; 383(5): 1081-96.
[http://dx.doi.org/10.1016/j.jmb.2008.07.071] [PMID: 18694760]

[338] Thorp EB, Boscarino JA, Logan HL, Goletz JT, Gallagher TM. Palmitoylations on murine coronavirus spike proteins are essential for virion assembly and infectivity. J Virol 2006; 80(3): 1280-9.
[http://dx.doi.org/10.1128/JVI.80.3.1280-1289.2006] [PMID: 16415005]

[339] Shulla A, Gallagher T. Role of spike protein endodomains in regulating coronavirus entry. J Biol Chem 2009; 284(47): 32725-34.
[http://dx.doi.org/10.1074/jbc.M109.043547] [PMID: 19801669]

[340] Akerström S, Gunalan V, Keng CT, Tan YJ, Mirazimi A. Dual effect of nitric oxide on SARS-CoV replication: viral RNA production and palmitoylation of the S protein are affected. Virology 2009; 395(1): 1-9.
[http://dx.doi.org/10.1016/j.virol.2009.09.007] [PMID: 19800091]

[341] McBride CE, Machamer CE. Palmitoylation of SARS-CoV S protein is necessary for partitioning into detergent-resistant membranes and cell-cell fusion but not interaction with M protein. Virology 2010; 405(1): 139-48.
[http://dx.doi.org/10.1016/j.virol.2010.05.031] [PMID: 20580052]

[342] Salaun C, Greaves J, Chamberlain LH. The intracellular dynamic of protein palmitoylation. J Cell Biol 2010; 191(7): 1229-38.
[http://dx.doi.org/10.1083/jcb.201008160] [PMID: 21187327]

[343] Lopez LA, Riffle AJ, Pike SL, Gardner D, Hogue BG. Importance of conserved cysteine residues in the coronavirus envelope protein. J Virol 2008; 82(6): 3000-10.
[http://dx.doi.org/10.1128/JVI.01914-07] [PMID: 18184703]

[344] Tseng YT, Wang SM, Huang KJ, Wang CT. SARS-CoV envelope protein palmitoylation or nucleocapid association is not required for promoting virus-like particle production. J Biomed Sci 2014; 21: 34.
[http://dx.doi.org/10.1186/1423-0127-21-34] [PMID: 24766657]

[345] Surjit M, Kumar R, Mishra RN, Reddy MK, Chow VTK, Lal SK. The severe acute respiratory syndrome coronavirus nucleocapsid protein is phosphorylated and localizes in the cytoplasm by 14---3-mediated translocation. J Virol 2005; 79(17): 11476-86.
[http://dx.doi.org/10.1128/JVI.79.17.11476-11486.2005] [PMID: 16103198]

[346] Chen H, Gill A, Dove BK, et al. Mass spectroscopic characterization of the coronavirus infectious bronchitis virus nucleoprotein and elucidation of the role of phosphorylation in RNA binding by using surface plasmon resonance. J Virol 2005; 79(2): 1164-79.
[http://dx.doi.org/10.1128/JVI.79.2.1164-1179.2005] [PMID: 15613344]

[347] Wu CH, Chen PJ, Yeh SH. Nucleocapsid phosphorylation and RNA helicase DDX1 recruitment enables coronavirus transition from discontinuous to continuous transcription. Cell Host Microbe 2014; 16(4): 462-72.
[http://dx.doi.org/10.1016/j.chom.2014.09.009] [PMID: 25299332]

[348] McCormick C, Khaperskyy DA. Translation inhibition and stress granules in the antiviral immune response. Nat Rev Immunol 2017; 17(10): 647-60.

[http://dx.doi.org/10.1038/nri.2017.63] [PMID: 28669985]

[349] Shin GC, Chung YS, Kim IS, Cho HW, Kang C. Antigenic characterization of severe acute respiratory syndrome-coronavirus nucleocapsid protein expressed in insect cells: The effect of phosphorylation on immunoreactivity and specificity. Virus Res 2007; 127(1): 71-80.
[http://dx.doi.org/10.1016/j.virusres.2007.03.019] [PMID: 17499376]

[350] Álvarez E, DeDiego ML, Nieto-Torres JL, Jiménez-Guardeño JM, Marcos-Villar L, Enjuanes L. The envelope protein of severe acute respiratory syndrome coronavirus interacts with the non-structural protein 3 and is ubiquitinated. Virology 2010; 402(2): 281-91.
[http://dx.doi.org/10.1016/j.virol.2010.03.015] [PMID: 20409569]

[351] Keng CT, Akerström S, Leung CSW, *et al.* SARS coronavirus 8b reduces viral replication by down-regulating E *via* an ubiquitin-independent proteasome pathway. Microbes Infect 2011; 13(2): 179-88.
[http://dx.doi.org/10.1016/j.micinf.2010.10.017] [PMID: 21035562]

[352] Yu X, Chen S, Hou P, Wang M, Chen Y, Guo D. VHL negatively regulates SARS coronavirus replication by modulating nsp16 ubiquitination and stability. Biochem Biophys Res Commun 2015; 459(2): 270-6.
[http://dx.doi.org/10.1016/j.bbrc.2015.02.097] [PMID: 25732088]

[353] Harcourt BH, Jukneliene D, Kanjanahaluethai A, *et al.* Identification of severe acute respiratory syndrome coronavirus replicase products and characterization of papain-like protease activity. J Virol 2004; 78(24): 13600-12.
[http://dx.doi.org/10.1128/JVI.78.24.13600-13612.2004] [PMID: 15564471]

[354] Chen Z, Wang Y, Ratia K, Mesecar AD, Wilkinson KD, Baker SC. Proteolytic processing and deubiquitinating activity of papain-like proteases of human coronavirus NL63. J Virol 2007; 81(11): 6007-18.
[http://dx.doi.org/10.1128/JVI.02747-06] [PMID: 17392370]

[355] Mielech AM, Kilianski A, Baez-Santos YM, Mesecar AD, Baker SC. MERS-CoV papain-like protease has deISGylating and deubiquitinating activities. Virology 2014; 450-451: 64-70.
[http://dx.doi.org/10.1016/j.virol.2013.11.040] [PMID: 24503068]

[356] Yu L, Zhang X, Wu T, *et al.* The papain-like protease of avian infectious bronchitis virus has deubiquitinating activity. Arch Virol 2017; 162(7): 1943-50.
[http://dx.doi.org/10.1007/s00705-017-3328-y] [PMID: 28316013]

[357] Mielech AM, Chen Y, Mesecar AD, Baker SC. Nidovirus papain-like proteases: multifunctional enzymes with protease, deubiquitinating and deISGylating activities. Virus Res 2014; 194: 184-90.
[http://dx.doi.org/10.1016/j.virusres.2014.01.025] [PMID: 24512893]

[358] Devaraj SG, Wang N, Chen Z, *et al.* Regulation of IRF-3-dependent innate immunity by the papain-like protease domain of the severe acute respiratory syndrome coronavirus. J Biol Chem 2007; 282(44): 32208-21.
[http://dx.doi.org/10.1074/jbc.M704870200] [PMID: 17761676]

[359] Frieman M, Ratia K, Johnston RE, Mesecar AD, Baric RS. Severe acute respiratory syndrome coronavirus papain-like protease ubiquitin-like domain and catalytic domain regulate antagonism of IRF3 and NF-kappaB signaling. J Virol 2009; 83(13): 6689-705.
[http://dx.doi.org/10.1128/JVI.02220-08] [PMID: 19369340]

[360] Li SW, Wang CY, Jou YJ, *et al.* SARS coronavirus papain-like protease inhibits the TLR7 signaling pathway through removing Lys63-linked polyubiquitination of TRAF3 and TRAF6. Int J Mol Sci 2016; 17(5): E678.
[http://dx.doi.org/10.3390/ijms17050678] [PMID: 27164085]

[361] Matthews K, Schäfer A, Pham A, Frieman M. The SARS coronavirus papain like protease can inhibit IRF3 at a post activation step that requires deubiquitination activity. Virol J 2014; 11: 209.
[http://dx.doi.org/10.1186/s12985-014-0209-9] [PMID: 25481026]

[362] Ma-Lauer Y, Carbajo-Lozoya J, Hein MY, *et al.* p53 down-regulates SARS coronavirus replication and is targeted by the SARS-unique domain and PLpro *via* E3 ubiquitin ligase RCHY1. Proc Natl Acad Sci USA 2016; 113(35): E5192-201.
[http://dx.doi.org/10.1073/pnas.1603435113] [PMID: 27519799]

[363] Hu Y, Li W, Gao T, *et al.* The severe acute respiratory syndrome coronavirus nucleocapsid inhibits type i interferon production by interfering with trim25-mediated rig-i ubiquitination. J Virol 2017; 91(8): e02143-16.
[http://dx.doi.org/10.1128/JVI.02143-16] [PMID: 28148787]

[364] Cheng W, Chen S, Li R, Chen Y, Wang M, Guo D. Severe acute respiratory syndrome coronavirus protein 6 mediates ubiquitin-dependent proteosomal degradation of N-Myc (and STAT) interactor. Virol Sin 2015; 30(2): 153-61.
[http://dx.doi.org/10.1007/s12250-015-3581-8] [PMID: 25907116]

[365] El Hajjaji H, Collet J-F. Disulfide Bond Formation. In: Walsh PDG, Ed. Post-translational Modification of Protein Biopharmaceuticals. Wiley-Blackwell 2009; pp. 277-94.
[http://dx.doi.org/10.1002/9783527626601.ch11]

[366] de Marco A. Strategies for successful recombinant expression of disulfide bond-dependent proteins in *Escherichia coli*. Microb Cell Fact 2009; 8: 26.
[http://dx.doi.org/10.1186/1475-2859-8-26] [PMID: 19442264]

[367] Ceaglio N, Etcheverrigaray M, Kratje R, Oggero M. Novel long-lasting interferon alpha derivatives designed by glycoengineering. Biochimie 2008; 90(3): 437-49.
[http://dx.doi.org/10.1016/j.biochi.2007.10.013] [PMID: 18039474]

[368] Garcia-Quintanilla F, Iwashkiw JA, Price NL, Stratilo C, Feldman MF. Production of a recombinant vaccine candidate against *Burkholderia pseudomallei* exploiting the bacterial N-glycosylation machinery. Front Microbiol 2014; 5: 381.
[http://dx.doi.org/10.3389/fmicb.2014.00381] [PMID: 25120536]

[369] Xu D, You G. Loops and layers of post-translational modifications of drug transporters. Adv Drug Deliv Rev 2017; 116: 37-44.
[http://dx.doi.org/10.1016/j.addr.2016.05.003] [PMID: 27174152]

[370] Stelzl T, Baranov T, Geillinger KE, Kottra G, Daniel H. Effect of N-glycosylation on the transport activity of the peptide transporter PEPT1. Am J Physiol Gastrointest Liver Physiol 2016; 310(2): G128-41.
[http://dx.doi.org/10.1152/ajpgi.00350.2015] [PMID: 26585416]

[371] Stelzl T, Geillinger-Kästle KE, Stolz J, Daniel H. Glycans in the intestinal peptide transporter PEPT1 contribute to function and protect from proteolysis. Am J Physiol Gastrointest Liver Physiol 2017; 312(6): G580-91.
[http://dx.doi.org/10.1152/ajpgi.00343.2016] [PMID: 28336547]

[372] Czuba LC, Hillgren KM, Swaan PW. Post-translational modifications of transporters. Pharmacol Ther 2018; 192: 88-99.
[http://dx.doi.org/10.1016/j.pharmthera.2018.06.013] [PMID: 29966598]

[373] An S, Fu L. Small-molecule PROTACs: An emerging and promising approach for the development of targeted therapy drugs. EBioMedicine 2018; 36: 553-62.
[http://dx.doi.org/10.1016/j.ebiom.2018.09.005] [PMID: 30224312]

[374] Xue G, Chen J, Liu L, *et al.* Protein degradation through covalent inhibitor-based PROTACs. Chem Commun (Camb) 2020; 56(10): 1521-4.
[http://dx.doi.org/10.1039/C9CC08238G] [PMID: 31922153]

[375] Su MG, Weng JTY, Hsu JBK, Huang KY, Chi YH, Lee TY. Investigation and identification of functional post-translational modification sites associated with drug binding and protein-protein interactions. BMC Syst Biol 2017; 11 (Suppl. 7): 132.

[http://dx.doi.org/10.1186/s12918-017-0506-1] [PMID: 29322920]

[376]   Walsh G. Post-translational modifications of protein biopharmaceuticals. Drug Discov Today 2010; 15(17-18): 773-80.
[http://dx.doi.org/10.1016/j.drudis.2010.06.009] [PMID: 20599624]

[377]   Weake VM. Histone ubiquitylation control of gene expression. Fundamentals of Chromatin 2014.
[http://dx.doi.org/10.1007/978-1-4614-8624-4_6]

[378]   Hu H, Sun SC. Ubiquitin signaling in immune responses. Cell Res 2016; 26(4): 457-83.
[http://dx.doi.org/10.1038/cr.2016.40] [PMID: 27012466]

[379]   Chuikov S, Kurash JK, Wilson JR, *et al.* Regulation of p53 activity through lysine methylation. Nature 2004; 432(7015): 353-60.
[http://dx.doi.org/10.1038/nature03117] [PMID: 15525938]

[380]   Zhang W, Bailey-Elkin BA, Knaap RCM, *et al.* Potent and selective inhibition of pathogenic viruses by engineered ubiquitin variants. PLoS Pathog 2017; 13(5): e1006372.
[http://dx.doi.org/10.1371/journal.ppat.1006372] [PMID: 28542609]

[381]   Hui KF, Ho DN, Tsang CM, Middeldorp JM, Tsao GSW, Chiang AKS. Activation of lytic cycle of Epstein-Barr virus by suberoylanilide hydroxamic acid leads to apoptosis and tumor growth suppression of nasopharyngeal carcinoma. Int J Cancer 2012; 131(8): 1930-40.
[http://dx.doi.org/10.1002/ijc.27439] [PMID: 22261816]

[382]   Zhao J, Meyerkord CL, Du Y, Khuri FR, Fu H. 14-3-3 proteins as potential therapeutic targets. Semin Cell Dev Biol 2011; 22(7): 705-12.
[http://dx.doi.org/10.1016/j.semcdb.2011.09.012] [PMID: 21983031]

[383]   Fu H, Subramanian RR, Masters SC. 14-3-3 proteins: structure, function, and regulation. Annu Rev Pharmacol Toxicol 2000; 40: 617-47.
[http://dx.doi.org/10.1146/annurev.pharmtox.40.1.617] [PMID: 10836149]

[384]   Obsilová V, Silhan J, Boura E, Teisinger J, Obsil T. 14-3-3 proteins: a family of versatile molecular regulators. Physiol Res 2008; 57 (Suppl. 3): S11-21.
[PMID: 18481918]

[385]   Nathan KG, Lal SK. The multifarious role of 14-3-3 family of proteins in viral replication. Viruses 2020; 12(4): E436.
[http://dx.doi.org/10.3390/v12040436] [PMID: 32294919]

[386]   Aoki H, Hayashi J, Moriyama M, Arakawa Y, Hino O, Hepatitis C. Hepatitis C virus core protein interacts with 14-3-3 protein and activates the kinase Raf-1. J Virol 2000; 74(4): 1736-41.
[http://dx.doi.org/10.1128/JVI.74.4.1736-1741.2000] [PMID: 10644344]

[387]   Diao J, Khine AA, Sarangi F, *et al.* X protein of hepatitis B virus inhibits Fas-mediated apoptosis and is associated with up-regulation of the SAPK/JNK pathway. J Biol Chem 2001; 276(11): 8328-40.
[http://dx.doi.org/10.1074/jbc.M006026200] [PMID: 11099494]

[388]   Chan YK, Gack MU. A phosphomimetic-based mechanism of dengue virus to antagonize innate immunity. Nat Immunol 2016; 17(5): 523-30.
[http://dx.doi.org/10.1038/ni.3393] [PMID: 26998762]

[389]   Petrosillo N, Viceconte G, Ergonul O, Ippolito G, Petersen E. COVID-19, SARS and MERS: are they closely related? Clin Microbiol Infect 2020; 26(6): 729-34.
[http://dx.doi.org/10.1016/j.cmi.2020.03.026] [PMID: 32234451]

[390]   Keyser P, Elofsson M, Rosell S, Wolf-Watz H. Virulence blockers as alternatives to antibiotics: type III secretion inhibitors against Gram-negative bacteria. J Intern Med 2008; 264(1): 17-29. [Internet].
[http://dx.doi.org/10.1111/j.1365-2796.2008.01941.x] [PMID: 18393958]

[391]   Langdon A, Crook N, Dantas G. The effects of antibiotics on the microbiome throughout development and alternative approaches for therapeutic modulation. Genome Med 2016; 8(1):

39.https://pubmed.ncbi.nlm.nih.gov/27074706 [Internet].
[http://dx.doi.org/10.1186/s13073-016-0294-z] [PMID: 27074706]

[392]   Schjørring S, Krogfelt KA. Assessment of bacterial antibiotic resistance transfer in the gut. Int J
        Microbiol 2011; 312956.
        [http://dx.doi.org/10.1155/2011/312956]

[393]   Boudaher E, Shaffer CL. Inhibiting bacterial secretion systems in the fight against antibiotic
        resistance. MedChemComm 2019; 10(5): 682-92. [Internet].
        [http://dx.doi.org/10.1039/C9MD00076C] [PMID: 31741728]

[394]   Duncan MC, Linington RG, Auerbuch V. Chemical inhibitors of the type three secretion system:
        disarming   bacterial   pathogens.   Antimicrob   Agents   Chemother   2012;   56(11):
        5433-41.https://pubmed.ncbi.nlm.nih.gov/22850518
        [http://dx.doi.org/10.1128/AAC.00975-12]

[395]   Felise HB, Nguyen HV, Pfuetzner RA, *et al.* An inhibitor of gram-negative bacterial virulence protein
        secretion. Cell Host Microbe 2008; 4(4): 325-36. https://pubmed.ncbi.nlm.nih.gov/18854237
        [Internet].
        [http://dx.doi.org/10.1016/j.chom.2008.08.001] [PMID: 18854237]

[396]   Harmon DE, Davis AJ, Castillo C, Mecsas J. Identification and characterization of small-molecule
        inhibitors of yop translocation in pseudotuberculosis. Antimicrob Agents Chemother 2010; 54(8):
        3241-54.http://aac.asm.org/content/54/8/3241

[397]   Charpentier X, Gabay JE, Reyes M, Zhu JW, Weiss A, Shuman HA. Chemical genetics reveals
        bacterial and host cell functions critical for type IV effector translocation by *Legionella pneumophila.*
        PLoS Pathog 2009; 7(7): e1000501. https://pubmed.ncbi.nlm.nih.gov/19578436

[398]   He W, Elizondo-Riojas M-A, Li X, Lokesh GLR, Somasunderam A, Thiviyanathan V, *et al.* X-
        aptamers: a bead-based selection method for random incorporation of druglike moieties onto next-
        generation   aptamers   for   enhanced   binding.   Biochemistry   2012;   51(42):
        8321-3.https://pubmed.ncbi.nlm.nih.gov/23057694

[399]   Hamula CLA, Peng H, Wang Z, *et al.* The effects of SELEX conditions on the resultant aptamer pools
        in the selection of aptamers binding to bacterial cells. J Mol Evol 2015; 81(5-6): 194-209. [Internet].
        [http://dx.doi.org/10.1007/s00239-015-9711-y] [PMID: 26538121]

[400]   Darkoh C, Deaton M, DuPont HL. Nonantimicrobial drug targets for Clostridium difficile infections.
        Future Microbiol 2017; 12(11): 975-85.
        [PMID: 28759258] [http://dx.doi.org/10.2217/fmb-2017-0024]

[401]   Darkoh C, Brown EL, Kaplan HB, DuPont HL. Bile salt inhibition of host cell damage by Clostridium
        difficile toxins. PLoS One 2013; 8(11): e79631-1.
        [PMID: 24244530] [http://dx.doi.org/10.1371/journal.pone.0079631] [PMID: 24244530]

[402]   Louie TJ, Peppe J, Watt CK, *et al.* Tolevamer Study Investigator Group. Tolevamer, a novel
        nonantibiotic polymer, compared with vancomycin in the treatment of mild to moderately severe
        Clostridium difficile-associated diarrhea. Clin Infect Dis 2006; 43(4): 411-20.
        [http://dx.doi.org/10.1086/506349] [PMID: 16838228]

[403]   Bem AE, Velikova N, Pellicer MT, Baarlen Pv, Marina A, Wells JM. Bacterial histidine kinases as
        novel antibacterial drug targets. ACS Chem Biol 2015; 10(1): 213-24.
        [http://dx.doi.org/10.1021/cb5007135] [PMID: 25436989]

[404]   Rosales-Hurtado M, Meffre P, Szurmant H, Benfodda Z. Synthesis of histidine kinase inhibitors and
        their biological properties. Med Res Rev 2020; 40(4): 1440-95. [Internet].
        [http://dx.doi.org/10.1002/med.21651] [PMID: 31802520]

[405]   Tiwari S, Jamal SB, Hassan SS, *et al.* Two-component signal transduction systems of pathogenic
        bacteria as targets for antimicrobial therapy: an overview. Front Microbiol 2017; 8: 1878.
        [http://dx.doi.org/10.3389/fmicb.2017.01878] [PMID: 29067003]

[406] Velikova N, Fulle S, Manso AS, *et al.* Putative histidine kinase inhibitors with antibacterial effect against multi-drug resistant clinical isolates identified by *in vitro* and *in silico* screens. Sci Rep 2016; 6(1): 26085.
[http://dx.doi.org/10.1038/srep26085] [PMID: 27173778]

[407] Boibessot T, Zschiedrich CP, Lebeau A, *et al.* The rational design, synthesis, and antimicrobial properties of thiophene derivatives that inhibit bacterial histidine kinases. J Med Chem 2016; 59(19): 8830-47.
[http://dx.doi.org/10.1021/acs.jmedchem.6b00580] [PMID: 27575438]

[408] Lewallen DM, Sreelatha A, Dharmarajan V, *et al.* Inhibiting AMPylation: a novel screen to identify the first small molecule inhibitors of protein AMPylation. ACS Chem Biol 2014; 9(2): 433-42. [Internet].
[http://dx.doi.org/10.1021/cb4006886] [PMID: 24274060]

[409] Maculins T, Fiskin E, Bhogaraju S, Dikic I. Bacteria-host relationship: ubiquitin ligases as weapons of invasion. Cell Res 2016; 26(4): 499-510.
[http://dx.doi.org/10.1038/cr.2016.30] [PMID: 26964724]

[410] Rossi M, Rotblat B, Ansell K, *et al.* High throughput screening for inhibitors of the HECT ubiquitin E3 ligase ITCH identifies antidepressant drugs as regulators of autophagy. Cell Death Dis 2014; 5(5): e1203.
[http://dx.doi.org/10.1038/cddis.2014.113] [PMID: 24787015]

[411] Maculins T, Carter N, Dorval T, *et al.* A generic platform for cellular screening against ubiquitin ligases. Sci Rep 2016; 6(1): 18940.
[http://dx.doi.org/10.1038/srep18940] [PMID: 26743172]

[412] Zurawski DV, McLendon MK. Monoclonal antibodies as an antibacterial approach against bacterial pathogens. Antibiotics (Basel) 2020; 9(4): 155.
[http://dx.doi.org/10.3390/antibiotics9040155] [PMID: 32244733]

[413] Iwamoto R, Senoh H, Okada Y, Uchida T, Mekada E. An antibody that inhibits the binding of diphtheria toxin to cells revealed the association of a 27-kDa membrane protein with the diphtheria toxin receptor. J Biol Chem 1991; 266(30): 20463-9.
[http://dx.doi.org/10.1016/S0021-9258(18)54947-4] [PMID: 1939101]

[414] Aguilar JL, Varshney AK, Pechuan X, Dutta K, Nosanchuk JD, Fries BC. Monoclonal antibodies protect from *staphylococcal enterotoxin* K (SEK) induced toxic shock and sepsis by USA300 *Staphylococcus aureus*. Virulence 2016; 8(6): 741-50.

[415] Storek KM, Auerbach MR, Shi H, Garcia NK, Sun D, Nickerson NN, *et al.* Monoclonal antibody targeting the β-barrel assembly machine of *Escherichia coli* is bactericidal. Proc Natl Acad Sci 2018; 115(14): 3692-7.

[416] Vij R, Lin Z, Chiang N, *et al.* A targeted boost-and-sort immunization strategy using *Escherichia coli* BamA identifies rare growth inhibitory antibodies. Sci Rep 2018; 8(1): 7136.
[http://dx.doi.org/10.1038/s41598-018-25609-z] [PMID: 29740124]

[417] Novotny LA, Jurcisek JA, Goodman SD, Bakaletz LO. Monoclonal antibodies against DNA-binding tips of DNABII proteins disrupt biofilms in vitro and induce bacterial clearance *in vivo*. EBioMedicine 2016; 10: 33-44.

[418] Tursi SA, Puligedda RD, Szabo P, *et al. Salmonella typhimurium* biofilm disruption by a human antibody that binds a pan-amyloid epitope on curli. Nat Commun 2020; 11(1): 1007.
[http://dx.doi.org/10.1038/s41467-020-14685-3] [PMID: 32081907]

[419] Singh KV, Pinkston KL, Gao P, Harvey BR, Murray BE. Anti-ace monoclonal antibody reduces *Enterococcus faecalis* aortic valve infection in a rat infective endocarditis model. Pathog Dis 2018; 76(8).
[http://dx.doi.org/10.1093/femspd/fty084] [PMID: 30445491]

[420] Aye R, Weldearegay YB, Lutta HO, *et al.* Identification of targets of monoclonal antibodies that inhibit adhesion and growth in Mycoplasma mycoides subspecies mycoides. Vet Immunol Immunopathol 2018; 204: 11-8.
[http://dx.doi.org/10.1016/j.vetimm.2018.09.002]

[421] Chin Y-W, Balunas MJ, Chai HB, Kinghorn AD. Drug discovery from natural sources. AAPS J2006; 8(2): E239-53. https://link.springer.com/article/10.1007/BF02854894
[http://dx.doi.org/10.1007/BF02854894]

[422] Katz L, Baltz RH. Natural product discovery: past, present, and future. J Ind Microbiol Biotechnol 2016; 43(2-3): 155-76.
[http://dx.doi.org/10.1007/s10295-015-1723-5] [PMID: 26739136]

[423] Jhong JH, Chi YH, Li WC, Lin TH, Huang KY, Lee TY. dbAMP: an integrated resource for exploring antimicrobial peptides with functional activities and physicochemical properties on transcriptome and proteome data. Nucleic Acids Res 2019; 47(D1): D285-97.
[http://dx.doi.org/10.1093/nar/gky1030] [PMID: 30380085]

[424] Letzel A-C, Pidot SJ, Hertweck C. Genome mining for ribosomally synthesized and post-translationally modified peptides (RiPPs) in anaerobic bacteria. BMC Genomics 2014; 15(1): 983.http://www.biomedcentral.com/1471-2164/15/983

[425] Mwangi J, Hao X, Lai R, Zhang ZY. Antimicrobial peptides: new hope in the war against multidrug resistance. Zoological Research NLM (Medline). 2019; 40: pp. 488-505.

[426] Lázár V, Martins A, Spohn R, *et al.* Antibiotic-resistant bacteria show widespread collateral sensitivity to antimicrobial peptides. Nat Microbiol 2018; 3(6): 718-31.
[http://dx.doi.org/10.1038/s41564-018-0164-0] [PMID: 29795541]

[427] Hudson GA, Mitchell DA. RiPP antibiotics: biosynthesis and engineering potential. Current Opinion in Microbiology. Elsevier Ltd 2018; 45: pp. 61-9.

[428] Pan SJ, Rajniak J, Maksimov MO, Link AJ. The role of a conserved threonine residue in the leader peptide of lasso peptide precursors. Chem Commun (Camb) 2012; 48(13): 1880-2.
[http://dx.doi.org/10.1039/c2cc17211a] [PMID: 22222556]

[429] Hegemann JD, Zimmermann M, Xie X, Marahiel MA. Lasso peptides: an intriguing class of bacterial natural products. Acc Chem Res 2015; 48(7): 1909-19.
[http://dx.doi.org/10.1021/acs.accounts.5b00156] [PMID: 26079760]

[430] Li Y, Ducasse R, Zirah S, *et al.* Characterization of sviceucin from streptomyces provides insight into enzyme exchangeability and disulfide bond formation in lasso peptides. ACS Chem Biol 2015; 10(11): 2641-9.
[http://dx.doi.org/10.1021/acschembio.5b00584] [PMID: 26343290]

[431] Lin PF, Samanta H, Bechtold CM, *et al.* Characterization of siamycin I, a human immunodeficiency virus fusion inhibitor. Antimicrob Agents Chemother 1996; 40(1): 133-8.
[http://dx.doi.org/10.1128/AAC.40.1.133] [PMID: 8787894]

[432] Wilson KA, Kalkum M, Ottesen J, *et al.* Structure of microcin J25, a peptide inhibitor of bacterial RNA polymerase, is a lassoed tail. J Am Chem Soc 2003; 125(41): 12475-83.
[http://dx.doi.org/10.1021/ja036756q] [PMID: 14531691]

[433] Potterat O, Wagner K, Gemmecker G, *et al.* BI-32169, a bicyclic 19-peptide with strong glucagon receptor antagonist activity from Streptomyces sp. J Nat Prod 2004; 67(9): 1528-31.
[http://dx.doi.org/10.1021/np040093o] [PMID: 15387654]

[434] Sumida T, Dubiley S, Wilcox B, Severinov K, Tagami S. Structural basis of leader peptide recognition in lasso peptide biosynthesis pathway. ACS Chem Biol 2019; 14(7): 1619-27.
[http://dx.doi.org/10.1021/acschembio.9b00348] [PMID: 31188556]

[435] Maksimov MO, Pan SJ, James Link A. Lasso peptides: structure, function, biosynthesis, and

engineering. Nat Prod Rep 2012; 29(9): 996-1006.
[http://dx.doi.org/10.1039/c2np20070h] [PMID: 22833149]

[436] Romano M, Fusco G, Choudhury HG, *et al.* Structural basis for natural product selection and export by bacterial ABC transporters. ACS Chem Biol 2018; 13(6): 1598-609.
[http://dx.doi.org/10.1021/acschembio.8b00226] [PMID: 29757605]

[437] Martin-Gómez H, Linne U, Albericio F, Tulla-Puche J, Hegemann JD. Investigation of the biosynthesis of the lasso peptide chaxapeptin using an *E. coli*-based production system. J Nat Prod 2018; 81(9): 2050-6.
[http://dx.doi.org/10.1021/acs.jnatprod.8b00392] [PMID: 30178995]

[438] Zhang Y, Chen M, Bruner SD, Ding Y. Heterologous production of microbial ribosomally synthesized and post-translationally modified peptides. Front Microbiol 2018; 9(AUG): 1801.
[http://dx.doi.org/10.3389/fmicb.2018.01801] [PMID: 30135682]

[439] Pavlova O, Mukhopadhyay J, Sineva E, Ebright RH, Severinov K. Systematic structure-activity analysis of microcin J25. J Biol Chem 2008; 283(37): 25589-95.
[http://dx.doi.org/10.1074/jbc.M803995200] [PMID: 18632663]

[440] Tan S, Moore G, Nodwell J. Put a bow on it: Knotted antibiotics take center stage. Antibiotics (Basel) 2019; 8(3): 117.

[441] Helynck G, Dubertret C, Mayaux JF, Leboul J. Isolation of RP 71955, a new anti-HIV-1 peptide secondary metabolite. J Antibiot (Tokyo) 1993; 46(11): 1756-7.
[http://dx.doi.org/10.7164/antibiotics.46.1756] [PMID: 8270499]

[442] Fréchet D, Guitton JD, Herman F, *et al.* Solution structure of RP 71955, a new 21 amino acid tricyclic peptide active against HIV-1 virus. Biochemistry 1994; 33(1): 42-50.
[http://dx.doi.org/10.1021/bi00167a006] [PMID: 8286361]

[443] Coley W, Kehn-Hall K, Van Duyne R, Kashanchi F. Novel HIV-1 therapeutics through targeting altered host cell pathways. Expert Opin Biol Ther 2009; 9(11): 1369-82.
[http://dx.doi.org/10.1517/14712590903257781] [PMID: 19732026]

[444] Tan S, Ludwig KC, Müller A, Schneider T, Nodwell JR. The lasso peptide siamycin-I targets lipid II at the gram-positive cell surface. ACS Chem Biol 2019; 14(5): 966-74.
[http://dx.doi.org/10.1021/acschembio.9b00157] [PMID: 31026131]

[445] Kaweewan I, Hemmi H, Komaki H, Harada S, Kodani S. Isolation and structure determination of a new lasso peptide specialicin based on genome mining. Bioorg Med Chem 2018; 26(23-24): 6050-5.
[http://dx.doi.org/10.1016/j.bmc.2018.11.007] [PMID: 30448257]

[446] Salomón RA, Farías RN. The peptide antibiotic microcin 25 is imported through the TonB pathway and the SbmA protein. J Bacteriol 1995; 177(11): 3323-5.
[http://dx.doi.org/10.1128/JB.177.11.3323-3325.1995] [PMID: 7768835]

[447] Delgado MA, Rintoul MR, Farías RN, Salomón RA. *Escherichia coli* RNA polymerase is the target of the cyclopeptide antibiotic microcin J25. J Bacteriol 2001; 183(15): 4543-50.
[http://dx.doi.org/10.1128/JB.183.15.4543-4550.2001] [PMID: 11443089]

[448] Mazaheri Tehrani M, Erfani M, Amirmozafari N, Nejadsattari T. Synthesis of a peptide derivative of microcinJ25 and evaluation of antibacterial and biological activities. Iran J Pharm Res 2019; 18(3): 1264-76.
[PMID: 32641937]

[449] Zhu S, Su Y, Shams S, Feng Y, Tong Y, Zheng G. Lassomycin and lariatin lasso peptides as suitable antibiotics for combating mycobacterial infections: current state of biosynthesis and perspectives for production. Appl Microbiol Biotechnol 2019; 103(10): 3931-40.
[http://dx.doi.org/10.1007/s00253-019-09771-6] [PMID: 30915503]

[450] Gavrish E, Sit CS, Cao S, *et al.* Lassomycin, a ribosomally synthesized cyclic peptide, kills mycobacterium tuberculosis by targeting the ATP-dependent protease ClpC1P1P2. Chem Biol 2014;

21(4): 509-18.
[http://dx.doi.org/10.1016/j.chembiol.2014.01.014] [PMID: 24684906]

[451]   Vinogradov AA, Suga H. Introduction to thiopeptides: biological activity, biosynthesis, and strategies for functional reprogramming. Cell Chem Biol 2020; 27(8): 1032-51.
[http://dx.doi.org/10.1016/j.chembiol.2020.07.003] [PMID: 32698017]

[452]   Just-Baringo X, Albericio F, Álvarez M. Thiopeptide antibiotics: retrospective and recent advances. Marine Drugs. 2014; 12: pp. 317-51.

[453]   Fabbretti A, He CG, Gaspari E, *et al.* A derivative of the thiopeptide GE2270A highly selective against propionibacterium acnes. Antimicrob Agents Chemother 2015; 59(8): 4560-8.
[http://dx.doi.org/10.1128/AAC.05155-14] [PMID: 25987631]

[454]   Travin DY, Bikmetov D, Severinov K. Translation-targeting ripps and where to find them. Front Genet 2020; 11: 226.

[455]   Walter JD, Hunter M, Cobb M, Traeger G, Spiegel PC. Thiostrepton inhibits stable 70S ribosome binding and ribosome-dependent GTPase activation of elongation factor G and elongation factor 4. Nucleic Acids Res 2012; 40(1): 360-70.
[http://dx.doi.org/10.1093/nar/gkr623] [PMID: 21908407]

[456]   Lau RCM, Rinehart KL, Berninamycin B. C and D, minor metabolites from the fermentation extract of S. bernensis. J Antibiot (Tokyo) 1994; 47(12): 1466-72.
[http://dx.doi.org/10.7164/antibiotics.47.1466] [PMID: 7844041]

[457]   Akasapu S, Hinds AB, Powell WC, Walczak MA. Total synthesis of micrococcin P1 and thiocillin I enabled by Mo(vi) catalyst. Chem Sci (Camb) 2018; 10(7): 1971-5.
[http://dx.doi.org/10.1039/C8SC04885A] [PMID: 30881626]

[458]   Mikolajka A, Liu H, Chen Y, *et al.* Differential effects of thiopeptide and orthosomycin antibiotics on translational GTPases. Chem Biol 2011; 18(5): 589-600.
[http://dx.doi.org/10.1016/j.chembiol.2011.03.010] [PMID: 21609840]

[459]   Heffron SE, Jurnak F. Structure of an EF-Tu complex with a thiazolyl peptide antibiotic determined at 2.35 A resolution: atomic basis for GE2270A inhibition of EF-Tu. Biochemistry 2000; 39(1): 37-45.
[http://dx.doi.org/10.1021/bi9913597] [PMID: 10625477]

[460]   Walsh CT, Acker MG, Bowers AA. Thiazolyl peptide antibiotic biosynthesis: a cascade of post-translational modifications on ribosomal nascent proteins. J Biol Chem 2010; 285(36): 27525-31.
[http://dx.doi.org/10.1074/jbc.R110.135970] [PMID: 20522549]

[461]   Wieland Brown LC, Acker MG, Clardy J, Walsh CT, Fischbach MA. Thirteen posttranslational modifications convert a 14-residue peptide into the antibiotic thiocillin. Proc Natl Acad Sci USA 2009; 106(8): 2549-53.
[http://dx.doi.org/10.1073/pnas.0900008106] [PMID: 19196969]

[462]   Burkhart BJ, Schwalen CJ, Mann G, Naismith JH, Mitchell DA. YcaO-dependent posttranslational amide activation: biosynthesis, structure, and function. Chem Rev 2017; 117(8): 5389-456.
[http://dx.doi.org/10.1021/acs.chemrev.6b00623] [PMID: 28256131]

[463]   Melby JO, Li X, Mitchell DA. Orchestration of enzymatic processing by thiazole/oxazole-modified microcin dehydrogenases. Biochemistry 2014; 53(2): 413-22.
[http://dx.doi.org/10.1021/bi401529y] [PMID: 24364559]

[464]   Bothwell IR, Cogan DP, Kim T, Reinhardt CJ, van der Donk WA, Nair SK. Characterization of glutamyl-tRNA-dependent dehydratases using nonreactive substrate mimics. Proc Natl Acad Sci USA 2019; 116(35): 17245-50.
[http://dx.doi.org/10.1073/pnas.1905240116] [PMID: 31409709]

[465]   Zhang Z, Hudson GA, Mahanta N, Tietz JI, van der Donk WA, Mitchell DA. Biosynthetic timing and substrate specificity for the thiopeptide thiomuracin. J Am Chem Soc 2016; 138(48): 15511-4.
[http://dx.doi.org/10.1021/jacs.6b08987] [PMID: 27700071]

[466]   Vinogradov AA, Shimomura M, Goto Y, *et al.* Minimal lactazole scaffold for *in vitro* thiopeptide bioengineering. Nat Commun 2020; 11(1): 2272.
[http://dx.doi.org/10.1038/s41467-020-16145-4] [PMID: 32385237]

[467]   Cogan DP, Hudson GA, Zhang Z, *et al.* Structural insights into enzymatic [4+2] *aza*-cycloaddition in thiopeptide antibiotic biosynthesis. Proc Natl Acad Sci USA 2017; 114(49): 12928-33.
[http://dx.doi.org/10.1073/pnas.1716035114] [PMID: 29158402]

[468]   LaMarche MJ, Leeds JA, Amaral K, *et al.* Antibacterial optimization of 4-aminothiazolyl analogues of the natural product GE2270 A: identification of the cycloalkylcarboxylic acids. J Med Chem 2011; 54(23): 8099-109.
[http://dx.doi.org/10.1021/jm200938f] [PMID: 21999529]

[469]   Singh SB, Xu L, Meinke PT, *et al.* Thiazomycin, nocathiacin and analogs show strong activity against clinical strains of drug-resistant Mycobacterium tuberculosis. J Antibiot (Tokyo) 2017; 70(5): 671-4.
[http://dx.doi.org/10.1038/ja.2016.165] [PMID: 28096545]

[470]   PharmaVet. Nystatin, neomycin sulfate, thiostrepton, & triamcinolone topical ointment, plumb's® veterinary medication guide. PharmaVet 2019; p. 3.

[471]   Benazet F, Cartier JR. Effect of nosiheptide as a feed additive in chicks on the quantity, duration, prevalence of excretion, and resistance to antibacterial agents of *Salmonella typhimurium*; on the proportion of *Escherichia coli* and other coliforms resistant to antibacterial agents; and on their degree and spectrum of resistance. Poult Sci 1980; 59(7): 1405-15.
[http://dx.doi.org/10.3382/ps.0591405] [PMID: 6994088]

[472]   LaMarche MJ, Leeds JA, Amaral A, *et al.* Discovery of LFF571: an investigational agent for clostridium difficile infection. J Med Chem 2012; 55(5): 2376-87.
[http://dx.doi.org/10.1021/jm201685h] [PMID: 22315981]

[473]   Haste NM, Thienphrapa W, Tran DN, *et al.* Activity of the thiopeptide antibiotic nosiheptide against contemporary strains of methicillin-resistant *Staphylococcus aureus*. J Antibiot (Tokyo) 2012; 65(12): 593-8.
[http://dx.doi.org/10.1038/ja.2012.77] [PMID: 23047246]

[474]   Vinogradov AA, Shimomura M, Kano N, Goto Y, Onaka H, Suga H. Promiscuous enzymes cooperate at the substrate level en route to lactazole A. J Am Chem Soc 2020; 142(32): 13886-97.
[http://dx.doi.org/10.1021/jacs.0c05541] [PMID: 32664727]

[475]   Malcolmson SJ, Young TS, Ruby JG, Skewes-Cox P, Walsh CT. The posttranslational modification cascade to the thiopeptide berninamycin generates linear forms and altered macrocyclic scaffolds. Proc Natl Acad Sci USA 2013; 110(21): 8483-8.
[http://dx.doi.org/10.1073/pnas.1307111110] [PMID: 23650400]

[476]   Arnison PG, Bibb MJ, Bierbaum G, *et al.* Ribosomally synthesized and post-translationally modified peptide natural products: overview and recommendations for a universal nomenclature. Nat Prod Rep 2013; 30(1): 108-60.
[http://dx.doi.org/10.1039/C2NP20085F] [PMID: 23165928]

[477]   Ebner P, Reichert S, Luqman A, Krismer B, Popella P, Götz F. Lantibiotic production is a burden for the producing staphylococci. Sci Rep 2018; 8(1): 7471.
[http://dx.doi.org/10.1038/s41598-018-25935-2] [PMID: 29749386]

[478]   Cheigh CI, Pyun YR. Nisin biosynthesis and its properties. Biotechnol Lett 2005; 27(21): 1641-8.
[http://dx.doi.org/10.1007/s10529-005-2721-x] [PMID: 16247668]

[479]   Wiedemann I, Benz R, Sahl HG. Lipid II-mediated pore formation by the peptide antibiotic nisin: a black lipid membrane study. J Bacteriol 2004; 186(10): 3259-61.
[http://dx.doi.org/10.1128/JB.186.10.3259-3261.2004] [PMID: 15126490]

[480]   Ortega MA, Hao Y, Zhang Q, Walker MC, van der Donk WA, Nair SK. Structure and mechanism of the tRNA-dependent lantibiotic dehydratase NisB. Nature 2015; 517(7535): 509-12.

[http://dx.doi.org/10.1038/nature13888] [PMID: 25363770]

[481] Garg N, Salazar-Ocampo LMA, van der Donk WA. *In vitro* activity of the nisin dehydratase NisB. Proc Natl Acad Sci USA 2013; 110(18): 7258-63.
[http://dx.doi.org/10.1073/pnas.1222488110] [PMID: 23589847]

[482] Kluskens LD, Kuipers A, Rink R, *et al.* Post-translational modification of therapeutic peptides by NisB, the dehydratase of the lantibiotic nisin. Biochemistry 2005; 44(38): 12827-34.
[http://dx.doi.org/10.1021/bi050805p] [PMID: 16171398]

[483] Li Q, Montalban-Lopez M, Kuipers OP. Feasability of introducing a thioether ring in vasopressin by nisBTC co-expression in *Lactococcus lactis*. Front Microbiol 2019; 10(JUL): 1508.
[http://dx.doi.org/10.3389/fmicb.2019.01508] [PMID: 31333616]

[484] Okeley NM, Paul M, Stasser JP, Blackburn N, van der Donk WA. SpaC and NisC, the cyclases involved in subtilin and nisin biosynthesis, are zinc proteins. Biochemistry 2003; 42(46): 13613-24.
[http://dx.doi.org/10.1021/bi0354942] [PMID: 14622008]

[485] Li B, van der Donk WA. Identification of essential catalytic residues of the cyclase NisC involved in the biosynthesis of nisin. J Biol Chem 2007; 282(29): 21169-75.
[http://dx.doi.org/10.1074/jbc.M701802200] [PMID: 17513866]

[486] Montalbán-López M, Deng J, van Heel AJ, Kuipers OP. Specificity and application of the lantibiotic protease NisP. Front Microbiol 2018; 9(FEB): 160.
[http://dx.doi.org/10.3389/fmicb.2018.00160] [PMID: 29479343]

[487] Velásquez JE, Zhang X, van der Donk WA. Biosynthesis of the antimicrobial peptide epilancin 15X and its N-terminal lactate. Chem Biol 2011; 18(7): 857-67.
[http://dx.doi.org/10.1016/j.chembiol.2011.05.007] [PMID: 21802007]

[488] Huang E, Yousef AE. Biosynthesis of paenibacillin, a lantibiotic with N-terminal acetylation, by *Paenibacillus polymyxa*. Microbiol Res 2015; 181: 15-21.
[http://dx.doi.org/10.1016/j.micres.2015.08.001] [PMID: 26640048]

[489] Götz F, Perconti S, Popella P, Werner R, Schlag M. Epidermin and gallidermin: staphylococcal lantibiotics. Int J Med Microbiol 2014; 304(1): 63-71.
[http://dx.doi.org/10.1016/j.ijmm.2013.08.012] [PMID: 24119540]

[490] Ortega MA, Cogan DP, Mukherjee S, *et al.* Two flavoenzymes catalyze the post-translational generation of 5-chlorotryptophan and 2-aminovinyl-cysteine during NAI-107 biosynthesis. ACS Chem Biol 2017; 12(2): 548-57.
[http://dx.doi.org/10.1021/acschembio.6b01031] [PMID: 28032983]

[491] Cruz JCS, Iorio M, Monciardini P, *et al.* Brominated variant of the lantibiotic NAI-107 with enhanced antibacterial potency. J Nat Prod 2015; 78(11): 2642-7.
[http://dx.doi.org/10.1021/acs.jnatprod.5b00576] [PMID: 26512731]

[492] Foulston LC, Bibb MJ. Microbisporicin gene cluster reveals unusual features of lantibiotic biosynthesis in actinomycetes. Proc Natl Acad Sci USA 2010; 107(30): 13461-6.
[http://dx.doi.org/10.1073/pnas.1008285107] [PMID: 20628010]

[493] Siezen RJ. Comparison of lantibiotic gene clusters and encoded proteins. Antonie van Leeuwenhoek, Int J Gen. Mol Microbiol 1996; 69(2): 171-84.

[494] Chatterjee C, Miller LM, Leung YL, *et al.* Lacticin 481 synthetase phosphorylates its substrate during lantibiotic production. J Am Chem Soc 2005; 127(44): 15332-3.
[http://dx.doi.org/10.1021/ja0543043] [PMID: 16262372]

[495] You YO, van der Donk WA. Mechanistic investigations of the dehydration reaction of lacticin 481 synthetase using site-directed mutagenesis. Biochemistry 2007; 46(20): 5991-6000.
[http://dx.doi.org/10.1021/bi602663x] [PMID: 17455908]

[496] Begley M, Cotter PD, Hill C, Ross RP. Identification of a novel two-peptide lantibiotic, lichenicidin,

following rational genome mining for LanM proteins. Appl Environ Microbiol 2009; 75(17): 5451-60.
[http://dx.doi.org/10.1128/AEM.00730-09] [PMID: 19561184]

[497] Morgan SM, O'connor PM, Cotter PD, Ross RP, Hill C. Sequential actions of the two component peptides of the lantibiotic lacticin 3147 explain its antimicrobial activity at nanomolar concentrations. Antimicrob Agents Chemother 2005; 49(7): 2606-11.
[http://dx.doi.org/10.1128/AAC.49.7.2606-2611.2005] [PMID: 15980326]

[498] Cox CR, Coburn PS, Gilmore MS. Enterococcal cytolysin: a novel two component peptide system that serves as a bacterial defense against eukaryotic and prokaryotic cells. Curr Protein Pept Sci 2005; 6(1): 77-84.
[http://dx.doi.org/10.2174/1389203053027557] [PMID: 15638770]

[499] Cotter PD, O'Connor PM, Draper LA, *et al.* Posttranslational conversion of L-serines to D-alanines is vital for optimal production and activity of the lantibiotic lacticin 3147. Proc Natl Acad Sci USA 2005; 102(51): 18584-9.
[http://dx.doi.org/10.1073/pnas.0509371102] [PMID: 16339304]

[500] Ökesli A, Cooper LE, Fogle EJ, van der Donk WA. Nine post-translational modifications during the biosynthesis of cinnamycin. J Am Chem Soc 2011; 133(34): 13753-60.
[http://dx.doi.org/10.1021/ja205783f] [PMID: 21770392]

[501] Gao SS, Naowarojna N, Cheng R, Liu X, Liu P. Recent examples of α-ketoglutarate-dependent mononuclear non-haem iron enzymes in natural product biosyntheses. Nat Prod Rep 2018; 35(8): 792-837.
[http://dx.doi.org/10.1039/C7NP00067G] [PMID: 29932179]

[502] Boakes S, Cortés J, Appleyard AN, Rudd BAM, Dawson MJ. Organization of the genes encoding the biosynthesis of actagardine and engineering of a variant generation system. Mol Microbiol 2009; 72(5): 1126-36.
[http://dx.doi.org/10.1111/j.1365-2958.2009.06708.x] [PMID: 19400806]

[503] Hegemann JD, Süssmuth RD. Matters of class: coming of age of class III and IV lanthipeptides. RSC Chem Biol 2020; 1(3): 110-27.
[http://dx.doi.org/10.1039/D0CB00073F]

[504] Repka LM, Chekan JR, Nair SK, van der Donk WA. Mechanistic understanding of lanthipeptide biosynthetic enzymes. Chem Rev 2017; 117(8): 5457-520.
[http://dx.doi.org/10.1021/acs.chemrev.6b00591] [PMID: 28135077]

[505] Smith GK, Ke Z, Hengge AC, Xu D, Xie D, Guo H. Active-site dynamics of SpvC virulence factor from *Salmonella typhimurium* and density functional theory study of phosphothreonine lyase catalysis. J Phys Chem B 2009; 113(46): 15327-33.
[http://dx.doi.org/10.1021/jp9052677] [PMID: 19715325]

[506] Hegemann JD, Shi L, Gross ML, van der Donk WA. Mechanistic studies of the kinase domains of class iv lanthipeptide synthetases. ACS Chem Biol 2019; 14(7): 1583-92.
[http://dx.doi.org/10.1021/acschembio.9b00323] [PMID: 31243957]

[507] Field D, Cotter PD, Hill C, Ross RP. Bioengineering lantibiotics for therapeutic success. Front Microbiol 2015; 6: 1363.
[PMID: 26640466]

[508] Wang H, van der Donk WA. Biosynthesis of the class III lantipeptide catenulipeptin. ACS Chem Biol 2012; 7(9): 1529-35.
[http://dx.doi.org/10.1021/cb3002446] [PMID: 22725258]

[509] Sambeth GM, Süssmuth RD. Synthetic studies toward labionin, a new α,α-disubstituted amino acid from type III lantibiotic labyrinthopeptin A2. J Pept Sci 2011; 17(8): 581-4.
[http://dx.doi.org/10.1002/psc.1378] [PMID: 21644246]

[510] Yu Y, Zhang Q, van der Donk WA. Insights into the evolution of lanthipeptide biosynthesis. Protein

Sci 2013; 22(11): 1478-89.
[http://dx.doi.org/10.1002/pro.2358] [PMID: 24038659]

[511] Meindl K, Schmiederer T, Schneider K, *et al.* Labyrinthopeptins: a new class of carbacyclic lantibiotics. Angew Chem Int Ed Engl 2010; 49(6): 1151-4.
[http://dx.doi.org/10.1002/anie.200905773] [PMID: 20082397]

[512] Iorio M, Sasso O, Maffioli SI, *et al.* A glycosylated, labionin-containing lanthipeptide with marked antinociceptive activity. ACS Chem Biol 2014; 9(2): 398-404.
[http://dx.doi.org/10.1021/cb400692w] [PMID: 24191663]

[513] Walker LM, Burton DR. Passive immunotherapy of viral infections: 'super-antibodies' enter the fray. Nat Rev Immunol 2018; 18(5): 297-308. [Internet].
[http://dx.doi.org/10.1038/nri.2017.148] [PMID: 29379211]

[514] Vogt E, Künzler M. Discovery of novel fungal RiPP biosynthetic pathways and their application for the development of peptide therapeutics. Applied Microbiology and Biotechnology. Springer Verlag 2019; 103: pp. 5567-81.
[http://dx.doi.org/10.1007/s00253-019-09893-x]

[515] Scott LJ, Curran MP, Figgitt DP. Rosuvastatin: a review of its use in the management of dyslipidemia. Am J Cardiovasc Drugs 2004; 4(2): 117-38.
[http://dx.doi.org/10.2165/00129784-200404020-00005] [PMID: 15049723]

[516] Kong W, Lu T. Cloning and optimization of a nisin biosynthesis pathway for bacteriocin harvest. ACS Synth Biol 2014; 3(7): 439-45.
[http://dx.doi.org/10.1021/sb500225r] [PMID: 24847677]

[517] Chen S, Xu B, Chen E, *et al.* Zn-dependent bifunctional proteases are responsible for leader peptide processing of class III lanthipeptides. Proc Natl Acad Sci USA 2019; 116(7): 2533-8.
[http://dx.doi.org/10.1073/pnas.1815594116] [PMID: 30679276]

[518] Rubin GM, Ding Y. Recent advances in the biosynthesis of RiPPs from multicore-containing precursor peptides. J Ind Microbiol Biotechnol 2020; 47(9-10): 659-74.

CHAPTER 3

Scope and Limitations on the Potent Antimicrobial Activities of Hydrazone Derivatives

Jean Michel Brunel[1,*]

[1] Aix Marseille University, INSERM, SSA, MCT, Marseille, France

Abstract: Antimicrobial resistance of Gram-negative bacteria is a major concern, and no new classes of antibiotics that are effective against this type of bacteria have been discovered since the 1960s. During the last decades, multiple approaches have been developed to combat such bacterial resistance. However, the combination of antibiotic resistance mechanisms by bacteria and the limited number of effective antibiotics available, decreases the number of interventions for the treatment of current bacterial infections. The solution to emerging antibiotic resistance will likely involve new therapies or new classes of antibacterial agents. For a few years now, there was a real interest in the design and synthesis of hydrazones possessing an azometine -NHN=CH- proton and constituting an important class of compounds for new drugs development as anticonvulsants, antidepressants, antitumoral agents. In this context, the design and antimicrobial evaluation of hydrazone derivatives have constituted one of the new strategies developed to fight bacterial resistance. As pointed out, the range of biological activities is very broad, and this review will deal exclusively with the synthesis and use of hydrazones as antimicrobial agents and will not cover the other biological properties already well depicted in literature. Thus, we will report herein the scope and limitation of such an approach providing numerous examples demonstrating structure-activity relationships and potent interesting antimicrobial activities against both fungi, Gram-positive and/or Gram-negative bacteria.

Keywords: Aldehydes, Antimicrobial agents, Antifungal activity, Antimicrobial resistance, Azomethine, Gram-positive bacteria, Gram-negative bacteria, Heterocycles, Hydrazones, Hydrazine, Ketones.

INTRODUCTION

An important interest in the design and synthesis of hydrazones possessing an azometine -NHN=CH- proton and constituting an important class of compounds for new drugs development has recently emerged [1, 2]. Since the range of biological activities is very broad, this review will deal exclusively with the synt-

---

[*] **Corresponding author Jean Michel Brunel:** Aix Marseille University, INSERM, SSA, MCT, Marseille, France; Tel: (+33) 689271645; E-mail: bruneljm@yahoo.fr

Atta-ur-Rahman, *FRS* and M. Iqbal Choudhary (Eds.)

hesis and use of hydrazones as antimicrobial agents, excluding the other well depicted biological properties [1 - 7].

Hydrazones, which general formula is R-NH-N=C, have been widely used and studied in organic chemistry. There are easily produced by condensation of a hydrazine (NH_2-NHR) with a ketone or an aldehyde (Scheme **1**).

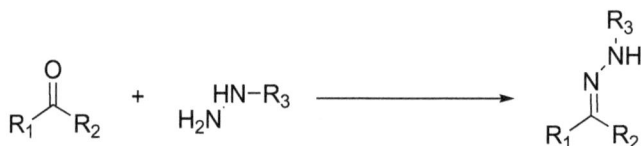

Scheme 1.

During numerous decades, this condensation has been the only way of detecting the presence of a ketone or an aldehyde group in a molecule. Moreover, hydrazones have also been involved in many reactions such as:

• The Bamford-Stevens reaction allowing the formation of a dual-link Z (Scheme **2**) [8].

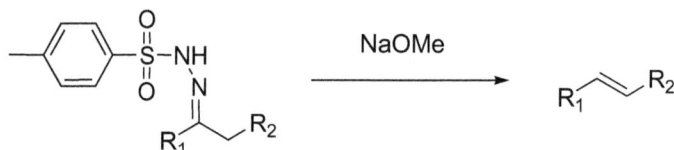

Scheme 2.

• The reaction of Shapiro [9] involves the elimination of a tosylhydrazone group and the formation of a double bond. It is noteworthy that during this reaction, the transitional carbanion can be used to graft different functional groups (Scheme **3**).

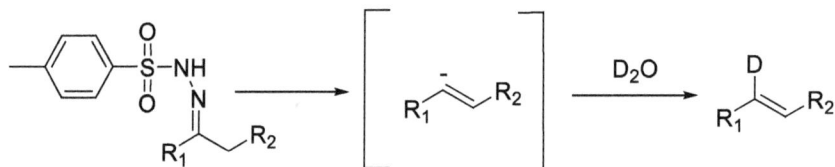

Scheme 3.

Nevertheless, although these hydrazones are well known in organic chemistry, it is only recently that researchers became interested in their biological potentialities, particularly for the treatment of infectious diseases [10].

Hydrazones as Potent Antimicrobial Agents

As already mentioned, hydrazones possess a general formula R-NH-N=C. In the following part, we will discuss on the antimicrobial activity of different classes of hydrazones depending on the nature of the R group attached to the nitrogen atom.

R is a Hydrogen

In 2005, Shinge *et al.* reported the reaction of 4-acetyl-3-arylsydnone derivatives [11] with hydrazine leading to the formation of hydrazones **1** and dimers **2** in good yields and the evaluation of their antimicrobial activities against various Gram-negative bacteria and fungi (Table **1**).

Table 1. Structure and antimicrobial activities of derivatives 1a-2f.

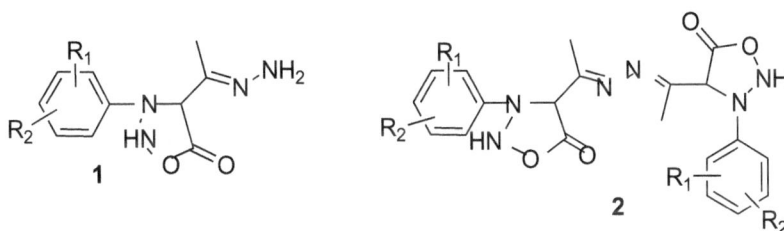

Compound	R_1	R_2	Diameter of Inhibition (mm)			
			E. coli	*P. pyocyanous*	*R. bataticola*	*A. niger*
1a	H	4-Cl	29	24	13	18
1b	H	4-Br	30	22	14	18
1c	3-CH$_3$	4-CH$_3$	19	18	18	21
1d	4-CH$_3$	3-Cl	29	21	12	13
1e	2-OCH$_3$	4-Cl	31	26	11	14
1f	4-Cl	3-F	29	23	13	16
2e	2-OCH$_3$	4-Cl	18	16	11	14
2f	4-Cl	3-F	21	15	13	16

Determination of the antifungal activity of derivatives **2** led to similar results that their parent monomers **1** (Table **1**, derivatives **1e-1f** and **2e-2f**) whereas weaker activities were encountered against bacteria. Moreover, compounds possessing a chloro, bromo or fluoro substituent group exhibited antibacterial activities greater than norfloxacin reference drug. Derivative **1c** with a methyl group substitution led to an increase of the antifungal activity compared to griseofulvin. Additionally, compound **1d** possessing a methyl and halogen substituent is slightly active against bacteria and less active against fungi compared to reference drugs.

In the same area, Sztanke *et al.* reported that derivatives **3a-3f** presented moderate to good antibacterial activities against both Gram-positive (*S. aureus, S. epidermidis, S. pyogenes)* and Gram-negative bacteria (*E. coli*) (Table **2**) [12]. Thus, compound **3d** bearing a 1-(4-methoxyphenyl) group appeared to be the most active compound of this series with MICs varying from 15 to 30 µM in all cases. Nevertheless, no mechanism of action of such derivatives has still been proposed to rationalize such observations.

Table 2. Antimicrobial activities of derivatives 3a-f.

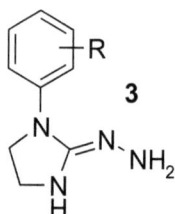

	-					
	MIC (µM)					
	3a	**3b**	**3c**	**3d**	**3e**	**3f**
R	H	2-CH$_3$	2-OCH$_3$	4-OCH$_3$	2,3-CH$_3$	4-Cl
S. aureus	41.1	39.3	37.4	29.9	37.6	29.5
S. epidermidis	41.1	31.4	37.4	18.7	18.8	18.4
S. pyogenes	65.8	78.6	74.8	59.8	75.2	59.1
E. coli	41.1	15.7	29.9	15.0	18.8	36.9

R is an Aryl Group

Most of the results presented in this part have been reported in the last twenty years demonstrating the interest and potentiality of such compounds. In 2002, Moreau *et al.* carried out the synthesis of new polyaromatic molecules **4a-4b** and have evaluated their antifungal properties against *C. albicans* and *C. krusei* strains [13]. Nevertheless, the results remain quite modest in terms of diversity with respect to the number and nature of the strains tested (Table **3**).

Table 3. Structure and biological activities of compounds 4.

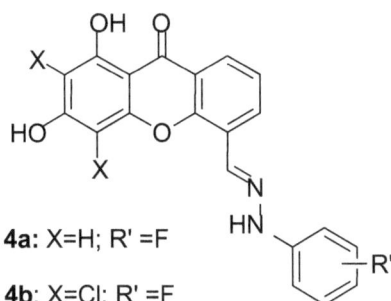

4a: X=H; R' =F

4b: X=Cl; R' =F

-	Inhibition Diameter (mm)	
Compounds	*C. krusei*	*C. albicans*
4a	15	10
4b	35	15

In the same context, Tyrkov *et al.* demonstrated that a double substitution at the nitrogen atom by two phenyl groups leads to molecules **5a-5c** possessing significant activities against Gram-positive bacteria such as *S. aureus* and *S. pneumoniae* as well as against Gram-negative *E. coli* and *P. aeruginosa* (Table **4**) [14].

Table 4. Antimicrobial activities of compounds 5a-5c.

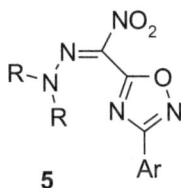

5

-			MIC (µg/mL)			
Cpds	R	Ar	*S. aureus*	*S. pneumoniae*	*E. coli*	*P. aeruginosa*
5a	C₆H₅	C₆H₅	7.8	7.8	3.9	7.8
5b	C₆H₅	4-CH₃OC₆H₄	7.8	7.8	3.9	7.8
5c	C₆H₅	2-ClC₆H₄	15.7	15.7	31.2	31.2

Some other compounds of interest were reported including derivatives **6a-6c**, **7a-7b** and **8a-8b** and demonstrating moderate to good biological activities

(Scheme **4**) [15 - 17]. Particularly, molecules **7** and **8** present anti *Trichophyton mentagrophytes* and *Microsporum gyptem* activities with MIC less than 10 µg/mL [15]. On the other hand, some of them possessing fluorine groups can inhibit the growth of *Mycobacterium tuberculosis* at a concentration of 3.12 µg/mL [17].

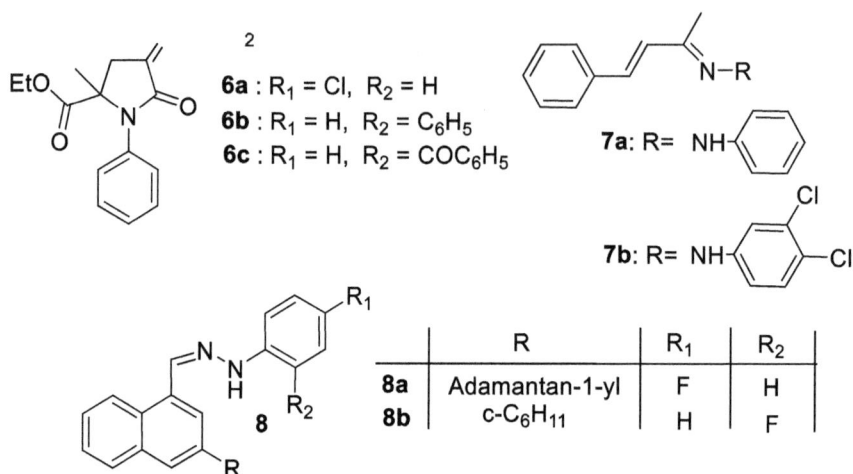

6a : R$_1$ = Cl, R$_2$ = H
6b : R$_1$ = H, R$_2$ = C$_6$H$_5$
6c : R$_1$ = H, R$_2$ = COC$_6$H$_5$

7a: R= NH—

7b: R= NH—

	R	R$_1$	R$_2$
8a	Adamantan-1-yl	F	H
8b	c-C$_6$H$_{11}$	H	F

Scheme 4.

R is a Heterocyclic Ring

In 2001, Oliveira *et al.* reported that hydrazones which are structurally more complex could possess specific antimicrobial activities.

Table 5. Antimicrobial activities of compounds 10-11.

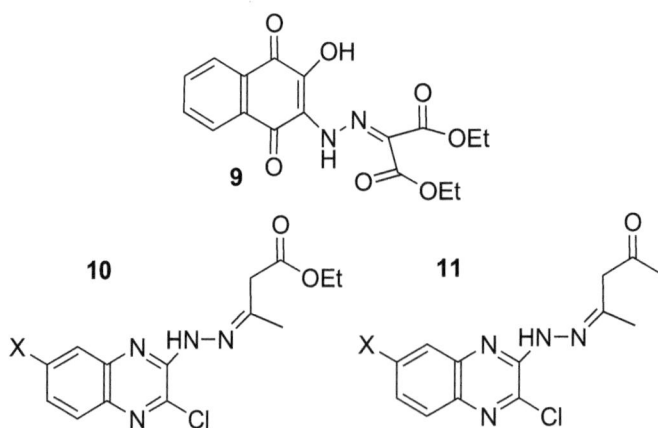

-		MIC (μg/mL)		
	X	*E. coli*	*S. aureus*	*C. albicans*
9	-	>128	64	>128
10a	H	1.8	12.3	12.3
10b	Cl	1.8	12.1	12.1
11a	H	6.25	6.25	6.25
11b	Cl	6.25	1.3	6.25

Thus, compound **9** can act against different strains of Gram-positive *S. aureus* sensitive or resistant to methicillin but with MICs ranging from 64 to 128 μg/mL [18]. On the other hand, molecules **10a**, **10b** and **11a**, **11b** present a wider spectrum of activity against both Gram-negative, Gram-positive bacteria as well as fungi (Table **5**) [19]. It is also noteworthy that the replacement of a hydrogen group by a chlorine one lead to an increase in terms of the activity of **11b** against *S. aureus* with a MIC of 1.3 μg/mL.

In another study, Savini *et al.* have described the design of quinolyl hydrazone derivatives **12a-c** and **13a-b**, presenting modest activities against *B. cereus*, *A. fumigatus* and *C. albicans* with MICs up to 100 μg/mL (Table **6**) [20].

Table 6. Structure of derivatives 12-13.

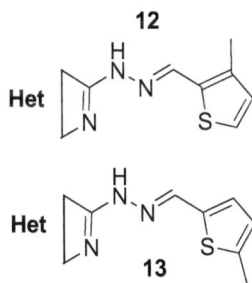

Compound	Het
12a	4-Methyl-2-quinolyl
12b	4,6-Dimethyl-2-quinolyl
12c	4-Methyl-7-methoxy-2-quinolyl
13a	4-Methyl-2-quinolyl
13b	4,6-Dimethyl-2-quinolyl

Additionally, 2-arylhydrazono-3-oxobutyrates **14** (Table **7**) presented antibacterial activities against Gram-positive bacteria *S. aureus* with a MIC value of 7.8 μg/mL whereas moderate ones (MICS ranging from 100 to 250 µg/mL) were encountered against Gram-negative bacteria and yeasts [21]. Surprisingly, arylhydrazone derivatives **15** and **16** possess MICs varying from 0.78 to 6.25 µg/mL against *M. tuberculosis* and present a low cytotoxicity ($120<IC_{50}$ (µg/mL) <180) suggesting a potent development for human therapeutic use [22].

Table 7. Structure of derivatives 14-15 and antituberculosis activities of compounds 16a-16e.

14a	S
14b	O

	R
15a	CH₃
15b	CH₃
15c	Cl

-	R	R'	Ar	*M. tuberculosis* MIC (µg/mL)
16a	H	7-OCH₃		0.78
16b		8-OCH₃		1.56
16c	CH₃	7-OC₂H₅	4-OCH₃-naphthyl	1.56
16d		6-n-OC₄H₉		0.78
16e		7-Cl		0.78

Another series of heterocyclic derivatives **17-18** was reported by Shaban [23] and El-Gazzar [24], demonstrating moderate activities against *C. albicans* and *C. glabrata* with diameter of inhibition of 8 mm. On the other hand, compound **18** appears highly active against bacteria such as *S. aureus* (16 mm), or Gram-negative bacteria *P. aeruginosa* (14 mm), *E. coli* (15 mm) or *K. pneumoniae* (18 mm) (Scheme 5).

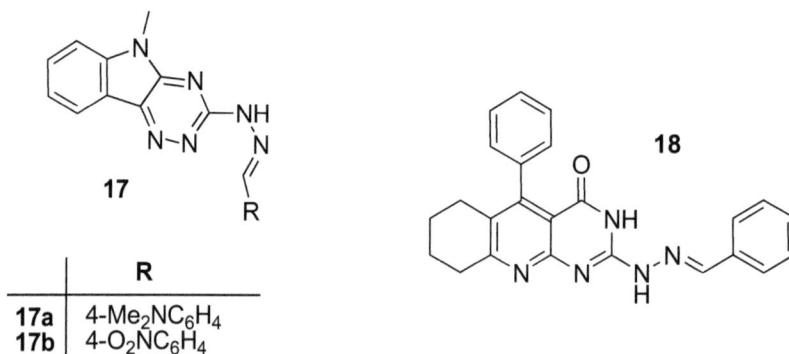

	R
17a	4-Me₂NC₆H₄
17b	4-O₂NC₆H₄

Scheme 5.

In the same context, Nassar *et al.* reported that uracil derivatives possess potent antimicrobial activities as illustrated by derivatives **19-21**, easily prepared as outlined in Table **8** [25]. The different compounds presented antibacterial activities against *L. monocytogenes* and were more potent than the reference drugs. Moreover, the antibacterial activity of **19** was significant against Gram-negative bacteria *E. coli*, with an inhibition zone of 13 mm compared to cefoperazone.

Table 8. Structure and antibacterial activities of derivatives 19-21.

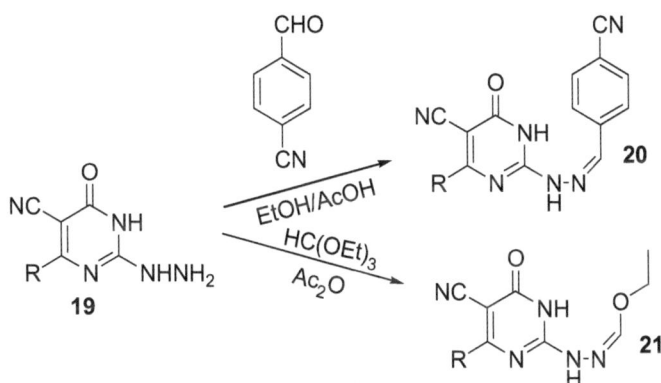

Bacteria	Zone of Inhibition (mm) Antibacterial Activity (1 mg/mL)			
	19	20	21	Cefoperazone
S. aureus	8	7.5	7.5	12
L. monocytogenes	14	12	12	11
E. coli	13	9	8.5	15
Y. enterolitica	-	9	-	12

Recently, quinoxaline derivatives were synthesized by the reaction of *o*-phenylenediamine with oxalic acid to yield 1,4-dihydro quinoxaline-2,3-dione and then treatment with thionyl chloride to yield 2,3-dichloro quinoxaline. This was further treated with hydrazine hydrate to produce 2,3-dihydrazinyl quinoxaline which reacted subsequently with the substituted aromatic aldehyde to afford 2,3-*bis*(2-(substituted benzylidine) hydrazinyl)quinoxaline **22**.

The Gram-positive and Gram-negative bacteria are sensitive to most of the tested compounds, and particularly **22c**, **22d**, and **22i** presenting significant activities against both type of microbial strains than others. Whereas the compound substituted with an electron-donating group or unsubstituted the phenyl ring offered a low to moderate activity against selected strains, derivatives bearing a methoxy group as a substituent of the phenyl ring has the least effect against selected bacterial strains (Table **9**) [26].

Table 9. Antimicrobial activities of quinoline derivatives expressed as MIC (mg/mL).

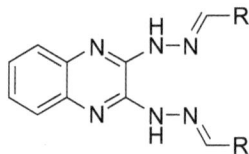

22a R=4FC$_6$H$_4$	22c R=3ClC$_6$H$_4$	22e R = 4OMeC$_6$H$_4$	22g R=3,4,5 (OMe)$_3$C$_6$H$_2$	22i R=4NO$_2$C$_6$H$_4$	22k R=4OH3OMeC$_6$H$_3$
22b R=2ClC$_6$H$_4$	22d R=4ClC$_6$H$_4$	22f R=3,4 (OMe)$_2$C$_6$H$_3$	22h R=2 NO$_2$C$_6$H$_4$	22j R=C$_6$H$_5$	22l R=2OHC$_6$H$_4$

Compounds	Gram-positive Bacteria		Gram-negative Bacteria	
	S. Pyogenes	**S. Aureus**	**E. Coli**	**P. Aeruginosa**
22a	1.1	1.28	1.89	1.97
22b	1.09	1.12	1.37	1.84
22c	0.97	0.92	0.93	0.98
22d	1.01	1.03	0.96	1.02
22e	2.87	3.28	3.17	3.14
22f	2.97	3.31	2.97	3.48
22g	3.03	3.43	3.23	3.17
22h	2.14	1.98	1.87	2.73
22i	1.04	1.06	1.10	1.01
22j	2.89	2.91	2.76	3.01
22k	1.87	2.12	2.28	1.98
22l	1.97	2.08	1.83	1.79
Ciprofloxacine	0.97	0.89	0.93	0.96

Another study dealing with the synthesis of benzenesulfonylurea and thiourea derivatives of 2*H*-pyran and 2*H*-pyridine-2-ones as antibacterial agents also needs to be mentioned. The results revealed that most of the tested compounds displayed greater inhibitory effect on the growth of the tested Gram-positive strain compared to Gram-negative ones such as *P. aeruginosa*. Moreover, few compounds were able to exert a potent antifungal activity against *C. albicans,* while all the tested compounds lacked antifungal activity against the *Aspergillus niger* fungus. A close examination of the structures of the active compounds revealed that the antimicrobial profile of the pyridine-2-one compounds seemed to be more interesting than their corresponding pyran-2-one isosteres, as evidenced by their MIC values (Table **10**) [27].

Table 10. Minimum Inhibitory Concentrations (µg/mL) of compounds 23a-23d.

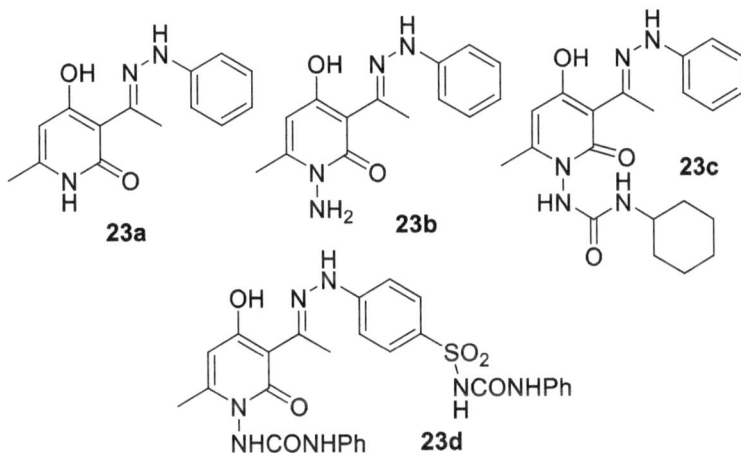

Compounds	Gram-positive Bacteria		Gram-negative Bacteria	
	B. Subtilis	*S. Aureus*	*E. Coli*	*P. Aeruginosa*
23a	100	50	>200	>200
23b	50	50	200	>200
23c	>200	>200	>200	>200
23d	50	12.5	50	200
ampicillin	25	12.5	25	50

Introduction of an amino group at position 1 of the pyridine ring as in compound **23b** resulted in significant changes in the overall antimicrobial spectrum. It showed two-fold improvement in the potency against *B. subtilis* when compared with **23a** (MIC 50 *vs* 100 µg/mL, respectively) whereas it revealed moderate activity against *E. coli* (MIC 200 µg/mL). Furthermore, compound **23d** produced the most potent antimicrobial activity in the current series of compounds (more potent than ampicillin (MIC 12.5 µg/mL)) against *S. aureus,* whereas its activity against *B. subtilis* and *E. coli* was 50% lower than that observed for ampicillin (MIC 50 *vs* 25 µg/mL, respectively).

Even if numerous of them presented a weak interest in terms of encountered biological activities, it is of interest to report the design of peculiar hydrazone compounds that we can find in literature. Thus, the synthesis and evaluation of antimicrobial activities of compounds **24-25** were achieved demonstrating low activities against both Gram-positive and Gram-negative bacteria (Table **11**) [28].

Table 11. Antimicrobial activities of hydrazones 24-25.

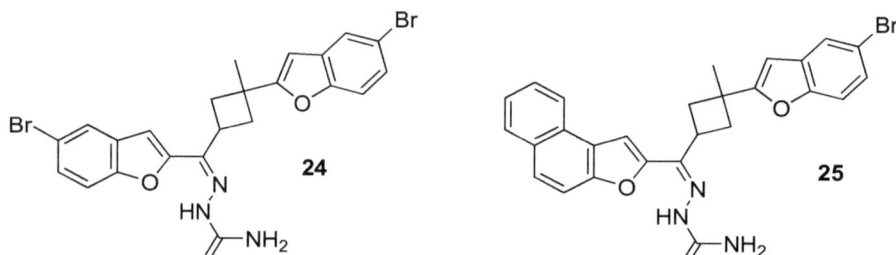

-	Diameter (mm)				
	B. subtilis	*P. aeruginosa*	*E. coli*	*L. monocytogenes*	*S. aureus*
24	9	6	9	9	9
25	8	10	8	10	-

More recently, steroid hydrazone derivatives **26-28** were designed and tested against various bacteria. The results indicated that compound **26a-26b** [29]are only active against *E. coli* whereas derivatives **27-28** [30] presented MICs ranging from 32 to 128 μg/mL against both Gram-positive and Gram-negative bacteria (Table **12**).

In 2008, new promising hydrazone anti-tuberculosis agents (**29-30**) were described in the literature (Scheme **6**). Thus, compounds **29** and **30** present MICs of 6.25 μg/mL against *M. tuberculosis* [31]. Furthermore, **30d** can inhibit the growth of this microorganism by 79% [32]. Nevertheless, no more results dealing with the mechanism of action or improvement of the design of such derivatives were reported until now.

Table 12. Antimicrobial activities of hydrazones 26-28.

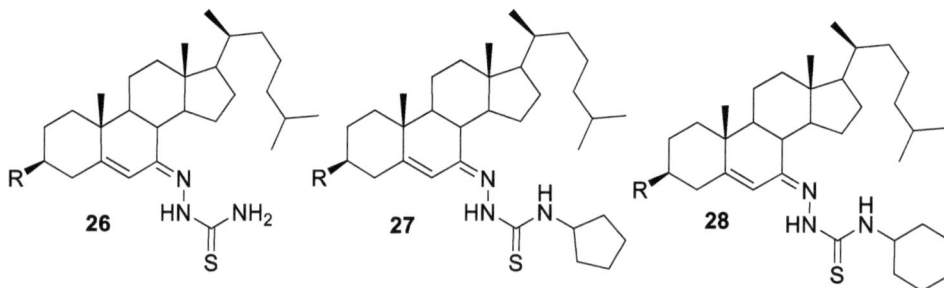

	MIC (µg/mL)					
-	**26a**	**26b**	**27a**	**27b**	**28a**	**28b**
R	CH₃COO	Cl	OAc	Cl	OAc	Cl
S. aureus	-	-	32	64	64	32
S. pyogenes	-	-	64	64	64	64
S. typhimurium	-	-	64	128	64	128
E. coli	128	64	32	64	32	64

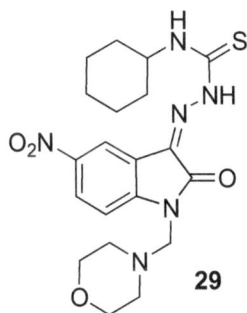

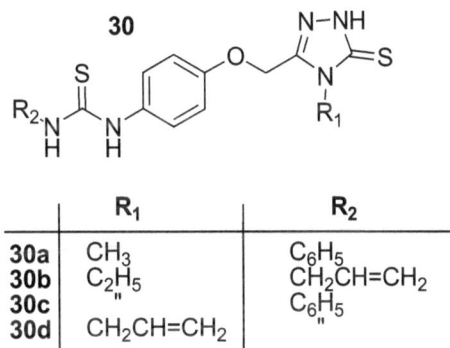

	R₁	R₂
30a	CH₃	C₆H₅
30b	C₂H₅	CH₂CH=CH₂
30c	"	C₆H₅
30d	CH₂CH=CH₂	"

Scheme 6.

In 2012, Karaca *et al.* reported the synthesis of compounds which contain hydrazone bridged thiazole and pyrrole rings easily obtained by directly reacting pyrrole-2-carboxaldehydes with thiosemicarbazide in ethanol and subsequently condensed them with α-bromoacetophenone derivatives (Hantzsch reaction) to afford 1-substituted pyrrole-2-carboxaldehyde [4-(4-substituted phenyl)-1,--thiazol-2-yl] hydrazones in good isolated yields (Scheme 7) [33]. All the compounds were screened for their antibacterial and antifungal activities against twelve different bacteria, but they only showed good activity against *S. aureus* and *E. faecalis* with MICs ranging from 6.25 to 25 µg/mL.

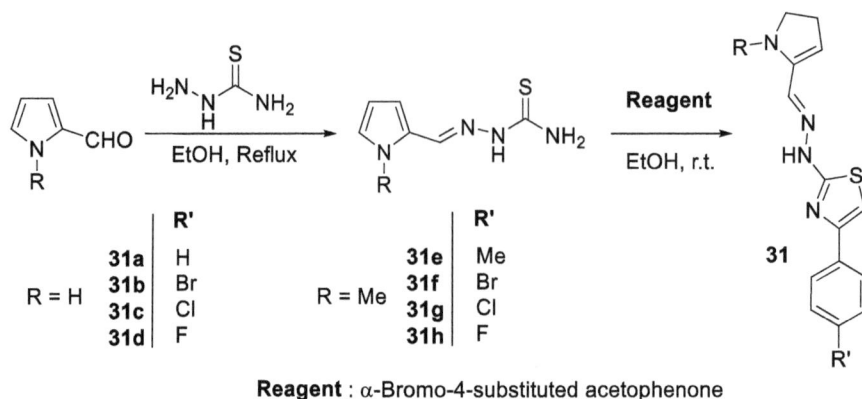

Reagent : α-Bromo-4-substituted acetophenone

Scheme 7.

Derivatives of 3-pyrazolylquinolinone, in three different types; enaminones **32**, enones **33**, and hydrazonones **34**, have also been investigated for their *In vitro* antimicrobial activity (Scheme **8**) [34, 35].

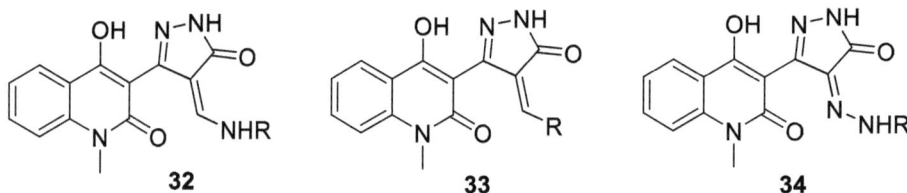

Scheme 8.

The compounds were screened for their biological activities and revealed that hydrazonones **34** possess desirable antimicrobial activity against both bacteria and fungi groups tested.

Recently, novel series of 4,6-disubstituted-1,3,5-triazines containing hydrazone derivatives **35-36** as well as fluorenyl-hydrazonothiazoles **37-38** were synthesized employing ultrasonic irradiation and conventional heating. The ultrasonication gave the target products in higher yields and purity in shorter reaction times compared with the conventional method [36, 37].

The biological results indicated that only compounds **35** and **36** displayed moderate biological activity against Gram-positive and Gram-negative bacteria, while fluorenyl-hydrazonothiazoles **37-38** present interesting antifungal activities (Table **13**).

Table 13. Antimicrobial activities of hydrazones 35-38.

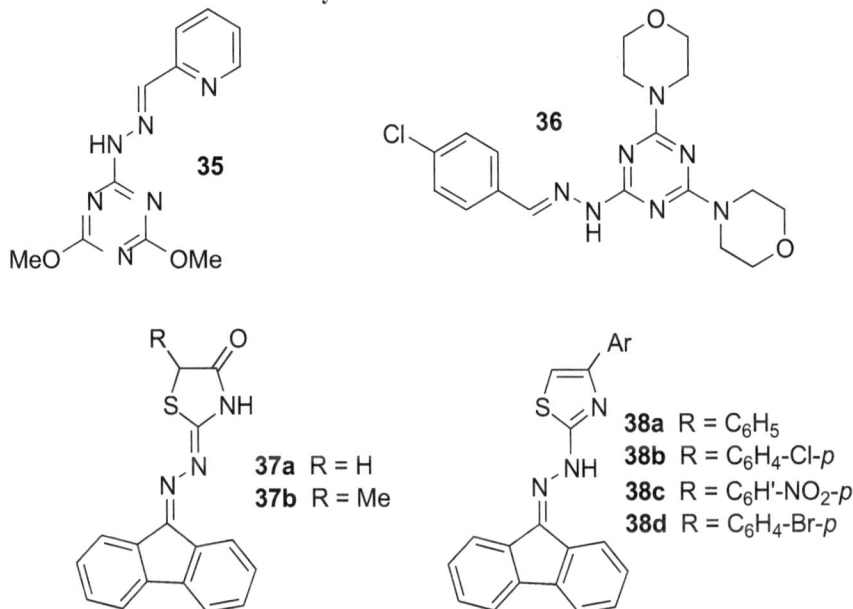

	MIC (µg/mL)							
-	**35**	**36**	**37a**	**37b**	**38a**	**38b**	**38c**	**38d**
S. aureus	100	100	50	25	25	12.5	25	12.5
B. laterosporus	50	50	NT	NT	NT	NT	NT	NT
E. coli	NA	NA	50	6.25	25	25	25	12.5
P. aeruginosa	NA	NA	25	25	25	12.5	12.5	25
A. niger	NA	NA	25	12.5	12.5	12.5	12.5	12.5
C. albicans	NA	NA	25	12.5	25	50	50	50

More recently, Chellamella *et al.* reported the synthesis and biological evaluation as antimicrobial agents of ethyl-2-(3-((2-(4-(4-aryl)thiazol-2-yl)hydrazono) methyl)-4-hydroxy/isobutoxyphenyl)-4-methylthiazole-5-carboxylate compounds (**39a-f** and **40a-f**) by employing a one-pot multi-component approach. The overall activity data revealed that the presence of a coumarin motif in their structure is essential for broad-spectrum antimicrobial activity. These compounds could bind the active site of the enzyme, DNA gyrase which is responsible for bacterial replication and thus leads to the inhibition of the bacterial growth (Table **14**) [38].

Table 14. Structure and antimicrobial activities of derivatives 39-40.

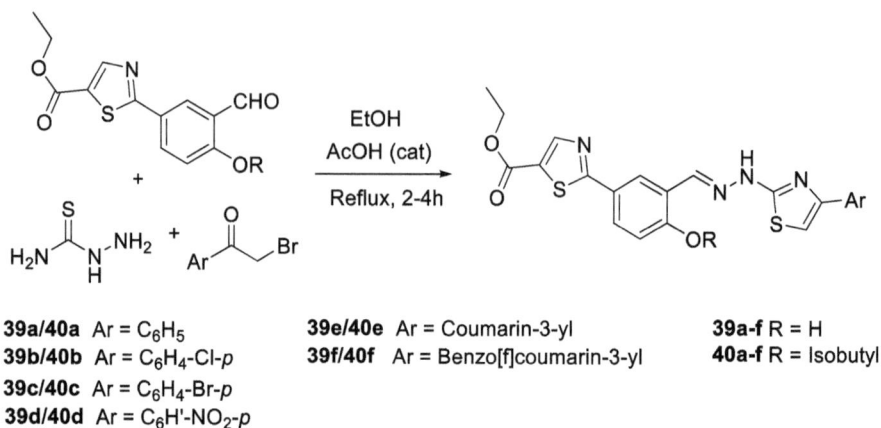

39a/40a Ar = C$_6$H$_5$ 39e/40e Ar = Coumarin-3-yl   39a-f R = H
39b/40b Ar = C$_6$H$_4$-Cl-*p*   39f/40f Ar = Benzo[f]coumarin-3-yl   40a-f R = Isobutyl
39c/40c Ar = C$_6$H$_4$-Br-*p*
39d/40d Ar = C$_6$H'-NO$_2$-*p*

-	MIC (µg/mL)				
	S. aureus	*B. subtilis*	*E. coli*	*C. albicans*	*A. niger*
39a	40	35	35	25	35
39b	35	30	25	25	50
39c	35	30	50	75	50
39d	40	30	50	50	25
39e	15	20	20	12.5	12.5
39f	15	25	20	12.5	12.5
40a	30	30	35	75	100
40b	25	25	20	75	75
40c	35	30	35	50	75
40d	25	25	30	75	75
40e	15	15	20	12.5	25
40f	20	20	20	12.5	12.5

Sulfonylhydrazones

Sulfonylhydrazones are hydrazones presenting the general formula: $R_1R_2C=N-NH-SO_2-R_3$.

In 1984, Bhatt *et al.* prepared the molecules **41a** and **41b** possessing antibacterial activity against *S. aureus* (inhibition diameter: 40mm) and *E. coli* (30mm), respectively [39]. In the same context, Salama *et al.* designed analogues of these molecules demonstrating the influence of the structure on their antimicrobial activities [40]. Thus, compounds **42a-42b** were identified as the best analogues active both against Gram-positive or negative bacteria and fungi (Scheme **9**).

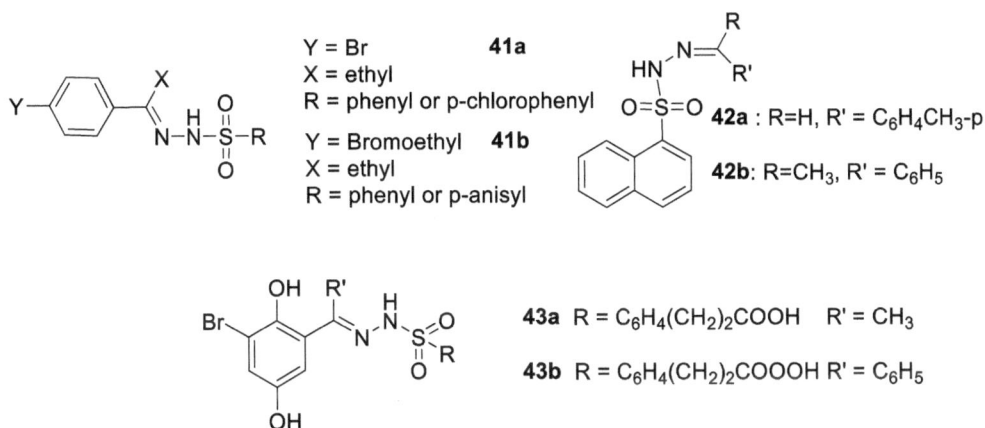

Scheme 9.

On the other hand, the group of Shad reported the synthesis of hydrazones **43a-43b** active against *E. coli* and *S. aureus* with a diameter of inhibition of 29 and 27 mm, respectively. Furthermore, they are less active against *B. negaterium* with only a 12 mm diameter of inhibition encountered (Scheme **9**) [41].

In 2004, The first cholesteryl hydrazone derivatives **44-45** were synthesized and tested for their antimicrobial activities demonstrating interesting antifungal activities especially against *C. albicans* with MICs ranging from 1.25 and 25 µg/mL (Scheme **10**) [42]. Recently, antiviral activities of hydrazones of 5α-steroids were reported highlighting the potent interest of such derivatives against polio, Rift Valley fever, and influenza A viruses [43].

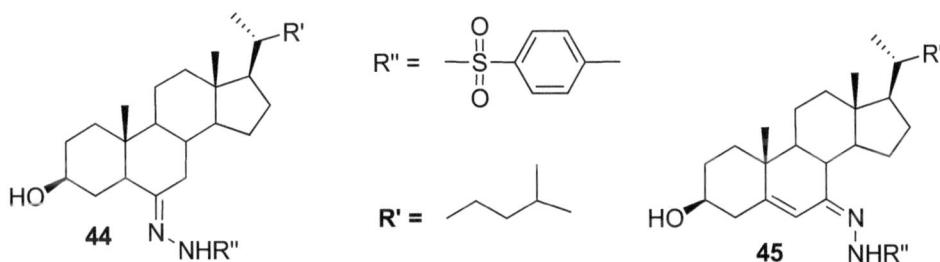

Scheme 10.

Ylidene Hydrazide Derivatives

Another class of hydrazones is constituted by ylidene hydrazide derivatives **46** possessing a hydrazone function and an amide group as illustrated in Scheme **11** and where R, R' and R'' could pertain to linear or cyclic alkyl or aryl substituents.

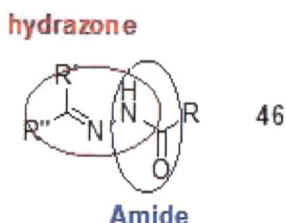

Scheme 11.

Metwally *et al.* reported the synthesis of derivatives **47** from quinoline and bearing various substituent groups (Table **15**) [44].

Table 15. Structures of hydrazone derivatives 47.

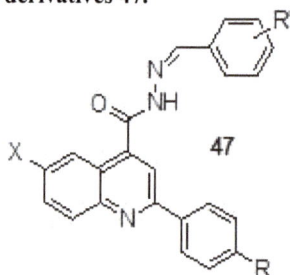

-	X	R	R'
47a	2-H	4-bromophenyl	2-nitrobenzylidene
47b	6-Cl	2-phenyl	4-bromobenzylidene
47c	6-Cl	4-bromophenyl	2-nitrobenzylidene
47d	6-Cl	4-bromophenyl	4-nitrobenzylidene
47e	6-Cl	4-methoxyphenyl	2-nitrobenzylidene
47f	6-Cl	4-methoxyphenyl	4-nitrobenzylidene

It has been observed that these compounds presented no activity against Gram-positive bacteria such as *S. aureus* (MIC > 200 µg/mL), while MICs are ranging from 25 to 50 µg/mL against *E. coli* and *C. albicans* (Table **15**). These activities against *E. coli* and *C. albicans* are as same as reference drugs. It may also point out that these molecules do not present any haemolytic activity. The authors concluded that the nature of the substituents and substitution pattern on the quinoline ring may have a considerable impact on the observed antibacterial and antifungal activities of the considered hydrazones, para substitution appearing to be more beneficial for activity compared to the ortho one (Table **16**). As an improvement of such studies, Shruthi *et al.* have recently reported that such compounds were found to be active against bacterial strains including *Acinetobacter baumannii, Escherichia coli* and *Staphylococcus aureus* [35].

Table 16. Antibacterial activities of hydrazone derivatives 47.

-	MIC (µg/mL)	
-	*E. coli*	*C. albicans*
47a	25-50	25-50
47b	100	25-50
47c	25-50	50-100
47d	25-50	50
47e	25-50	25-50
47f	25-50	25

Some other compounds **48-50** demonstrated antifungal activities (Table **17**). Particularly, compounds **48a** and **48d** possess a MIC of 128 µg/mL against three different *Candida* strains [45 - 47].

Table 17. Antifungal activities of compounds of 48-50.

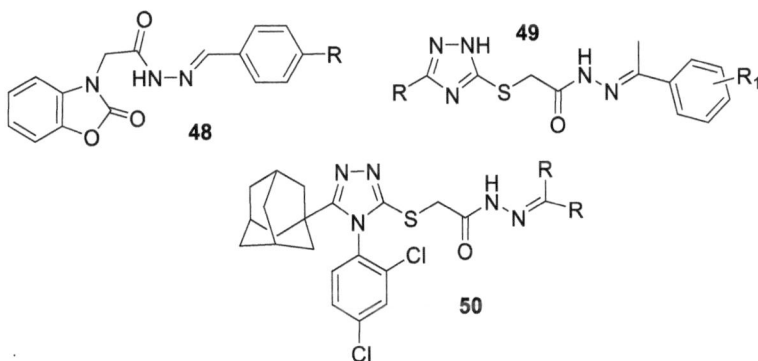

-		MIC (µg/mL)		
-	R	*C. albicans*	*C. krusei*	*C. parapsilosis*
48a	H	128	128	128
48b	Br	64	256	128
48c	Cl	128	256	256

48d	CH$_3$		128	128	128
48e	OCH$_3$		128	128	512
49a	H	4-NO$_2$	100	100	100
49b	CH$_3$	4-NO$_2$	100	100	200
49c	C$_2$H$_5$	4-Cl	100	100	200
49d	C$_2$H$_5$	4-NO$_2$	100	100	200
50a	(CH$_2$)$_3$		365	-	-
50b	(CH$_2$)$_4$		365	-	-
50c	(CH$_2$)$_5$		-	-	-

In 2001, Chornous *et al.* have synthesized hydrazone derivatives **51** possessing a hetero-nitrogen-ring but these molecules demonstrated moderate antibacterial activities against *S. aureus* and *E. coli* (Table **18**) [48].

Table 18. Antibacterial activities of compounds 51.

				MIC (µg/mL)	
			R	R'	*S. aureus*	*E. coli*
	51a	4-FC$_6$H$_4$	HOC$_6$H$_3$	62.5	250
	51b	4-FC$_6$H$_4$	5-nitrofur-2-yl	62.5	>500
	51c	4-C$_2$H$_5$C$_6$H$_4$	5-nitrofur-2-yl	31.2	>500
	51d	Thienyl-2-yl	5-nitrofur-2-yl	62.5	500

Rahman *et al.* also prepared hydrazones bearing long linear alkyl chains terminated by a carboxylic acid or allyl group. All these molecules do not possess any activity against *C. albicans* but are efficient against both Gram-positive and Gram-negative bacteria with diameters of inhibition varying from 10 to 20 mm (Table **19**) [49].

Another study of interest needs to be mentioned reported by Rollas *et al.* who performed the synthesis of analogues **55a-c** possessing nitroaryl or furyl groups. These compounds are very active against Gram-positive *S. aureus* bacteria with MICs ranging from 2 to 8 µg/mL whereas high MICS were encountered against yeasts and Gram-negative bacteria (Table **20**) [50].

Table 19. Antibacterial activities of compounds 52-54.

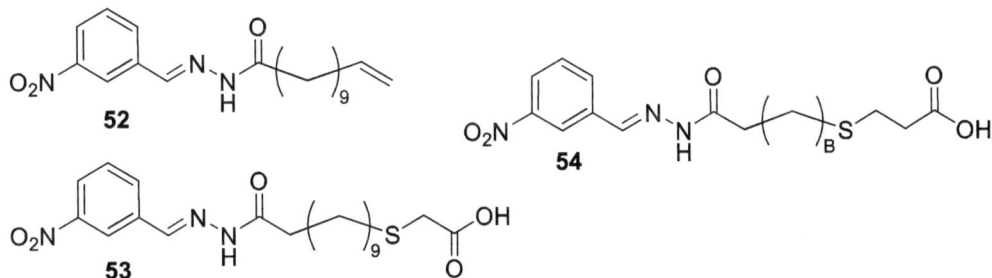

-	Diameters of Inhibition (mm)				
-	*S. aureus*	*B. subtilis*	*E. coli*	*P. aeruginosa*	*C. albicans*
52	-	-	19	-	-
53	12	12	10	14	-
54	18	15	14	20	-

Table 20. Antimicrobial activities of compounds 55a-55c.

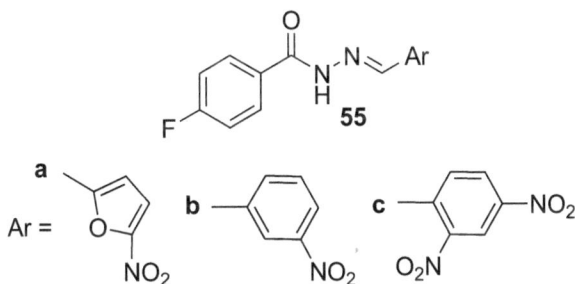

-	MIC (µg/mL)			
-	*S. aureus*	*C. albicans*	*E. coli*	*P. aeruginosa*
55a	2	62.5	250	250
55b	8	125	125	125
55c	4	125	125	125

In the same area of research, Rao [51], Kursun [52] and Fahmy [53] performed the synthesis of various analogues of derivatives **56a-d** demonstrating also moderate to good antibacterial and antifungal activities against Gram-positive bacteria and fungi with diameter of inhibition ranging from 0 to 17 mm depending on the considered microorganisms (Table **21**).

Table 21. Antimicrobial activities of compounds 56a-d.

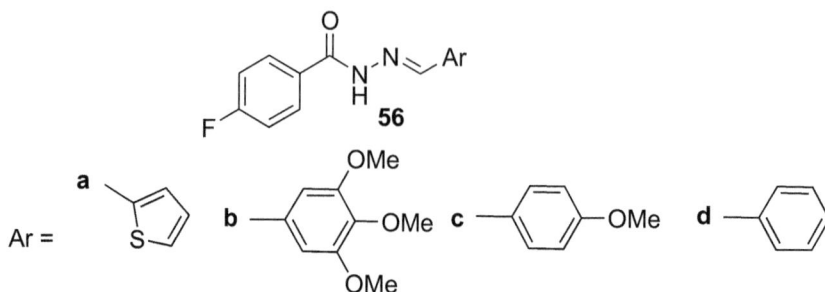

-	Diameter of inhibition (mm)				
	B. subtilis	*S. aureus*	*P. notatum*	*A. niger*	*C. utilis*
56a	8*	7*	0	0	0
56b	0	0	10*	0	12*
56c	11*	11**	12*	16*	17*
56d	10	9	9	14	13

*significant **highly significant

In 2007, numerous parent derivatives such as **57a-c, 58** and **59** had been prepared presenting interesting antibacterial activities against a large panel of bacteria (Scheme **12**) [54].

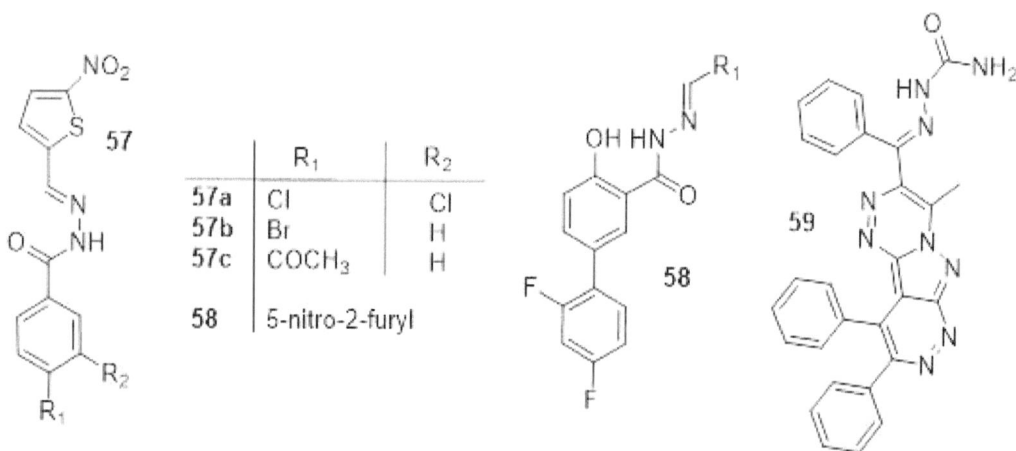

	R₁	R₂
57a	Cl	Cl
57b	Br	H
57c	COCH₃	H
58	5-nitro-2-furyl	

Scheme 12.

It is noteworthy that **57c** possesses the best MICS of 0.11 and 1.27 μg/mL against two different strains of *S. aureus*, respectively. Otherwise, the derivative **58** presents moderate activities against *B. subtilis* (75 μg/mL), *S. epidermis* (18.75

µg/mL), *E. coli* (75 µg/mL) and *S. aureus* (37.5 µg/mL), whereas hydrazone **59** presents a weak activity against all these pathogens [55]. Furthermore, **58** inhibits the growth of *M. tuberculosis* by 34% at a concentration of 6.25 µg/mL.

In 2007, Joshi *et al.* reported the synthesis of N'-(arylidene)-4-(1H-pyrrol-1-yl) benzohydrazide **60-61** and their moderate to good antimicrobial activities typically against *M. tuberculosis* with some derivatives **61b** and **61e** possessing MICs of 32.5 µg/mL (Table **22**) [56].

Table 22. Antibacterial activities of compounds 60-61.

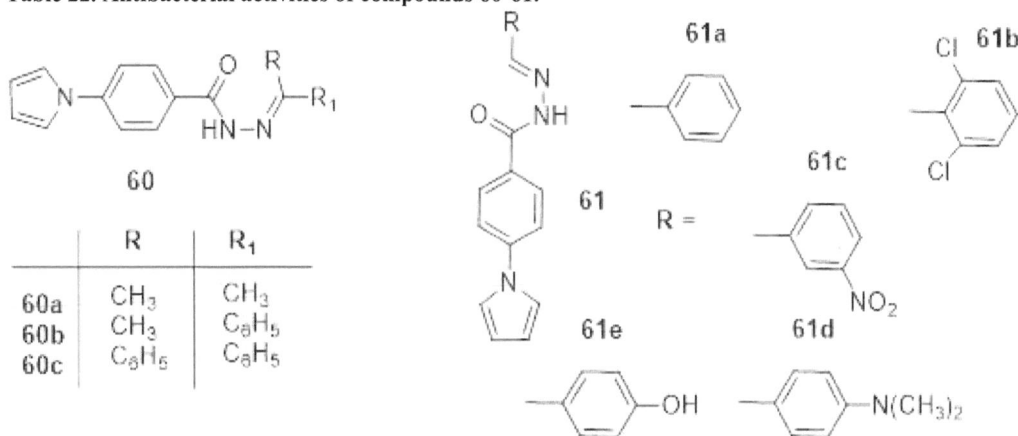

-	MIC (µg/mL)					
	S. aureus	*E. faecalis*	*M. tuberculosis*	*K. pneumoniae*	*E. coli*	*P. aeruginosa*
60a	250	125	62.5	250	125	62.5
60b	250	125	62.5	125	125	62.5
60c	500	250	62.5	125	125	62.5
61a	250	250	125	125	125	125
61b	125	125	31.25	125	62.5	62.5
61c	500	500	62.5	500	500	62.5
61d	250	125	62.5	125	250	125
61e	125	125	31.25	125	62.5	62.5

The design of derivatives **62** and **63** led to products active against *M. tuberculosis* with MICs varying from 0.39 to 15 µM, **63b** being the most active compound of this series (Scheme **13**) [57].

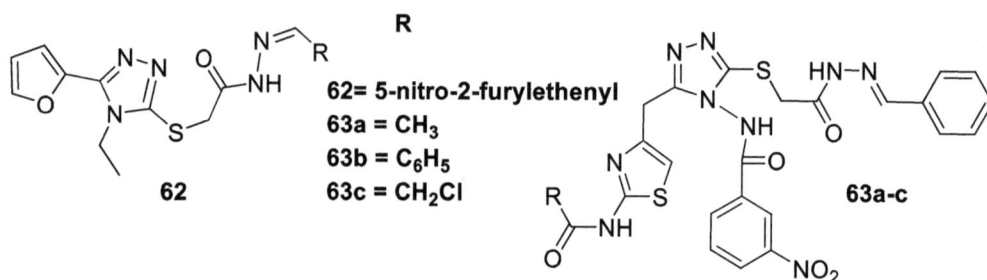

62= 5-nitro-2-furylethenyl
63a = CH₃
63b = C₆H₅
63c = CH₂Cl

Scheme 13.

Recently, Muluk *et al.* reported the synthesis of new pyridyl and thiazolyl clubbed hydrazone derivatives **64** displaying moderate antimicrobial activities and suggesting that the design of new parent derivatives could improve the selectivity and activity encountered (Table **23**) [58].

Table 23. Structure and antimicrobial activities of compounds 64a-64d.

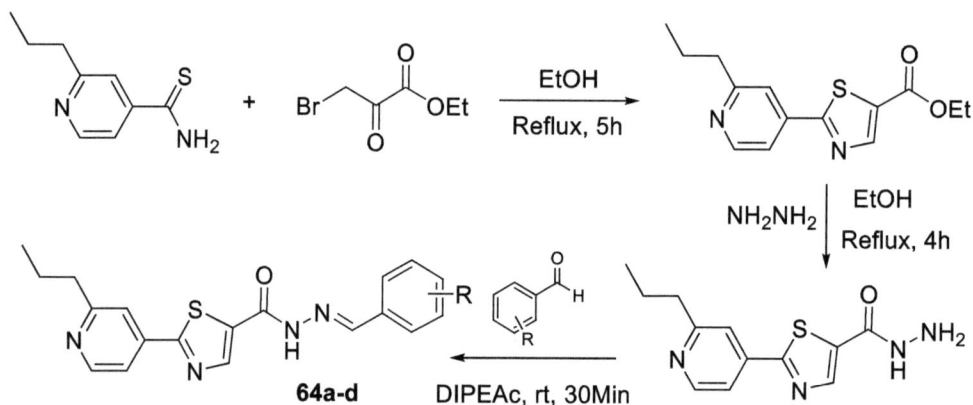

-		MIC (µg/mL)		
-	**R**	**B. subtilis**	**E. aerogenes**	**C. albicans**
64a	3, 5-Cl	90	170	150
64b	4-Cl	260	120	280
64c	3-Cl	120	150	250
64d	2-NO₂	75	85	210
Streptomycin	-	25	30	NA
Fluconazole	-	NA	NA	30

To further dissect the structural features necessary to inhibit azole-resistant fungal species, Backes *et al.* have recently performed the synthesis of a new class of modified salicylaldehyde derivatives and subsequently identified a series of modified pyridine-based hydrazones **65a-f** possesing fungicidal and antifungal activities against numerous *Candida* spp (Table **24**) [59].

Table 24. Structure and antimicrobial activities of compounds 65a-65f.

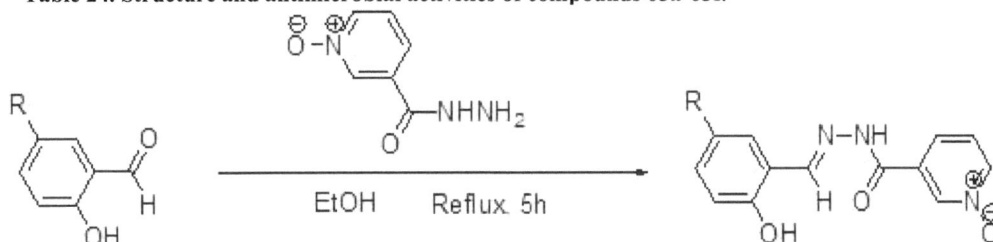

-	-	MIC$_{80}$ (µg/mL)			
-	**R**	*TW1*	*TW17*	*C. albicans* ATCC10231	*C. albicans* ATCC48435
65a	H	31	31	31	16
65b	Me	16	16	16	31
65c	MeO	62	31	16	4
65d	Cl	31	31	16	4
65e	Br	8	8	16	4
65f	NO$_2$	4	2	8	4

Condensation of 5,6,7,8-tetrahydroimidazo[1,2-a]-pyrimidine-2-carbohydrazide with various aromatic aldehydes in ethanol at reflux led to the generation of hydrazone derivatives **66** in 80–92% yield. Compounds **66d**, **66e** and **66f** exhibited excellent antibacterial activity with zone of inhibition 30–33 mm against *E. coli* and *S. aureus*. These compounds also exhibited excellent antibacterial activity with zone of inhibition ranging from 22 to 25 mm against *P. aeruginosa* and *S. pyogenes* (Table **25**) [60].

Table 25. Structure and antimicrobial activities of compounds 66a-66h.

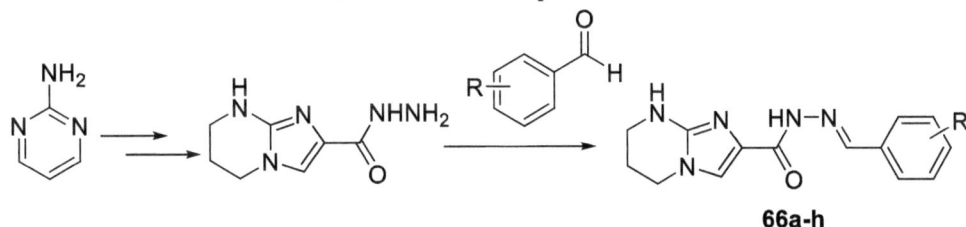

66a-h

-	-	Zone of inhibition of compounds 66a-f Concentration used 250µg/mL of DMSO			
-	R	*E. coli* MTCCC443	*P. aeruginosa* MTCC424	*S. aureus* MTCC96	*S. pyogenes* MTCC442
66a	4-F	25	19	24	17
66b	2-CF$_3$	27	20	23	18
66c	3-CF$_3$	26	19	23	17
66d	4-CF$_3$	33	24	29	24
66e	4-OCF$_3$	30	25	30	22
66f	4-OCHF$_2$	30	23	31	22
66g	2,4-F	20	16	19	13
66h	3,4-F	21	15	19	14

In another work, the synthesis of imidazole hydrazone derivatives **67a-m** and their evaluation against *A. niger, S. aureus, S. pyogenes, E. coli* and *P. aeruginosa* resulted in moderate to good antimicrobial activities (Table **26**) [61].

Table 26. Structure and antimicrobial activities of compounds 67a-m.

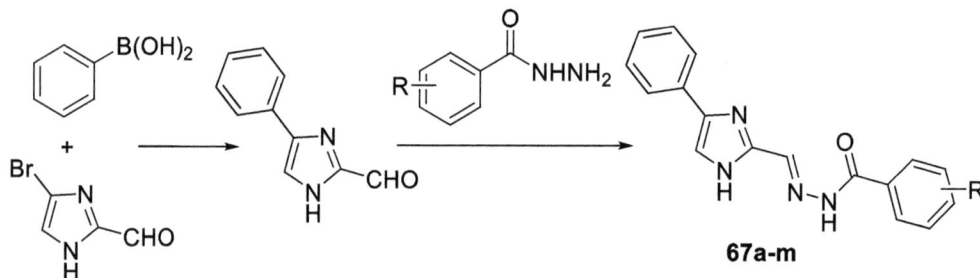

-		Zone of inhibition of compounds 67a-m Concentration used 250µg/mL of DMSO				
-	R	*E. coli* MTCCC443	*P. aeruginosa* MTCC424	*S. aureus* MTCC96	*S. pyogenes* MTCC442	*A. niger* MTCC282
67a	H	26	24	18	17	26
67b	4-OH	28	27	24	25	30
67c	4-Br	15	13	-	-	22
67d	4-Cl	14	12	-	-	21
67e	4-F	25	23	25	23	28
67f	4-SO$_2$CH$_3$	30	30	26	25	31
67g	3-NO$_2$	25	24	18	19	28
67h	3-Cl	14	12	-	-	21

(Table 26) cont.....

67i	2-Br	13	13	-	-	20
67j	2-I	15	14	-	-	18
67k	2,5-F	28	27	20	20	30
67l	3,5-Cl	15	15	-	-	17
67m	2,4-Cl	14	13	-	-	16

Pilai *et al.* have recently described the steroselective synthesis of a series of novel cyanoacetyl hydrazones of 3-alkyl-2,6-diarylpiperidin-4-ones **68a-j** demonstrating interesting antibacterial activities against *E. aerogenes* and some fungal strains (Table **27**) [62].

Table 27. Structure and antimicrobial activities of compounds 68a-j.

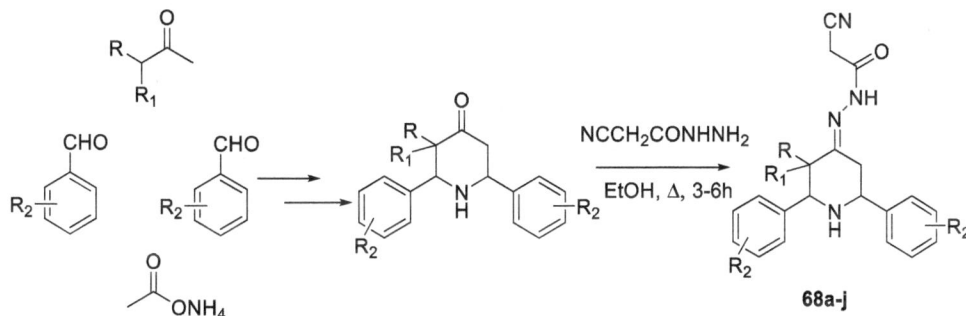

-	-	Zone of inhibition of compounds 68a-j Concentration used 250µg/mL of DMSO			
-	R/R$_1$/R$_2$	*E. coli*	*E. aerogenes*	*S. aureus*	*C. albicans*
68a	Me/H/H	-	34	-	9
68b	Et/H/H	-	-	-	6
68c	Me/Me/H	-	14	-	19
68d	Me/H/*p*-Me	11	11	12	-
68e	Me/H/*p*-OMe	9	12	-	12
68f	Me/H/*o*-Cl	12	9	-	-
68g	Me/H/*m*-NO$_2$	14	11	-	12
68h	Me/H/*p*-F	-	-	16	8
68i	Me/H/*p*-Cl	-	-	-	7
68j	Me/H/*p*-Br	-	-	16	28

Another example to be cited deals with the synthesis of hydrazone derivatives of anacardic acid linked with 1,2,3-triazole ring and exhibiting strong antifungal activity against *A. niger* and *C. albicans* (Table **28**) [63].

Table 28. Structure and antimicrobial activities of compounds 69a-j.

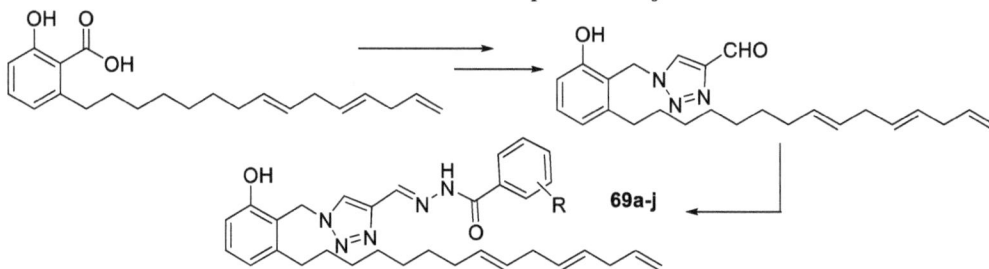

-	R	Zone of inhibition of compounds 69a-j Concentration used 250 µg/mL of DMSO	
-	R	*A. niger*	*C. albicans*
69a	H	16	15
69b	4-OMe	13	12
69c	4-Cl	17	18
69d	4-OH	26	23
69e	3,4,5-OMe	27	24
69f	2,5-Cl	19	19
69g	3,5-Cl	20	20
69h	Me/H/*m*-NO$_2$	25	24
69i	4-F	24	22
69j	2,5-F	26	24

CONCLUDING REMARKS

Numerous different approaches have been depicted for the design and synthesis of hydrazones presenting interesting antimicrobial activities. It also remains clear that this class of compounds is still too neglected, as outlined in a previous review highlighting their use as metal ligands for the formation of hydrazone-transition metal complexes possessing interesting biological, analytical and catalytic applications [64].

CONSENT FOR PUBLICATION

Not applicable.

CONFLICT OF INTEREST

The author declares no conflict of interest, financial or otherwise.

ACKNOWLEDGEMENTS

Declared none.

REFERENCES

[1] Chaudhary T, Varshney S, Singh A. An updated review on biological activities of hydrazone derivatives. World J Pharm Pharm Sci 2018; 7(10): 1532-69.

[2] Narang R, Narasimhan B, Sharma S. A review on biological activities and chemical synthesis of hydrazide derivatives. Curr Med Chem 2012; 19(4): 569-612.
[http://dx.doi.org/10.2174/092986712798918789] [PMID: 22204327]

[3] Negi VJ, Sharma AK, Negi JS, Ram V. Biological activities of hydrazone derivatives in the new millennium. Int J Pharm Chem 2012; 2(4): 100-9.

[4] Popiołek Ł. Hydrazide-hydrazones as potential antimicrobial agents: overview of the literature since 2010. Med Chem Res 2017; 26(2): 287-301.
[http://dx.doi.org/10.1007/s00044-016-1756-y] [PMID: 28163562]

[5] Sayed AR, Ali SH, Gomha SM, Al-Faiyz YS. Review of the synthesis and biological activity of hydrazonoyl halides. Synth Commun 2020; 50(21): 3175-203.
[http://dx.doi.org/10.1080/00397911.2020.1799016]

[6] Omidi S, Kakanejadifard A. A review on biological activities of Schiff base, hydrazone, and oxime derivatives of curcumin. RSC Advances 2020; 10(50): 30186-202.
[http://dx.doi.org/10.1039/D0RA05720G]

[7] de Oliveira Carneiro Brum J, França TCC, LaPlante SR, Villar JDF. Synthesis and biological activity of hydrazones and derivatives: A review. Mini Rev Med Chem 2020; 20(5): 342-68.
[http://dx.doi.org/10.2174/1389557519666191014142448] [PMID: 31612828]

[8] Bamford WR, Stevens TS. The decomposition of toluene-p-sulphonylhydrazones by alkali. J Chen Soc 1952; 55: 4735-40.
[http://dx.doi.org/10.1039/jr9520004735]

[9] Shapiro RH, Lipton MF, Kolondo KJ, Buswell RL, Capuano LA. Tosylhydrazones and alkyllithium reagents: More on the regiospecificity of the reaction and the trapping of three intermediates. Tetrahedron Lett 1975; 22: 1811-4.
[http://dx.doi.org/10.1016/S0040-4039(00)75263-4]

[10] Rollas S, Küçükgüzel SG. Biological activities of hydrazone derivatives. Molecules 2007; 12(8): 1910-39.
[http://dx.doi.org/10.3390/12081910] [PMID: 17960096]

[11] Shinge PS, Mallur SG, Badami BV. Termolecular one-pot synthesis of symmetrical azines of 4-acety--3-arylsydnones. Hydrazone and azine derivatives of 4-acetyl-3-arylsydnones, their spectral characterization and biological properties. J Indian Chem Soc 2005; 82(7): 659-64.

[12] Sztanke K, Pasternak K, Rzymowska J, *et al.* Identification of antitumour activity of novel derivatives of 8-aryl-2,6,7,8-tetrahydroimidazo[2,1-c][1,2,4]triazine-3,4-dione and 8-aryl-4-imino-2,3-7,8-tetrahydroimidazo[2,1-c][1,2,4]triazin-3(6H)-one. Bioorg Med Chem 2007; 15(8): 2837-49.
[http://dx.doi.org/10.1016/j.bmc.2007.02.024] [PMID: 17331732]

[13] Moreau S, Varache-Lembège M, Larrouture S, *et al.* (2-Arylhydrazonomethyl)-substituted xanthones as antimycotics: synthesis and fungistatic activity against Candida species. Eur J Med Chem 2002;

37(3): 237-53.
[http://dx.doi.org/10.1016/S0223-5234(01)01332-0] [PMID: 11900868]

[14]   Tyrkov AG, Sukhenko LT. Synthesis and antimicrobial activity of substituted nitro-1,2,4-oxadiazo-e-5-carbaldehyde hydrazones. Pharm Chem J 2004; 38(7): 376-8.
[http://dx.doi.org/10.1023/B:PHAC.0000048437.00540.6a]

[15]   Dimmock JR, Kirkpatrick DL, Negrave LE, Russell KL, Pannekoek WJ. Preparation of some hydrazones of conjugated styryl ketones and related compounds for evaluation principally as antineoplastic agents. Can J Pharm Sci 1981; 16(1): 1-7.
[PMID: 6262476]

[16]   Gein VL, Gein LF, Chirkova MV, Mikhalev VA, Voronina EV. Synthesis, properties, and antimicrobial activity of 3-hydrazones of 1-aryl-5-methyl-1,5-ethoxycarbonylpyrrolidine-2,3-diones. Pharm Chem J 2005; 39(8): 413-7.
[http://dx.doi.org/10.1007/s11094-005-0170-4]

[17]   Nayyar A, Malde A, Coutinho E, Jain R. Synthesis, anti-tuberculosis activity, and 3D-QSAR study of ring-substituted-2/4-quinolinecarbaldehyde derivatives. Bioorg Med Chem 2006; 14(21): 7302-10.
[http://dx.doi.org/10.1016/j.bmc.2006.06.049] [PMID: 16843663]

[18]   Oliveira CGT, Miranda FF, Ferreira VF, Freitas CC, Rabello RF, Carballido JM, *et al.* Synthesis and antimicrobial evaluation of 3-hydrazino-naphthoquinones as analogs of lapachol. J Braz Chem Soc 2001; 12(3): 339-45.
[http://dx.doi.org/10.1590/S0103-50532001000300004]

[19]   El-Bendary ER, Goda FE, Maarouf AR, Badria FA. Synthesis and antimicrobial evaluation of 3-hydrazino-quinoxaline derivatives and their cyclic analogues. Sci Pharm 2004; 72(2): 175-85.
[http://dx.doi.org/10.3797/scipharm.aut-04-15]

[20]   Savini L, Chiasserini L, Travagli V, *et al.* New alpha-(N)-heterocyclichydrazones: evaluation of anticancer, anti-HIV and antimicrobial activity. Eur J Med Chem 2004; 39(2): 113-22.
[http://dx.doi.org/10.1016/j.ejmech.2003.09.012] [PMID: 14987820]

[21]   Küçükgüzel ŞG. S. R, H. E, M. K. Synthesis, characterization and antimicrobial evaluation of ethyl 2-arylhydrazono-3-oxobutyrates. Eur J Med Chem 1999; 34: 153-60.
[http://dx.doi.org/10.1016/S0223-5234(99)80048-8]

[22]   Turan-Zitoun G, Saglik BN, Cevik UA, Levent S, Ilgin S, Hussein W. Synthesis and antimicrobial activity of new 2-((1-furan-2-yl)ethylidene)hydrazono)-4-phenylthiazol-3(2H)-amine derivatives and their schiff bases with 4-nitrobenzaldehyde. Phosphorus Sulfur Silicon Relat Elem 2018; 193(11): 744-51.
[http://dx.doi.org/10.1080/10426507.2018.1513512]

[23]   Shaban MAE, Nasr AZ, Morgaan AE. Sterically controlled regiospecific heterocyclization of 3-hydrazino-5-methyl-1,2,4-triazino[5,6-b]indole to 10-methyl-1,2,4-triazolo[4',3':2,3]1,2,4-triazino-5,6-b]indoles. Farmaco 1999; 54: 800-9.
[http://dx.doi.org/10.1016/S0014-827X(99)00107-X] [PMID: 10668182]

[24]   El-Gazzar A-RBA, El-Enany MM, Mahmoud MN. Synthesis, analgesic, anti-inflammatory, and antimicrobial activity of some novel pyrimido[4,5-b]quinolin-4-ones. Bioorg Med Chem 2008; 16(6): 3261-73.
[http://dx.doi.org/10.1016/j.bmc.2007.12.012] [PMID: 18158248]

[25]   Nassar IF, Farargy AFE, Abdelrazek FM, Hamza Z. Synthesis of new uracil derivatives and their sugar hydrazones with potent antimicrobial, antioxidant and anticancer activities 2020.
[http://dx.doi.org/10.1080/15257770.2020.1736300]

[26]   Dewangan D, Nakhate K, Mishra A, Thakur AS, Rajak H, Dwivedi J, *et al.* Design, synthesis, and characterization of quinoxaline derivatives as a potent antimicrobial agent. J Heterocycl Chem 2019; 56(2): 566-78.
[http://dx.doi.org/10.1002/jhet.3431]

[27] Faidallah HM, Khan KA, Asiri AM. Synthesis and characterization of a novel series of benzenesulfonyl urea and thiourea derivatives of 2H-pyran and 2H-pyridine-2-ones as antibacterial, antimycobacterial and antifungal agents. Eur J Chem 2011; 2(2): 243-50.
[http://dx.doi.org/10.5155/eurjchem.2.2.243-250.257]

[28] Koca M, Ahmedzade M, Cukurovali A, Kazaz C. Studies on the synthesis and reactivity of novel benzofuran-2-yl-[3-methyl-3-phenylcyclobutyl] methanones and their antimicrobial activity. Molecules 2005; 10(7): 747-54.
[http://dx.doi.org/10.3390/10070747] [PMID: 18007342]

[29] Khan SA, Saleem K, Khan Z. Synthesis, structure elucidation and antibacterial evaluation of new steroidal -5-en-7-thiazoloquinoxaline derivatives. Eur J Med Chem 2008; 43(10): 2257-61.
[http://dx.doi.org/10.1016/j.ejmech.2007.09.022] [PMID: 18440096]

[30] Khan SA, Kumar P, Joshi R, Iqbal PF, Saleem K. Synthesis and *In vitro* antibacterial activity of new steroidal thiosemicarbazone derivatives. Eur J Med Chem 2008; 43(9): 2029-34.
[http://dx.doi.org/10.1016/j.ejmech.2007.12.004] [PMID: 18450330]

[31] Karali N, Gürsoy A, Kandemirli F, *et al.* Synthesis and structure-antituberculosis activity relationship of 1H-indole-2,3-dione derivatives. Bioorg Med Chem 2007; 15(17): 5888-904.
[http://dx.doi.org/10.1016/j.bmc.2007.05.063] [PMID: 17561405]

[32] Küçükgüzel I, Tatar E, Küçükgüzel ŞG, Rollas S, De Clercq E. Synthesis of some novel thiourea derivatives obtained from 5-[(4-aminophenoxy)methyl]-4-alkyl/aryl-2,4-dihydro-3H-1,2,4--riazole-3-thiones and evaluation as antiviral/anti-HIV and anti-tuberculosis agents. Eur J Med Chem 2008; 43(2): 381-92.
[http://dx.doi.org/10.1016/j.ejmech.2007.04.010] [PMID: 17583388]

[33] Yurttaş L, Özkay Y, Kaplancıklı ZA, Tunalı Y, Karaca H. Synthesis and antimicrobial activity of some new hydrazone-bridged thiazole-pyrrole derivatives. J Enzyme Inhib Med Chem 2013; 28(4): 830-5.
[http://dx.doi.org/10.3109/14756366.2012.688043] [PMID: 22651798]

[34] Abass M, Othman ES. Substituted quinolinones. Part 22. *In vitro* antimicrobial evaluation of some 4-hydroxy-1-methyl-3-pyrazolinylquinolin-2(1H)-ones as useful antibiotic intermediates. Res Chem Intermed 2015; 41(1): 117-25.
[http://dx.doi.org/10.1007/s11164-013-1174-4]

[35] Shruthi TG, Subramanian S, Eswaran S. Design, synthesis and study of antibacterial and antitubercular activity of quinoline hydrazone hybrids. Heterocycl Commun 2020; 26(1): 137-47.
[http://dx.doi.org/10.1515/hc-2020-0109]

[36] Al-Rasheed HH, Al Alshaikh M, Khaled JM, Alharbi NS, El-Faham A. Ultrasonic irradiation: Synthesis, characterization, and preliminary antimicrobial activity of novel series of 4, 6-disubstitute--1, 3, 5-triazine containing hydrazone derivatives. J Chem 2016; 2016: 1-9.

[37] Kaur AP, Gautam D. Ultrasound aided expedient synthesis, characterization and antimicrobial studies of fluorenyl-hydrazono-thiazole derivatives. Asian J Chem 2019; 31(10): 2245-8.
[http://dx.doi.org/10.14233/ajchem.2019.22118]

[38] Deshineni R, Velpula R, Koppu S, Pilli J, Chellamella G. One-pot multi-component synthesis of novel ethyl-2-(3-((2-(4-(4-aryl)thiazol-2-yl)hydrazono)methyl)-4-hydroxy/isobuto-yphenyl)-4-methylthiazole-5-carboxylate derivatives and evaluation of their *In vitro* antimicrobial activity. J Heterocycl Chem 2020; 57(3): 1361-7.
[http://dx.doi.org/10.1002/jhet.3872]

[39] Bhatt DJ, Kamdar GC, Parikh AR. Studies on sulfonylhydrazones: preparation and antimicrobial activity of arylsulfonyl-(4-substituted)-aceto/propiophenone hydrazones. J Indian Chem Soc 1984; 61(9): 788-9.

[40] Salama MA, Farrag HA. Some new naphthalenesulfonyl hydrazones and their antimicrobial activity. Egypt J Pharm Sci 1995; 36(1-6): 407-13.

[41] Shad RR, Shad VH, Parikh AR. Studies or arylsulfonyl hydrazones: preparation and antimicrobial

activity of arylsulfonyl-(2,5-dihydroxy-3-bromo)-aceto/enzophenone hydrazones. Indian J Pharm Sci 1993; 55: 204-6.

[42]   Loncle C, Brunel JM, Vidal N, Dherbomez M, Letourneux Y. Synthesis and antifungal activity of cholesterol-hydrazone derivatives. Eur J Med Chem 2004; 39(12): 1067-71.
[http://dx.doi.org/10.1016/j.ejmech.2004.07.005] [PMID: 15571868]

[43]   Nadaraia NS, Barbakadze NN, Kakhabrishvili ML, Mshvildadze VD. Synthesis and biological activity of hydrazones of 5α-steroids. Res J Pharm Biol Chem Sci 2019; 10(1): 238-43.

[44]   Metwally KA, Abdel-Aziz LM, Lashine SM, Husseiny MI, Badawy RH. Hydrazones of 2-ary--quinoline-4-carboxylic acid hydrazides: synthesis and preliminary evaluation as antimicrobial agents. Bioorg Med Chem 2006; 14(24): 8675-82.
[http://dx.doi.org/10.1016/j.bmc.2006.08.022] [PMID: 16949294]

[45]   Salgin-Gökşen U, Gökhan-Kelekçi N, Göktaş O, *et al.* 1-Acylthiosemicarbazides, 1,2,4-triazol--5(4H)-thiones, 1,3,4-thiadiazoles and hydrazones containing 5-methyl-2-benzoxazolinones: synthesis, analgesic-anti-inflammatory and antimicrobial activities. Bioorg Med Chem 2007; 15(17): 5738-51.
[http://dx.doi.org/10.1016/j.bmc.2007.06.006] [PMID: 17587585]

[46]   Ersan S, Nacak S, Berkem R. Synthesis and antimicrobial activity of N-[(alpha-methyl)benzyliden-]-(3-substituted-1,2,4-triazol-5-yl-thio) acetohydrazides. Farmaco 1998; 53(12): 773-6.
[http://dx.doi.org/10.1016/S0014-827X(98)00095-0] [PMID: 10230058]

[47]   Papakonstantinou-Garoufalias S, Pouli N, Marakos P, Chytyroglou-Ladas A. Synthesis antimicrobial and antifungal activity of some new 3 substituted derivatives of 4-(2,4-dichlorophenyl)-5-adama-tyl-1H-1,2,4-triazole. Farmaco 2002; 57(12): 973-7.
[http://dx.doi.org/10.1016/S0014-827X(02)01227-2] [PMID: 12564470]

[48]   Chornous VA, Bratenko MK, Vovk MV, Sidorchuk II. Synthesis and antimicrobial activity of pyrazole-4-carboxylic acid hydrazides and N-(pyrazol-4-ylcarbonyl)hydrazones of aromatic and heteroaromatic aldehydes. Pharm Chem J 2001; 35(4): 203-5.
[http://dx.doi.org/10.1023/A:1010432029236]

[49]   Rahman VPM, Mukhtar S, Ansari WH, Lemiere G. Synthesis, stereochemistry and biological activity of some novel long alkyl chain substituted thiazolidin-4-ones and thiazan-4-one from 10-undecenoic acid hydrazide. Eur J Med Chem 2005; 40(2): 173-84.
[http://dx.doi.org/10.1016/j.ejmech.2004.10.003] [PMID: 15694652]

[50]   Rollas S, Gulerman N, Erdeniz H. Synthesis and antimicrobial activity of some new hydrazones of 4-fluorobenzoic acid hydrazide and 3-acetyl-2,5-disubstituted-1,3,4-oxadiazolines. Farmaco 2002; 57(2): 171-4.
[http://dx.doi.org/10.1016/S0014-827X(01)01192-2] [PMID: 11902660]

[51]   Rao NR. Synthesis and antimicrobial evaluation of fluorinated chalcones. Asian J Chem 2004; 16(1): 525-7.

[52]   Kursun Aktar BS, Sicak Y, Tok TT, Oruc-Emre EE, Yaglioglu AS, Iyidogan AK, *et al.* Designing heterocyclic chalcones, benzoyl/sulfonyl hydrazones: An insight into their biological activities and molecular docking study. J Mol Struct 2020; 1211: 128059.
[http://dx.doi.org/10.1016/j.molstruc.2020.128059]

[53]   Fahmy HH, Kassem EMM, Abdou WAM, Mahmoud SA. Synthesis of some new indole derivatives of possible antimicrobial activity. Egypt J Pharm Sci 1998; 38(1-3): 13-22.

[54]   Masunari A, Tavares LC. A new class of nifuroxazide analogues: synthesis of 5-nitrothiophene derivatives with antimicrobial activity against multidrug-resistant *Staphylococcus aureus*. Bioorg Med Chem 2007; 15(12): 4229-36.
[http://dx.doi.org/10.1016/j.bmc.2007.03.068] [PMID: 17419064]

[55]   Küçükgüzel ŞG, Mazi A, Şahin F, Oztürk S, Stables J. Synthesis and biological activities of diflunisal hydrazide-hydrazones. Eur J Med Chem 2003; 38(11-12): 1005-13.

[http://dx.doi.org/10.1016/j.ejmech.2003.08.004] [PMID: 14642333]

[56]   Joshi SD, Vagdevi HM, Vaidya VP, Gadaginamath GS. Synthesis of new 4-pyrrol-1-yl benzoic acid hydrazide analogs and some derived oxadiazole, triazole and pyrrole ring systems: a novel class of potential antibacterial and antitubercular agents. Eur J Med Chem 2008; 43(9): 1989-96.
       [http://dx.doi.org/10.1016/j.ejmech.2007.11.016] [PMID: 18207286]

[57]   Shiradkar MR, Murahari KK, Gangadasu HR, *et al.* Synthesis of new S-derivatives of clubbed triazolyl thiazole as anti-Mycobacterium tuberculosis agents. Bioorg Med Chem 2007; 15(12): 3997-4008.
       [http://dx.doi.org/10.1016/j.bmc.2007.04.003] [PMID: 17442576]

[58]   Muluk MB, Ubale AS, Dhumal ST, Rehman NNMA, Dixit PP, Kharat KK, *et al.* Synthesis, anticancer and antimicrobial evaluation of new pyridyl and thiazolyl clubbed hydrazone scaffolds. Synth Commun 2020; 50(2): 243-55.
       [http://dx.doi.org/10.1080/00397911.2019.1692870]

[59]   Backes GL, Jursic BS, Neumann DM. Potent antimicrobial agents against azole-resistant fungi based on pyridinohydrazide and hydrazomethylpyridine structural motifs. Bioorg Med Chem 2015; 23(13): 3397-407.
       [http://dx.doi.org/10.1016/j.bmc.2015.04.040] [PMID: 25943854]

[60]   Kethireddy S, Eppakayala L, Maringanti TC. Synthesis and antibacterial activity of novel 5,6,7,8-tetrahydroimidazo[1,2-a]pyrimidine-2-carbohydrazide derivatives. Chemistry Central Journal 2015; 9(51).

[61]   Prasanna VL, Narender R. Synthesis and antimicrobial activity of new imidazole-hydrazone derivatives. Asian J Chem 2015; 27(10): 3605-8.
       [http://dx.doi.org/10.14233/ajchem.2015.18886]

[62]   Velayutham Pillai M, Rajeswari K, Vidhyasagar T. Stereoselective synthesis, spectral and antimicrobial studies of some cyanoacetyl hydrazones of 3-alkyl-2,6-diarylpiperidin-4-ones. J Mol Struct 2014; 1076: 174-82.
       [http://dx.doi.org/10.1016/j.molstruc.2014.07.050]

[63]   Rambabu N, Dubey PK, Ram B, Balram B. Synthesis, characterization and antimicrobial evaluation of (E)-N'-[(1-(2-methoxy-6-pentadecylbenzyl)-1H-1, 2, 3-triazol-4-yl]- methylene)benzohydrazide derivatives. Asian J Chem 2016; 28(1): 175-80.
       [http://dx.doi.org/10.14233/ajchem.2016.19310]

[64]   Shakdofa MME, Shtaiwi MH, Morsy N, Abdel-rassel TMA. Metal complexes of hydrazones and their biological, analytical and catalytic applications: A review. Main Group Chem 2014; 13(3): 187-218.
       [http://dx.doi.org/10.3233/MGC-140133]

CHAPTER 4

Current Scenario of Anti-Leishmanial Drugs and Treatment

Priyanka H. Mazire[1] and **Amit Roy**[1,*]

[1] *Department of Biotechnology, Savitribai Phule Pune University, Ganeshkhind Road, Pune-411007, India*

Abstract: Leishmaniasis is a neglected tropical disease caused by a protozoan parasite of the genus *Leishmania*, mainly associated with the lack of community hygiene and poverty in the developing countries. Leishmaniasis can be cured but the emergence of drug resistance makes it difficult to completely eradicate the disease. Even after so many years, there is still no vaccine available against leishmaniasis. Therefore, treatment of the disease is mainly dependent on the available therapeutic drugs. However, the current chemotherapeutic drugs have several drawbacks such as high toxicity, less efficacy, high cost and emergence of drug resistance, *etc*. So, to boost the elimination of disease, development of newer therapeutic agents is imperative. As all this is very well-known, including the current anti-leishmanial drugs with their adverse effects, the authors state that the main objective of this book chapter is to present an overview of the disease, its different clinical forms and the diagnostic tools available for the detection of the disease. Natural sources such as plants and microorganisms have shown great results against *Leishmania* species over the years, indicating that they may be considered as therapeutic agents. Hereafter, potent investigational drugs obtained from the natural sources such as medicinal plants and microorganisms are also discussed in this book chapter.

Keywords: Amastigotes, Amphotericin B, Cutaneous leishmaniasis, Endophytes, Immunological tests, Kinetoplast, Leishmaniasis, Macroalgae, Miltefosine, Molecular diagnostic methods, Mucocutaneous leishmaniasis, Paromomycin, Pentamidine, Pentavalent antimonials, Post Kala-azar Dermal Leishmaniasis (PKDL), Promastigotes, Secondary metabolites, Serological diagnosis, Visceral leishmaniasis or Kala-azar.

INTRODUCTION

Leishmaniasis, a vector-borne disease caused by Trypanosomatid protozoans of the genus *Leishmania,* is classified as a neglected tropical disease having high

---
* **Corresponding author Amit Roy:** Department of Biotechnology, Savitribai Phule Pune University, Ganeshkhind Road, Pune-411007, India; Tel: 000 0000 0000; E-mail:amitavik@gmail.com

Atta-ur-Rahman, *FRS* and M. Iqbal Choudhary (Eds.)

epidemiological and clinical diversity [1, 2]. The disease is endemic and more prevalent in developing countries. The disease is widely spread in about 98 countries located in South and the Central America; Southern Europe, Africa, Middle East, Central Asia and Indian subcontinent. However, more than 90% of the new cases are mainly reported in 13 countries; namely, Afghanistan, Algeria, Bangladesh, Bolivia, Brazil, Columbia, Ethiopia, India, Iran, Perú, South Sudan, Sudan and Syria [1, 3]. Approximately 700,000 to 1 million new cases occur annually. In accordance with WHO (2018), both visceral leishmaniasis (VL) and cutaneous leishmaniasis (CL) are endemic in 68 countries. VL is found to be endemic in 9 countries and CL is endemic in 21 countries. The disease is primarily associated with developing countries that have poor socio-economic status and where problems such as malnutrition, lack of resources, poor housing and sanitary conditions, *etc.* are a major concern. Environmental changes and population mobility are also considered as major risk factors (WHO, 2020) [4].

More than 20 species of *Leishmania* are known to be responsible for the disease in humans [5]. Leishmaniasis is reported to be endemic in Asia, Africa, the Mediterranean, Europe and Middle East. The five-common species of *Leishmania*, responsible for leishmaniasis are *Leishmania tropica, Leishmania major, Leishmania aethiopica, Leishmania infantum* and *Leishmania donovani* in Asia, Africa, Middle East and Southern Europe. While, more than six species are responsible for leishmaniasis including *Leishmania mexicana, Leishmania braziliensis, Leishmania amazonensis, Leishmania infantum (Leishmania chagasi), Leishmania panamensis, Leishmania guyanensis, etc.* in South and the Central America [5]. The three known clinical forms of the disease are i) cutaneous leishmaniasis (CL); ii) mucocutaneous leishmaniasis (MCL) and iii) visceral leishmaniasis (VL) [4]. In accordance with WHO, more than 95% of global VL cases were reported in 10 countries: Brazil, Ethiopia, China, India, Iraq, Nepal, Kenya, Somalia, Sudan and South Sudan in the year 2018. While, 11 countries such as Afghanistan, Algeria, Bolivia, Brazil, Colombia, the Islamic Republic of Iran, Iraq, Pakistan, Perú, the Syrian Arab Republic and Tunisia reported more than 5000 cases of CL, this together accounts for 85% of global reported CL incidence [4, 6]. India, Bangladesh and Nepal have established a collaborative association for elimination of this disease in 2005. It was renewed in 2017 and as the goal was not fulfilled, the program has been extended. The disease is still persistent with high endemicity, mainly in certain regions of India. Moreover, the incidence of VL has increased in Latin America; migration has been one of the sources for increase in number of cases. In accordance to the recent report by the Pan American Health Organization (PAHO) and the World Health Organization (WHO), incidence of VL is expanding geographically. Therefore, the VL elimination program has been extended up to 2020 to facilitate the complete eradication of the disease from the South-Asia region. In addition to the three mentioned clinical forms of the disease, two major complications are associated with this disease. Post Kala-azar Dermal Leishmaniasis (PKDL) is a complication of VL that mainly occurs in East Africa and India. It is reported that about 5-10% of VL patients develop PKDL [6]. Moreover, HIV-VL co-infection is another complication associated with this disease. In the last few years, reported cases of *Leishmania*-HIV co-infection in endemic areas have increased. VL is considered as an opportunistic infection associated with HIV. Individuals with HIV are particularly more prone to VL infection due to suppressed immune response, leading to higher relapse and mortality rates. HIV-VL co-infection rates are high in Brazil, Ethiopia and Bihar in India. Thus, PKDL and HIV-VL co-infection are major complications of VL that affect the control of leishmaniasis (WHO, 2020).

At present, there is no effective vaccine against leishmaniasis. Therefore, treatment of leishmaniasis is entirely dependent on chemotherapeutic drugs. Pentavalent antimonials, miltefosine, paromomycin, pentamidine and liposomal amphotericin B are widely used drugs for treatment of leishmaniasis [2, 7]. However, the available drugs are toxic; have severe adverse effects and drug resistance is another problem which limits the use of these drugs [2, 7]. Therefore, the development of novel, effective, and less toxic anti-leishmanial agents having reduced side effects is the major priority. Thus, in this chapter an overview of the disease, existing treatment options, diagnostic assays currently available for leishmaniasis and the status of present anti-leishmanial drugs are highlighted.

History of Leishmaniasis

The history of leishmaniasis dates to 2,500 B.C. based on the primitive evidences reported in the ancient writings and recent molecular findings from ancient archaeological material. These reports suggest that the origin of genus *Leishmania* can be traced back in the Mesozoic era. Moreover, subsequent geographical distribution and initial evidence of the disease were reported in ancient times. First account of the infection was identified in the Middle Age, and the discovery of *Leishmania* parasites as causative agents of leishmaniasis was reported in modern times. After observing *Leishmania* organism for the first time in 1885, Russian military surgeon Peter Borovsky found out that the organism was a protozoan which was also confirmed by Wright in 1903. During this time, William Leishman and Charles Donovan described the agent responsible for VL. Leishman observed that VL-infected patients had fever and an enlarged spleen. Further, he also observed the samples from the patients under the microscope using Romanowsky method for staining and he stated that it was something he had never seen before [8]. *L. donovani* was the first identified *Leishmania* species taking its name from William Leishman (genera) and Charles Donovan (species), which was given by Ross with the aim to give credit to their studies [8, 9]. The detailed history of *Leishmania* with timeline is as follows (Table **1**) [9, 10]:

Table 1. History of leishmaniasis.

Century/Year	Major Event
2,500 to 1,500 B.C	First description of conspicuous lesions similar to current CL lesions.
First century A.D	Evidence for the presence of cutaneous form of the disease and cutaneous lesions called Balakh sore were described. During 15th -16th century, the CL was notified as "valley sickness", "Andean sickness", or "white leprosy".
1571	One of the first accounts of MCL was given by the Spanish chronicler Pedro Pizarro.
1756	Scottish physician and naturalist, Alexander Russell published a detailed clinical description of the disease providing details about the development of lesion.
1764	Cosme Bueno first reported the probable role of phlebotomine sand flies in disease transmission.
19th century	The first outbreak of kala-azar was recorded in 1824/25 in the village of Mahomedpore, Bengal, India. Description of clinical symptoms kala-azar by Indian physicians was reported. The term kala-azar (meaning 'back disease') was coined in the late 19th century.
1898	First accurate description of the causative agent of oriental sore, with reference to Protozoa was given by Borovsky.
1901	William Boog Leishman identified the organisms as "trypanosomes" from the spleen smears of Indian patients who died of Dum-dum fever. Charles Donovan confirmed the presence of what became known as Leishman-Donovan bodies in the smears from Indian patients.
1903	Ronald Ross published a paper in 1903 about the discovery of the ovoid bodies found by Leishman and Donovan in spleen pulp of patients with chronic pyrexia and splenomegaly. He proposed the name of the parasite as *Leishmania donovani* for Leishman-Donovan bodies.
1907	Patton provided evidence of the presence of Leishman-Donovan bodies in peripheral blood lymphocytes and its flagellated forms in the sand-fly's gut.
1909	*Leishmania* parasites were first described independently.
1914	Russian physicians Wassily L. Yakimoff and Nathan I. Schokhor suggested classifying *L. tropica* into the two subspecies *L. tropica minor* and *L. tropica major* based on the size of the parasites found in skin lesions.
1916	*Leishmania brazilienses* was corrected as *L. braziliensis* by Alfredo A. da Matta.
1942	Swaminath and colleagues demonstrated the process of *Leishmania* transmission to humans by sand-flies using a group of volunteers.
1948	Hoare demonstrated *Leishmania* circulation in sand-flies, indicating the flagellates being set free and multiplying in the sand-fly intestine.

(Table 1) cont.....

Century/Year	Major Event
1949	Kirk classified *Leishmania* according to their morphology, culture characteristics, clinical and epidemiological aspects of infections in human and other natural hosts, cross-immunity, serological tests, and xeno-differentiation. He proposed a complete nomenclature of the *Leishmania* genus and their synonyms.
1953	*Leishmania* species were characterized, like *L. mexicana*.
1972	Localized cutaneous leishmaniasis (LCL) and MCL causing species *L. amazonensis* and *L. panamensis* were characterized.
1990	WHO categorized the *Leishmania* species into three subgenera: *Leishmania*, *Sauroleishmania*, and *Viannia*.
1994	Shaw proposed that the genus *Leishmania* encompasses 30 species infecting mammals and 21 species infecting humans.
2002	New *Leishmania* species *L. lindenbergi* was characterized.
2011	Research carried out by Kuhls *et al*. (2011) and Leblois *et al* (2011) *et al*. led to import of *L. infantum* to Latin America as a suitable vector was identified over there.
2014	Lukeš and colleagues stated that Trypanosomatidae family consists of 13 genera: *Trypanosoma, Phytomonas, Leishmania, Leptomonas, Crithidia, Blastocrithidia, Herpetomonas, Sergeia, Wallacemonas, Blechomonas, Angomonas, Strigomonas, and Kentomonas*.

Morphology of *Leishmania* Parasites

Morphologically, there are two forms of *Leishmania* parasites, the promastigote form is present in sand-fly vector and the amastigote form in the mammalian host. Promastigotes are elongated with a central nucleus and a terminal kinetoplast, measuring up to 15-30 μm in length and 5 μm in width. The kinetoplast DNA (kDNA) is a dense network of circular DNA within the large mitochondrion. The promastigotes are characterized by the presence of flagellum, required for forward movement of parasites and for its attachment to the microvilli in the gut of sand-fly. Promastigotes are sub-classified into five types: procyclic, nectomonad, leptomonad, haptomonad and metacyclic promastigotes. Metacyclic promastigotes are the infective stage and are successfully transmitted within the human host [7, 11]. On the other hand, there is absence of flagellum in amastigotes. Amastigotes are round-shaped, have a nucleus and a kinetoplast, measuring about 3-6 μm in length and 1-3 μm in breadth. Amastigotes are intracellular forms that reside within macrophages and other mononuclear phagocytic cells such as dendritic cells, neutrophils and fibroblasts. The amastigotes divide within host immune cells [7, 11] (Fig. **1**).

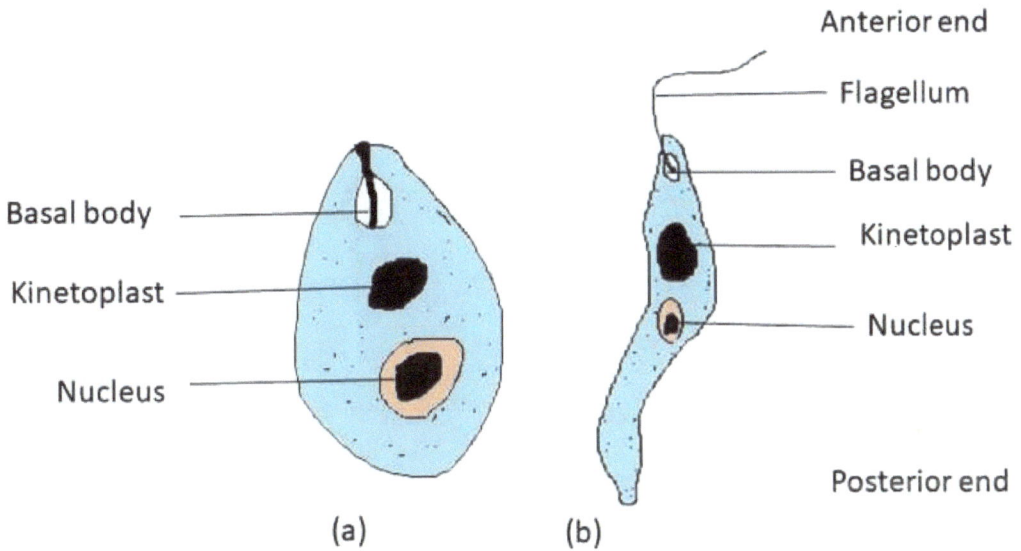

Fig. (1). Diagrammatic representation of morphology of Leishmania parasites: **(a)** amastigote form – a flagellar and round in shape **(b)** promastigote form: it has flagellum and is elongated in shape.

Lifecycle of *Leishmania* Parasite

The female sand-fly of genus *Phlebotomus* or *Lutzomyia* is the only vector responsible for transmission of leishmaniasis [12]. During the host-infective stage, the sand-fly takes a blood meal and injects the metacyclic promastigotes into the mammalian host. The metacyclic promastigotes are then phagocytosed by macrophages. On the other hand, the diagnostic stage involves the transformation of the metacyclic promastigotes into amastigotes inside macrophages. Within the macrophage phagolysosome, metacyclic promastigotes transform into non-motile amastigotes. Amastigotes multiply and subsequently invade the immune cells such as dendritic cells, neutrophils and fibroblasts; therefore, the parasite's replication continues [7]. The amastigote-infected macrophages are ingested into the sand-fly after it takes a blood meal from an infected mammalian host. The amastigotes are then released from the cells, transforming into promastigotes in the midgut of the sand-fly. Promastigotes multiply in the midgut and then transform into infective metacyclic promastigotes. Ultimately, the metacyclic promastigotes are injected into the mammalian host and this cycle continues [7] (Fig. **2**). The period between the time of the initial infection and the appearance of clinical symptoms, generally varies from 3 to 6 months, but in certain cases it may exceed up to two years.

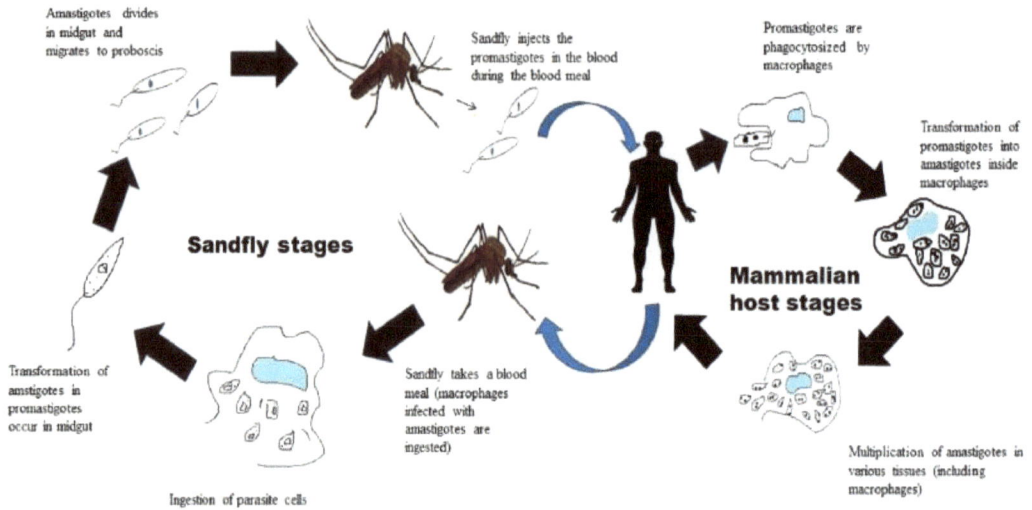

Fig. (2).   Lifecycle of Leishmania Parasites: The mammalian host stage includes ingestion of the promastigotes in the host blood, transformation of the promastigote into amastigote forms in the macrophage cells and finally multiplication of amastigotes inside various tissues. The conversion of amastigotes into promastigotes upon ingestion of infected macrophages with amastigotes occurs during the sand-fly stages.

Classification of Leishmaniasis

Leishmaniasis is a parasitic infection caused by flagellated parasitic protozoa of the *Leishmania* genus spread through the bite of sand-flies [7, 13]. Leishmaniasis mainly affects to poor people [14]. Clinical manifestations of leishmaniasis occur under three main categories *i.e.* cutaneous, mucocutaneous and visceral leishmaniasis (WHO, 2020).

I. **Cutaneous Leishmaniasis (CL):** CL is the most common form of leishmaniasis. It is caused by the *Leishmania* species such as, *Leishmania major* and *Leishmania tropica* in India, Ethiopia, Sudan and Iran. Multiple species such as *L. peruviana, L. braziliensis, L. amazonensis, L. venezuelensis, L. guyanensis and L. panamensis* are the causative agents of the disease in Central and South American countries [7, 12, 13]. It is reported that approximately between 600.000 to1 million new cases occur worldwide annually. The major characteristics of CL are skin lesions, papules which progresses to a nodule over the duration of weeks to months with a central crust underneath, skin thickening at multiple sites on the facial skin and the outer surface of the membranous tissue [12, 15]. The size of the lesions may vary from a few millimeters to centimeters in diameter. Healing of these lesions require several months or years and may leave a scar and permanent alterations in the skin pigmentation [4, 12].

II. **Mucocutaneous Leishmaniasis (MCL):** MCL is caused by *L. braziliensis, L. panamensis* and *L. amazonensis*. Individuals infected with *L. braziliensis* develop metastatic lesions, in which the amastigotes spread through the blood and lymphatic system from skin to the naso-oropharyngeal mucosa causing mucosal leishmaniasis. Incubation period persists from 1 to 3 months, but it may occur after many years of initial cutaneous ulcer has been healed [4, 12, 13]. More than 90% of MCL cases occur in Bolivia, Brazil, Ethiopia and Perú [4].

III. **Visceral Leishmaniasis (VL):** VL, also known as Kala-azar, is the most severe form of leishmaniasis, as the parasites disseminate to vital organs such as bone marrow, spleen and liver. In fact, it can be fatal if patients are not treated. It is caused by *L. donovani* and *L. infantum*. Considering that it results from systemic and progressive infection of macrophages in the reticuloendothelial systems or lymphoid organs, it is characterized by hepatosplenomegaly, fever, anemia, leucopenia and hypergammaglobulinemia [4, 7, 12]. The period between the time of the initial infection and the appearance of clinical symptoms generally varies from 3 to 6 months, but in certain cases it may exceed up to two years. There are evidences suggesting that pathogenesis is immunologically mediated; in fact, abnormal levels of interleukin IL-10 have been reported in the peripheral blood of VL patients [16]. Most cases occur in Brazil, East Africa and in India. About 50.000 to 90.000 new cases of VL occur worldwide annually. As reported by WHO (2018), more than 95% of new cases occurred in 10 countries: Brazil, China, Ethiopia, India, Iraq, Kenya, Nepal, Somalia, South Sudan and Sudan [4, 7, 12].

Post kala-azar dermal leishmaniasis (PKDL): This type of disease occurs after the treatment of VL. It is characterized by the presence of macular, papular or nodular rash usually on face, upper arms, and other parts of the body [4, 7, 12]. It occurs in East Africa and in India and 5-10% of patients with kala-azar are reported to develop the disease. It usually occurs 6 months to 1 year or more after kala-azar has apparently been cured, it can occur earlier too [4, 7]. Ganguly *et al.* (2010) and Katara *et al.* (2011) have reported that along with IL-10, immune regulator FoxP3, are responsible for the disease [17, 18]. It is also reported that macrophage polarization possesses phenotype M2 (alternatively activated macrophage) in human PKDL lesions [19]. PKDL is often described in three grades based on the density and spread of lesions. In grade one, the lesions are scattered but restricted to face, grade two is characterized by lesions on the face and upper part of the trunk and grade three is described with lesions all over the body [16]. There is spontaneous healing of patients with grade one and mild grade PKDL, with careful follow-up [20].

Clinical Symptoms

Cutaneous Leishmaniasis: The major symptom associated with CL is the presence of skin lesions.

Skin Lesions: A lesion develops at the site of sand-fly bite. Formation of plaques, papules and nodule lengthwise with skin thickening at multiple sites on face and the outer surface of the membranous tissue are the characteristics of CL [7, 21].

Diffuse Cutaneous Leishmaniasis: This is characterized by an initial skin lesion that spreads and affects multiple different areas of the body [21]. Another characteristic is a poor immune response [21, 22].

Leishmaniasis Recidivans: There is recurrence of a skin lesion years after the initial lesion healed. This illness often develops on the face, specifically the cheek, with a new ulcer or papule establishing over or near the scar of the old lesion [21, 22].

Mucocutaneous Leishmaniasis: Persistent stuffiness in nose or bleeding from the nose can be the first signs of the disease [21, 22].

Metastatic Lesions: The parasites spread through the blood and lymphatic system from the skin to the naso-oropharyngeal mucosa and cause mucosal leishmaniasis [21, 22].

Visceral Leishmaniasis: The major symptoms of this condition are repeated bouts of prolonged fever, weakness, significant pancytopenia (low levels of blood cells- red blood cells, white blood cells and platelets). The other symptoms are diarrhea, fatigue, paleness of the skin (pallor), shortness of breath, light-headedness, dizziness and a fast or irregular heartbeat [21, 22].

Pyrexia: Continuous or discontinuous fever during initial phase of the disease.

Skin: The skin over the entire body become dry, rough, and harsh with often darkened skin. Hair tends to be brittle and falls off, and in few cases, cutaneous lesions may appear.

Cachexia: Sudden weight loss or even severe wasting of the body.

Splenomegaly: The spleen shows various degrees of enlargement. In severe infection spleen, may extend below the level of the umbilicus and the capsule covering spleen is often thickened due to perisplenitis.

Hepatomegaly: Liver is less frequently enlarged as compared to the spleen in kala-azar. The Kuffer's cells are greatly enlarged both in size and number as their cytoplasm gets packed with large number of parasites. Normally jaundice does not appear in Kala-azar if the liver is greatly damage.

Changes in Bone Marrow: *Leishmania* infection causes hyperplasia, which is an anomalous increase in the number of normal cells and a profound disturbance in the hemopoietic activities of the bone marrow. Leucopenia (neutropenia) and monocytosis occur, which reduces the resistance of the body against other infectious agents.

Changes in Lymph Nodes: The lymphatic glands are frequently enlarged.

Changes in Intestine: Intestinal lesion may appear as a secondary infection.

Anaemia: Profound anemia may occur in kala-azar patients. The possible reason for this is hemolysis and destruction of Red Blood Cells (RBC) in spleen of the patient.

Post Kala-azar Dermal Leishmaniasis: Skin lesions with raised rashes on the face, buttocks, arms and legs are common. Presence of macules (multiple, flat discolored areas of skin) and nodules is the characteristic of PKDL. The skin lesions eventually turn into plaques or nodules on the face.

Diagnosis of Leishmaniasis

The important aspect for control of leishmaniasis involves early diagnosis and treatment of the disease. In addition, accurate diagnosis of the disease is important because other diseases might have similar clinical symptoms to that of CL and VL. For confirmed diagnosis of leishmaniasis, clinical signs and available serological tests (such as rapid diagnostic tests) are considered [14]. Following are the diagnostic measurements for the different forms of leishmaniasis.

Diagnosis of Cutaneous and Mucocutaneous leishmaniasis

Clinical Signs: The clinical signs of CL are broad and may be comparable to other skin conditions, such as staphylococcal or streptococcal infection, leprosy, fungal infection, sarcoidosis and tropical ulcer. Diagnostic confirmation is necessary in case of CL as clinical symptoms of CL lack specificity [14].

Parasitological/Serological Tests: These methods are widely used to visualize parasites in the infected tissues. Microscopic examination of Giemsa-stained lesion smears, scrapings or impression smears is the primary method for the detection of amastigotes. As the parasite load is usually low in CL and MCL, combination of PCR method with the microscopic examination may increase the sensitivity of detection. Parasites culture (obtained from the biopsy samples) in suitable conditions and culture medium is useful for confirming and is useful for species identification and characterization [14]. Inoculation of *Leishmania* parasites in animal models is another method used for diagnosis. In this method, parasites obtained from biological samples are inoculated into footpad, nose, or tail base of the mice [14].

Molecular Diagnostic Tools: Polymerase chain reaction (PCR) has been successfully used for the detection of *Leishmania* species [23 - 25]. Kumar *et al.* (2007) reported *L. tropica* as the causative agent for Indian CL through species characterization by internal transcribed spacer 1 (ITS1) PCR-restriction fragment length polymorphism (RFLP), kDNA-PCR, and immunofluorescence. They also showed that kDNA PCR was more sensitive (96.6%) as compared to ITS1 PCR (sensitivity: 82.75%), thus facilitating diagnosis and species identification [26]. Multilocus Enzyme Electrophoresis (MLEE) is a method that relies on isolation of parasites followed by culture. The different species are determined on set of proteins obtained in a pH-dependent gel electrophoresis [14].

Diagnosis of Visceral Leishmaniasis: An accurate diagnostic test that can identify active VL *versus* asymptomatic disease is an important determination that aims to control this serious disease [14].

Parasitological/Serological Tests: Microscopic observation of parasites is still considered as a standard method for VL diagnosis [27]. The main sources of samples selected for microscopic observation of parasites are lymph nodes, bone marrow and spleen. Spleen aspirate has highest sensitivity for microscopic detection [14]. *In vitro* cultivation of *Leishmania* promastigotes (obtained from tissue biopsies/whole blood) is another method for VL diagnosis and species identification by molecular methods [28]. Intravenous or intraperitoneal inoculation of parasites in mice or golden hamsters is another method for diagnosis of VL.

Molecular Diagnostic Tools : Different types of PCR assays such as species-specific PCR (29), single-strand conformation polymorphisms (SSCP) [30], and restriction fragment length polymorphism (RFLP) [31] analysis have been developed for the detection and differentiation of parasites. MLEE is thought to be the only method that can discriminate all species of human leishmaniasis. However, this method requires expertise and its use for VL diagnosis is restricted to few laboratories across the world [14].

Different target sequences for real time-PCR-based assays include Heat Shock Protein 70 kDa (HSP70) [32], DNA polymerase [33], glucose-6-phosphate dehydrogenase (G6PD) [34], glucose phosphate isomerase (GPI) [35], mannose phosphate isomerase (MPI), 6-phosphogluconate dehydrogenase (6PGD), tryparedoxin peroxidase [36], ribosomal RNA genes, kinetoplast DNA (kDNA) [37], mini exon-derived RNA (medRNA) [38], *etc.*

Another technique that is used for diagnosis purpose includes nucleic acid sequence-based amplification (NASBA); it is more sensitive than conventional PCR [39]. Loop mediated isothermal amplification (LAMP) is a recently developed rapid and highly specific assay, which has been validated for diagnosis of VL & PKDL in several countries [44, 41]. Recent study by Campos-Neto *et al.* (2020) discussed a novel test for VL detection. This protein-based test detects six proteins namely iron superoxide dismutase, tryparedoxin, nuclear transport factor 2, MaoC family dehydratase, peptidyl-prolyl cis-trans isomerase, and malate dehydrogenase from *L.* infantum (chagasi) and *L. donovani* from the urine sample.

Immunological Test: These tests detect antigen in the given sample. Tests such as rk39 dip test [42, 43], enzyme-linked immunosorbent assay (ELISA), western blot and indirect fluorescent antibody (IFA) and direct agglutination test (DAT) [44] have been extensively used in endemic areas for the diagnosis of the disease. The rapid diagnostic test rk39 is based on a recombinant 39-amino acid repeat antigen and is the preferred choice in diagnosis of VL due to its high specificity and sensitivity. K39 is a conserved epitope of amastigotes of *L. infantum* and is therefore employed for detection of parasite in the host body. However, there are several limitations for using this test. It cannot distinguish an active VL infection from those that have occurred in the past. Also, it did not yield good results with low infection intensity [14].

Treatment for Leishmaniasis

The treatment methods for leishmaniasis depend on various factors such as the host immune system, causative *Leishmania* species affecting the host and the mode of parasite transmission. Important determinants for disease treatment include the host immune response, some factors related to treatment such as dosage, period, and factors related to the parasite, such as intrinsic sensitivity of the species and lack of resistance to the medication [7]. The extent of concomitant infection should be found out, as this might influence the choice of therapy or supportive treatment. In accordance to the WHO guidelines, anti-leishmanial medicines and treatment regimens to be used in patients with leishmaniasis are described in Table **2** [21]:

Table 2. Treatment for Leishmaniasis.

Cutaneous leishmaniasis	
Drugs	**Doses**
Paromomycin ointments	Formulation of 15 % drug plus 12% ointment methyl benzethonium chloride, twice daily for up to 20 days.
Pentavalent antimonials	20 mg/kg Sb5+ per day for 20 days.
Pentamidine	Dose of 3–4 mg/kg on alternate days, for a total of three or four doses is reported to be effective.
Miltefosine	Dose of 2 mg/kg/day for 28 days is effective against cutaneous leishmaniasis caused by *L. panamensis* (70–90 % cure rate) but has limited effect against *L. braziliensis* and *L. mexicana*.
Ketoconazole	Effective (76–90 %) in certain regions when administered at a dose of 600 mg daily for 28 days in *L. panamensis* and *L. mexicana*.
Local Therapy	
Therapy	**Procedure**
Thermotherapy	One or two applications of localized heat (50 °C for 30 s) at the site of lesion. This treatment was reported to be as effective as intra-lesional pentavalent antimonials (Sb^{5+}) with CR of 70 % in Afghanistan (*L. tropica)* and more effective than pentavalent antimonials in *L. major* cutaneous leishmaniasis
Cryotherapy	Cryotherapy with liquid nitrogen (–195 °C) applied once or twice to the lesion weekly up to 6 weeks has also been reported to be effective.
Mucocutaneous leishmaniasis	
Drugs	**Doses**
Pentavalent antimonials	Treatment regimen consists of 20 mg/kg/day for 30 days
Miltefosine	Dose of 2.5–3.3 mg/kg/day for 4 weeks is reported to be effective.
AmB deoxycholate	Dose of 0.7–1.0 mg/kg is 80–90 % effective. It requires intravenous infusion and strict monitoring of renal function.
Liposomal amphotericin B	Dose of 2–3 mg/kg for at least 20 days gives similar results as AmB deoxycholate and also fewer adverse events compare to AmB deoxycholate
Visceral leishmaniasis	
Drugs	**Doses**
Pentavalent antimonials	Daily injection of 20 mg/kg/ body weight of Sb^{5+}. Injections were usually given for 28–30 days.
Miltefosine	A dose of 2.5 mg/kg per day for 28 days to children aged 2–11 years and for subjects aged 12 years and above at a daily dose of 50 mg, 100 mg and 150 mg for those with body weight < 25 kg, for 25–50 kg body weight and for > 50 kg body weight, respectively, during 28 days

(Table 2) cont.....

Cutaneous leishmaniasis	
Drugs	**Doses**
Paromomycin	Effective in Indian visceral leishmaniasis at a dose of 15 mg/kg paromomycin sulfate (11 mg base) for 21 days (cure rate of 93–95 %). In East Africa, the efficacy was 85 % when increased dose of 20 mg/kg/day (15 mg base) for 21 days was administered.
Amphotericin B deoxycholate	A dose of 0.75–1.0 mg/kg/day, daily or on alternate days for 15–20 doses was reported to be 99 % effective in India.
Liposomal amphotericin B	Most extensively used formulation in visceral leishmaniasis. It is given as a dose of 3–4 mg/kg/day to a total dose of 15–24 mg/kg. In India, a total dose of 10 mg/kg results in a cure rate of > 95 %.
Combination therapy	Combination therapy of two sequential administrations, with either L-AmB (5 mg/kg, single infusion) plus 7 days miltefosine (dosage as mentioned above) or L-AmB (5 mg/kg, single infusion) plus 10 days paromomycin (11 mg/kg base), and co-administration of 10 days miltefosine plus 10 days paromomycin have been reported to be effective in India.
Post kala-azar dermal leishmaniasis (PKDL)	
Drugs	**Doses**
Combination therapy	In India, clinical experience with treatment for up to 4 months with intermittent AmB deoxycholate (20 days on, 20 days off) or 3 months of continuous miltefosine has been effective.
Leishmaniasis-HIV co-infection	
Drugs	**Doses**
Liposomal amphotericin B (L-AmB)	As WHO guidelines recommends, a dose of 4 mg/kg of L-AmB is applied ten times reaching a total dose of 40 mg/kg.
Combination therapy	LAmB is given at doses of 30 mg/kg on alternate days, along with oral miltefosine for 14 days. A trial in Bihar, India demonstrated that a combination of L-AmB and miltefosine in HIV-VL co-infected patients reduced the relapse rate.

CURRENTLY USED ANTI-LEISHMANIAL DRUGS

Over the past several years, a very limited number of drugs have been available in the market for the treatment of leishmaniasis. These drugs are used as first and second line drugs. Those administered firstly during the treatment due to their less toxicity and high efficacy are known as first line drugs. Amphotericin B, miltefosine and pentavalent antimonials are first line drugs for the treatment of leishmaniasis. The overview of the currently used anti-leishmanial drugs is summarized in Table **3** and their chemical structure is mentioned in Fig. (**3**).

Table 3. Mechanism of action of the current antileishmanial drugs.

Drug	Mechanism of action	Toxicity	Resistance	Refs
Sodium stibogluconate **Meglumine antimoniate**	Affects fatty acid–oxidation, glycolysis and ATP formation. Causes oxidation of nitrogenous bases, leading to DNA damage, thus inhibiting the growth of parasites.	Severe cardiotoxicity, nephrotoxicity, pancreatitis and hepatotoxicity.	Common in Bihar, India (>65 %)	[7, 45]
Pentamidine	Inhibits active transport system as well as inhibits transcription process.	Severe hyperglycemia, myocarditis hypotension and tachycardia.	Not reported	[7, 46]
Paromomycin	Binds to 30S ribosomal subunit, interfering with the initiation of protein synthesis, leading to the accumulation of the initiation complex.	Severe ototoxicity, nephrotoxicity and seldom hepatotoxicity.	Reported in laboratory strains.	[7, 45, 46]
Miltefosine	Exact mechanism of miltefosine is not known. It inhibits the synthesis of phosphatidylcholine and cytochrome C is postulated.	Hepatotoxicity, nephrotoxicity and teratogenicity (in pregnant women)	Reported in laboratory strains	[7, 45 - 47]
Amphotericin B **Amphotericin B deoxycholate** **Liposomal amphotericin (L-AmB)**	Interacts with ergosterol, causes the formation of transmembrane AmB, resulting in membrane depolarization and in concentration-dependent cell killing. - It increases the bioavailability of AmB.	Infusion-related pyrexia and chills. Severe nephrotoxicity, thrombophlebitis and hypokalaemia. Mild nephrotoxicity, chills and fever during infusion.	Not reported Reported in laboratory strains. Not reported	[9, 45, 46, 48]

Amphotericin B

Amphotericin B (AmB) is a polyene antifungal that was first isolated from *Streptomyces nodosus*, in Venezuela, year 1955. It is used as a first line drug to treat VL throughout the world [49]. Among the different formulations of AmB, Liposomal Amphotericin B (L-AmB) is most widely used because of its efficacy and low toxicity. L-AmB is a formulation of a bilayer liposome, which is composed of phospholipids and cholesterol, where AmB is intercalated within the membrane.

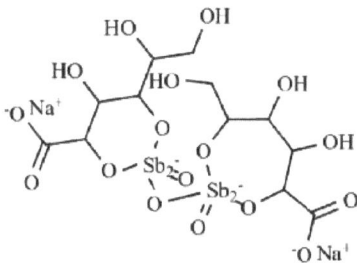

Sodium stibogluconate

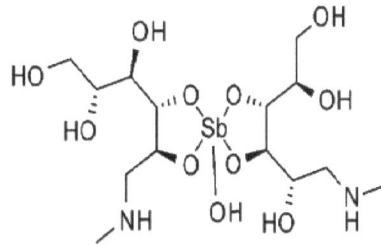

Meglumine antimoniate

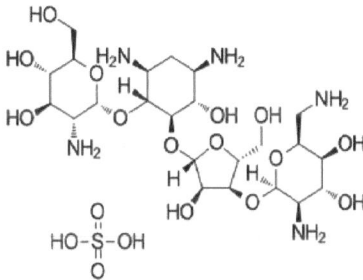

Paromomycin

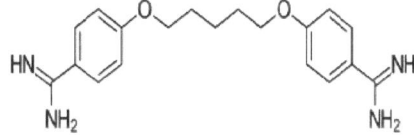

Pentamidine

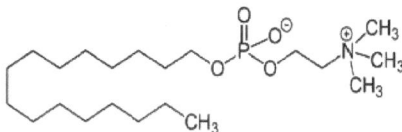

Miltefosine

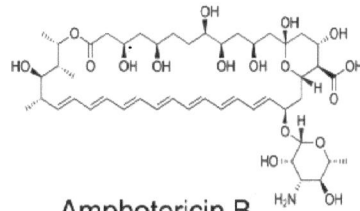

Amphotericin B

Fig. (3). Currently used anti-leishmanial drugs.

This formulation is beneficial due to increased efficacy with minimal toxicity, effective penetration and sustained levels in tissue, especially in liver and spleen. AmB is used in complex with deoxycholate or different lipids and all formulations are administered by intravenous infusion. In India, AmB was initially recommended for treatment of VL in patients who showed resistance to pentavalent antimonials (Sb^v) [46]. But, due to increasing resistance for Sb^v, it is being used as first line drug for VL treatment even in endemic areas [46]. The deoxycholate form of the drug has several adverse effects including infusion reactions, nephrotoxicity, hypokalemia, and myocarditis, and needs close monitoring and hospitalization for 4 to 5 weeks. Lipid formulations of AmB are more effective at lower doses and have reduced toxicity, but the high cost complicates treatment of patients with low income [50]. The lower rates of toxicity of L-AmB as compared to conventional AmB deoxycholate or AmB lipid complex (ABLC) have been previously reported by some researchers. However, the only drawback of liposomal AmB is the high cost [46, 49].

To make it affordable for patients, some of the scientists focused their research to reduce the extent of L-AmB whilst retaining its efficacy. Sundar *et al.* (2010) showed that 15 mg/kg of Ambisome®C (3 mg/kg on each of 5 doses) cured 96% patients [46]. Two separate studies performed by Thakur *et al.* (2001) and Sundar *et al.* (2010) have demonstrated the efficacy and safety of Ambisome®C, achieving maximum efficacy (rates more than 90%) in single doses of 5 to15 mg/kg, thus making it a better treatment option for VL in the Indian sub-continent [46]. In accordance with the study conducted in Indian and Ethiopian HIV-VL co-infected patients, AmBisome (30 mg/kg) in combination with miltefosine (100 mg/day) for 14 days and 28 days, respectively, was well tolerated and effective [51, 52].

The lipid formulations of AmB differ from each other with respect to efficacy, toxicity and dosage. The six different lipid formulations of AmB commercially available are: i) liposomal AmB (AmBisome®C; Gilead Sciences); ii) AmB lipid complex (Abelcet®C; ENZON Pharmaceuticals Inc.); iii) AmB cholesteryl sulfate complex, also called AmB colloidal dispersion [ABCD] (Amphocil; Sequus Pharmaceuticals); iv) FUNGISOME™ (Lifecare Innovation Pvt Ltd); v) AmB emulsion (Amphomul, Bharat Serum and Vaccines, India); and vi) amphiphilic L-AmB (KALSOME™10, Life care Innovation, Pvt. Ltd., India). Amongst all, Ambisome®C is probably the most efficacious, of all anti-leishmanial drugs currently available [46].

Combination therapies have been established as safe and effective treatment options. It involves the use of two different drugs, sequentially [50]. Recent trials in India established that a single infusion of 5 mg/kg of AmBisome followed by either 7 days of 50 mg/kg/day of miltefosine or 10 days of 11 mg/kg/day of paromomycin both yielded 97.5% of cure rates 6 months after the end of the treatment [50].

Mechanism of Action

Amphotericin B

The mechanism of AmB in most fungi is to bind to ergosterol in the cell membrane. After binding with ergosterol, it causes the formation of transmembrane AmB channels which induces altered permeability to monovalent cations, water, and glucose affecting membrane-bound enzymes [48]. Leakage of cations, results in membrane depolarization and concentration-dependent cell killing. However, in case of *Leishmania* parasites, the AmB interacts with both the ergosterol and cholesterol (of macrophages). It is known that the interaction of AmB with cholesterol is responsible for reducing the ability of cholesterol to interact with other membrane components such as receptors, thus inhibiting *Leishmania* infection [48].

Liposomal Amphotericin B (L-AmB)

The main purpose of L-AmB is effective delivery of the drug to the target site. Binding of AmB with liposomes results in liposomal disruption, which determines the external release of AmB. Thus, considering that free AmB exerts its fungicidal activity by binding to cell membrane, it is necessary to increase the bioavailability of the drug [48, 53].

Treatment Regimen

WHO guidelines use of AmB is described as follows: single dose of 10 mg/kg of L-AmB or combination therapy consisting of either single dose of 5 mg/kg L-AmB and 7-day 50 mg oral miltefosine or single shot of 5 mg/kg L-AmB and 10-day 11 mg/kg intramuscular paromomycin (PM) or 10 days each of miltefosine and PM are the preferred treatment options for VL.

Miltefosine

Miltefosine is an anti-cancer agent developed in 1980s. It is a phospholipid drug which was approved in India as the first oral treatment of VL in the year 2002 [50]. This drug was selected for the VL elimination program in India, Nepal, and Bangladesh in 2002, after the phase III trial in India resulted in a 94% cure rate on following a regimen of 50-100 mg/day for 28 days [50]. It showed to be the first effective oral drug for the treatment of CL, with greater accessibility and lower toxicity compared to pentavalent antimonials. At a dose of 2 mg/kg/day during 28 days, it is effective against CL in Colombia caused by *L. panamensis* (70-90% of cure rate), but has only shown a limited effect against the disease caused by *L. braziliensis* and *L. mexicana* (<60% of cure rate) [50]. The most common adverse effects that have been reported for this drug include gastrointestinal effects (such as diarrhea, vomiting, and dehydration) and occasional hepato- and nephrotoxicity. Another limitation presented is teratogenicity in pregnant women [50, 54]. Moreover, it seems to be ineffective in the treatment of infection by *L. major* and *L. braziliensis* [54].

Mechanism of Action

The precise mechanism of miltefosine is still not known. However, there are reports that suggest the mechanism of this drug in *Leishmania* species by different targets. Miltefosine is reported to inhibit the synthesis of phosphatidylcholine and affects the parasite mitochondrion by inhibiting the cytochrome c oxidase, this potent drug might produce its effect through other targets [47]. It has been reported that the disruption of the intracellular Ca^{2+} homeostasis represents an important object for the action of drugs in trypanosomatids. It is also known to activate the plasma membrane Ca^{2+} channel, strongly affecting the acidocalcisomes from *L. donovani* with rapid alkalization of the important organelles [47].

Treatment Regimen

In accordance with WHO guidelines the treatment course for miltefosine reported as a dose of 2.5 to 3.3 mg/kg/day during 4 weeks showed to be effective for MCL. On the other hand, treatment regimen for VL consists of a dose from 2.5 mg/kg/day during 28 days for children aged 2 to11 years old and for people aged 12 years and above of a dose from 50 mg/day for those weighting < 25 kg, 100 mg/day for 25 to 50 kg of body weight and 150 mg/day for > 50 kg of body weight, during 28 days.

Paromomycin (PM)

PM was first discovered during the 1950s and is produced by *Streptomyces rimosus* var. *Paromomycinus*. It is an aminoglycoside antibiotic which exists as PM sulfate [55]. A phase III study in Bihar (2003-2004) showed that intramuscularly PM regimen of 11 mg/kg (15 mg/kg as PM sulfate) during 21 days was non-inferior to AmB (1 mg/kg i.v. for 30 alternate days) with final cure rates of 94.6% *versus* 98.8%, respectively [50, 56]. Topical formulation of PM is used for treatment of CL by application to the lesion twice-a-day for 20 days [50]. The main disadvantage of PM is that its efficacy varies between and within regions, especially lack of efficacy in East Africa, while its affordability is the biggest advantage of PM [54]. The main adverse effects associated with PM are discomfort at injection site, elevated liver function tests (LFTs); fever, proteinuria, vomiting, and elevated alkaline phosphatase and bilirubin levels [46]. Parenteral formulations of paromomycin can cause serious adverse reactions, including nephrotoxicity and ototoxicity and infrequently hepatotoxicity, significantly lower in patients who are receiving PM as compared with patients receiving AmB [54, 55].

Mechanism of Action

PM is known to bind to the major groove in the A-site of 16S rRNA in *Escherichia coli* and induces misreading of mRNA. The mode of action of PM is not clear in case of *Leishmania* spp. It has been proposed that it might alter membrane fluidity, interact with ribosomes, interfere with the mitochondrial membrane potential and inhibit respiration process [57].

Treatment Regimen

In accordance with WHO guidelines the current treatment for CL includes the twice daily administration of PM of a formulation of 15% of the drug plus 12% methyl benzethonium chloride ointment during up to 20 days. For Indian VL treatment, a dose of 15 mg/kg PM sulfate (11 mg base) for 21 days (cure rate of 93 to 95%) is effective. In East Africa, the efficacy was 85% when the dose was increased to 20 mg/kg/day (15 mg base) and was administered during 21 days.

Pentavalent Antimonials (Sb^V)

Sb^V had been used as first line drugs for the treatment against all forms of leishmanial infections [57]. In 1925, the use of antimony for leishmaniasis treatment was discovered, saving millions of lives in India during the VL epidemics, especially in Assam state [50]. Sodium stibogluconate (100 mg antimony (Sb^{V+})/100 ml) and meglumine antimoniate (85 mg antimony/100 ml), are the two formulations used for treatment for leishmaniasis. Antimonials are administered *via* intramuscular injections or intravenous infusions, due to poor oral absorption. Common side effects of Sb^V include prolonged QTc interval, ventricular premature beats, ventricular tachycardia, ventricular fibrillation, and torsade of points. Prolongation of QTc interval (>0.5 s) is often associated with serious or even fatal cardiac arrhythmias [50, 54]. Other common adverse events associated with use of Sb^V are arthralgia and myalgia, elevated hepatic enzyme levels and pancreatitis [50]. Antimonial use causes more toxicity and mortality in HIV-positive patients compared to either patients treated with miltefosine, AmBisome, or HIV-negative patients treated with Sb^V [58].

Initially, in India, sodium stibogluconate was administered at low doses of 10 mg/kg/day during 6 to 10 days. These regimens successfully cured patients until the late seventies [59]. However, during the 1990s and 2000s, the clinical efficacy of Sb^V in Bihar state (where ~90% of VL cases in India occur) gradually declined due to high resistance to Sb^V [50]. Even so, the drug continues to be effective in surrounding areas (*e.g.*, Uttar Pradesh state of India) [50]. Resistance to this drug has become a major barrier in the treatment of VL in many endemic regions, particularly in India [57]. Generic stibogluconate remains the most important anti-leishmanial drug in most parts of the world as it enables the cost-effective treatment of all forms of leishmaniasis [60].

Mechanism of Action

The exact mechanism of inhibition of parasites growth by Sb^V is not clear. Berman *et al.* (1987) and Demicheli *et al.* (2002) proposed that Sb^V interfere with the bioenergetics process of *Leishmania* amastigotes, leading to the formation of stable complexes with ribonucleosides, which interfere with the parasite's fatty acid-oxidation and glycolysis, thus resulting in depletion of intracellular ATP levels [61, 62]. Moreira *et al.* (2017) reported that meglumine antimoniate causes oxidation of nitrogenous bases, leading to DNA damage, thus inhibiting the parasites growth [63].

Treatment Regimen

The current treatment regimen as per WHO guidelines for CL treatment consists of the administration from Sb^Vs at a dose of 20 mg/kg/day Sb^{5+} during 20 days. While, MCL treatment regimen requires 20 mg/kg/day during 30 days and VL treatment needs a daily injection of 20 mg/kg/ body weight of Sb^{5+} (Injections were usually given for 28 to 30 days).

Pentamidine

Pentamidine is an aromatic diamidine which emerged as a second line drug in Bihar, India to overcome the problems of Sb^V resistance in VL patients [46]. However, the use of this drug as monotherapy has been abandoned in endemic areas due to the lower cure rate compared to AmB and its toxicity issues (like-cardiac, hypotension, diabetes mellitus, and gastrointestinal effects) [46]. It is commercially available as Pentacarinat®C (Sanofi-Aventis) and is currently recommended as secondary prophylaxis in HIV-VL co-infection [46]. Most treatments are based on intramuscular injection or intravenous infusion of 4 mg/kg/day of pentamidine for a variable number of days (up to 30) [50]. It is highly toxic and shows adverse effects such as severe hypoglycemia, hypotension, myocarditis, and renal toxicity; and can ultimately cause death [54]. It has also been reported that the drug efficacy varies between *Leishmania* species [50, 54].

Mechanism of Action

Pentamidine is reported to inhibit active transport system as well as transcription process in *Leishmania* and other kinetoplastids [46].

Treatment Regimen

Most treatments are based on intramuscular injection or intravenous infusion of 4 mg/kg/day of pentamidine for a variable number of days (up to 30) for VL.

Anti-leishmanial Activity of Compounds from Natural Sources

In the recent years, a great emphasis has been focused on search of natural compounds from medicinal plants as leads for drug discovery to develop potent anti-leishmanial drugs and to overcome the drawbacks of the currently used drugs. Plant extracts or essential oils that have different phytochemicals such as alkaloids, saponins, flavonoids, terpenoids, quinines, naphthoquinones, *etc.* have shown promising results. Other than plants, secondary metabolites from endophytes and marine microorganisms have been also reported to have activity against *Leishmania* parasites.

Plants

Various plants extract or the essential oils from these plants have been reported to have leishmanicidal activity. Recently, Arencibia *et al.* (2019) showed that certain compounds from *Withania aristata* had anti-leishmanial activity. They reported that compounds 1 and 3 (withanolide-type metabolites) inhibit proliferation in both *L. amazonensis* promastigotes and *T. cruzi* epimastigotes in a dose-dependent manner. Also, these compounds were more potent than the reference drugs with IC_{50} value in the range of 0.055 to 0.663 µM against the intracellular amastigote stage of *L. amazonensis* and compound 1 had a high selectivity index (SI) in murine macrophage cells (SI=216.73). *Cryptocarya aschersoniana Mez.* is popular in Brazil as *Canela-nhutinga*, is an important native climax species of shade tolerant species. The extract of essential oil from this species mainly consists of monoterpene hydrocarbons (48.8%), limonene (42.3%), linalool (9.7%) and nerolidol (8.6%). The *in vitro* activity of this essential oil against the promastigote forms of *L. amazonensis* reported IC_{50} value of 4.46 µg/ml. However, it has also demonstrated relatively high cytotoxicity on mouse peritoneal macrophages (CC_{50} = 7.71 µg/ml) (64). The anti-leishmanial activity of medicinal plants native to North-West region of Morocco such as *Myrtus communis*, *Arbutus unedo*, *Origanum compactum* and *Cistus crispus* was evaluated by Bouyahya *et al* (2018). They reported that among all the tested extracts, n-hexane extract from *Cistus crispus* showed better inhibition of *L. major* (IC_{50} = 47.29 ± 2.25 µg/ml), while *Arbutus unedo* n-hexane extract showed anti-leishmanial effect against both *L. infantum* (IC_{50} = 64.05 ± 1.44 µg/ml) and *L. tropica* (IC_{50} = 79.57 ± 2.66 µg/ml) [65]. Recently, anti-leishmanial activity of a diprenylated flavonoid known as 5,7,3,4′-tetrahydroxy-6,8-diprenylisoflavone (CMt) has been investigated against *L. infantum* and *L. amazonensis* species, showing selectivity index (SI) of 70.0 and IC_{50} value of 6.36 ± 0.75 μg/ml against *L. infantum* while, SI and IC_{50} value against *L. amazonensis* promastigotes was 165.0 and 2.70 ± 0.67 μg/ml, respectively. Selectivity index of CMt against axenic amastigotes of *L. infantum* was 181.9 with an IC_{50} value of 2.45 ± 0.66 μg/ml. Whereas, SI against *L. amazonensis* axenic amastigotes was 397.8 with IC_{50} value of 1.12 ± 0.24μg/ml. It was reported that CMt developed a Th1-type cellular and humoral immune response after 1 and 15 days after the treatment in CMt/Mic-treated mice. Moreover, significant reductions in the parasite load in spleen, liver, bone marrow and draining lymph nodes, one and fifteen days-post treatment were observed. This suggests that CMt/Mic can be evaluated as a potential agent against VL [66]. The anti-leishmanial activity of *Moringa oleifera* against *L. donavani* has been already reported by Kaur *et al.* (2014). However, the effect of silver nanoparticles biosynthesized using *Moringa oleifera* extract against *L. major* has been reported. These nanoparticles significantly reduced the average lesion size in *L. major*-infected BALB/c mice, while, complete healing of the lesion was reported after 14 days of treatment. However, more studies on the stability of Ag-NPs biosynthesized by *Moringa oleifera* leaf extract need to be performed to establish it as a potential therapeutic measure for the treatment of CL [67]. The anti-leishmanial activity of 1,4- naphthoquinone derivative, the 2-(2,3,4-tri-Oacetyl-6-deoxy-β-L-galactopyranosyloxy)-1,4- naphthoquinone, namely Flau-A, was evaluated against *L. infantum* and *L. amazonensis* species. Flau-A inhibited *L. infantum* promastigotes and amastigotes with IC_{50} values of 0.73 μg/ml and 1.03 μg/ml, respectively. In addition, IC_{50} values against promastigotes and amastigotes form of L. *amazonensis* were 0.73 and 1.57 μg/ml, respectively [68]. Recently, Macêdo *et al.* (2020) reported the anti-leishmanial activity of *Piper marginatum Jacq.* They demonstrated that the essential oil and ethanol extracts had significant activity against amastigote form of *L. amazonensis*. Calvo *et al.* (2020) demonstrated anti-leishmanial activity of liposomal- berberine (LP-BER) against *L.infantum*. LP-BER presented anti-leishmanial activity against both *L. infantum* promastigotes (IC_{50} = 6.8 ± 0.6 μM) and amastigotes (IC_{50} = 1.4 ± 0.2 μM). When BALB/c mice infected with *L. infantum* parasites were daily administered intraperitoneally with LP-BER at a dose of 15 mg/kg during 10 days, a significant reduction of parasite burden was noted in liver and spleen by 99.2 and 93.5%, respectively.

Marine Macroalgae

Different species of brown macroalgae (*Phaeophyceae*) have been screened for their anti-leishmanial activity. Isopropyl alcohol-chloroform/methanol extracts of *B. bifurcata* and *H. siliquosa* extracts reported anti-leishmanial activity against *L. donovani* with IC_{50} of 6.4 and 8.6 μg/ml, respectively. However, these two extracts demonstrated cytotoxic effects against the mammalian skeletal myoblasts,

L6 cells having a CC_{50} value of 32.7 and 45.0μg/ml, respectively [69, 70]. Hydro alcoholic and ethyl acetate extract of *B. bifurcata, D. dichotoma* and *D. polypodioide* also exhibited anti-leishmanial activity. However, their extracts presented high cytotoxic effects, which indicated that the extracts were not suitable for the parasites. Brown macroalgae of *Dictyotaceae* family, namely *Canistrocarpus, Dictyota* and *Stypopodium* genera also had shown anti-leishmanial activity with less cytotoxicity. It has been reported that the organic extract of *T. turbinata* had IC_{50} value of 10.9 μg/ml with selectivity index of 70.41 [70].

Most of the anti-leishmanial compounds isolated from *Dictyotaceae* family belong to the family of diterpenes. Dolabellanediterpene, Dolabelladienetriol isolated from *Dictyota pfaffii* inhibited the replication of intracellular amastigote form of *L. amazonensis*. These compounds were also active against *Leishmania*-HIV co-infection with 56% of inhibition at 50 μM [70]. Elatol and obtusol are sesquiterpene compounds isolated from *Laurencia dendroidea,* which were active against the promastigotes and the intracellular amastigotes with less toxicity. Fucoidan, another compound found in many brown algae, is a polyanionic sulfated polysaccharide. Even though it contains inhibitory effect on intracellular amastigotes of *L. donovani,* it also displayed multiple disadvantages such as high hemorrhagic risk, poor solubility and bioavailability [70].

Endophytes

The drive for need of new treatment has led to the identification of several active metabolites for anti-leishmanial drug discovery. Extracts from endophytic fungi have been screened for their activity against *L. donovani*. Integracides H, and Integracides J, compounds isolated from *Fusarium sp.*, endophyte of *Mentha longifolia* were reported to inhibit *L. donovani* with IC_{50} values of 4.75 and 3.29 μM respectively [71, 72]. Compounds isolated from extract of *Aspergillus terreus,* an endophyte from the roots of *Carthamus lanatus* included terrenolide S, along with stigmast-4-ene3-one, (22E,24R)-stigmasta-5,7,22-trien-3-β-ol, stigmasta-4,6,8, 22-tetraen-3-one, terretonin A, terretonin, and butyrolactone VI. These compounds inhibited *L. donovani* with IC_{50} ranging from 11.24 to 87.34 μM [72, 73]. Compounds isolated from the fungus *Edenia* species such as preussomerin EG1, palmarumycin CP2, palmarumycin CP17, palmarumycin CP18, and CJ-12,371 showed activity against *L. donovani* amastigote, with IC_{50} values of 0.12, 3.93, 1.34, 0.62, and 8.40 μM, respectively. Palmarumycin CP18 was reported to inhibit *L. donovani* in macrophage cells with an IC_{50} value of 23.5 μM [72, 74]. This indicates that several compounds from different endophytes have anti-leishmanial activity and need to be studied in details to be considered as potential agents for the treatment of leishmaniasis.

CONCLUSION

The Asian elimination initiative of visceral leishmaniasis has raised global alertness about leishmaniasis. However, remains a major gap in effective treatment of leishmaniasis. Some of the main challenges of this neglected tropical disease are fewer therapeutic options, lack of diagnostics tools, and poor community awareness. The main limitations of the currently used anti-leishmanial drugs are high toxicity, low efficacy and emerging resistance to these drugs. Moreover, treatment options available for major complications of the disease such as PKDL and HIV-VL co-infection are scarce. Hence, due to low efficacy and high toxicity of the available drugs, up to date there is no satisfactory treatment of HIV-VL co-infection that results in an elevated deterioration rate. Hence, it is necessary to search for alternatives which are less expensive show low toxicity and have much better efficacy. Many natural compounds have been identified to have anti-leishmanial activity, but they need to be studied in detail before considering them as chemotherapeutic agents for the treatment of leishmaniasis. Recently, new anti-leishmanial lead compounds, such as bicyclic nitroimidazoles, amino pyrazoles and oxaboroles for VL and CpG ODN (D35) for CL have been selected for the drug development process (DNDi and WHO); they are still in initial stages of clinical trials and need to undergo the further development process to be established as a treatment option. This indicates that there are handful of drugs, which can be used for the effective treatment of the disease and there is an immediate need to find out less toxic and affordable novel drugs. Therefore, the search for new therapeutic drugs is urgently needed to treat the disease efficiently.

CONSENT FOR PUBLICATION

Not applicable.

CONFLICT OF INTEREST

The author declares no conflict of interest, financial or otherwise.

ACKNOWLEDGEMENTS

We are thankful to Prof. Nitin R. Karmalkar (Hon'ble Vice Chancellor, Savitribai Phule Pune University) for his interest on this topic and his valuable suggestions. This work was supported by Faculty Recharge Programme (FRP) under University Grants Commission (UGC), Govt. of India to AR.

REFERENCES

[1]   Karunaweera ND, Ferreira MU. Leishmaniasis: current challenges and prospects for elimination with special focus on the South Asian region. Parasitology 2018; 145(4): 425-9.

[http://dx.doi.org/10.1017/S0031182018000471] [PMID: 29642962]

[2]   Singh N, Kumar M, Singh RK. Leishmaniasis: current status of available drugs and new potential drug targets. Asian Pac J Trop Med 2012; 5(6): 485-97.
[http://dx.doi.org/10.1016/S1995-7645(12)60084-4] [PMID: 22575984]

[3]   Güran M. Chapter- An Overview of Leishmaniasis: Historic to Future Perspectives. Vectors and Vector-Borne Zoonotic Diseases 2018.

[4]   World Health Organization. Leishmaniasis. World Health Org Fact Sheet. 2020. http://www.who.int/mediacentre/factsheets/fs375/en/ Accessed on 06 April, 2020

[5]   Von Stebut E. Leishmaniasis. J Dtsch Dermatol Ges 2015; 13(3): 191-200.
[http://dx.doi.org/10.1111/ddg.12595_suppl] [PMID: 25721626]

[6]   Alvar J, Vélez ID, Bern C, *et al.* Leishmaniasis worldwide and global estimates of its incidence. PLoS One 2012; 7(5) : e35671.
[http://dx.doi.org/10.1371/journal.pone.0035671] [PMID: 22693548]

[7]   Zulfiqar B, Shelper TB, Avery VM. Leishmaniasis drug discovery: recent progress and challenges in assay development. Drug Discov Today 2017; 22(10): 1516-31.
[http://dx.doi.org/10.1016/j.drudis.2017.06.004] [PMID: 28647378]

[8]   Leishman WB. On the possibility of the occurrence of trypanosomiasis in India. BMJ 1903; 2(2238): 1376-7.
[http://dx.doi.org/10.1136/bmj.2.2238.1376-a]

[9]   Akhoundi M, Kuhls K, Cannet A, *et al.* A historical overview of the classification, evolution, and dispersion of *Leishmania* parasites and sandflies. PLoS Negl Trop Dis 2016; 10(3) : e0004349.
[http://dx.doi.org/10.1371/journal.pntd.0004349] [PMID: 26937644]

[10]   Steverding D. The history of leishmaniasis. Parasit Vectors 2017; 10(1): 82.
[http://dx.doi.org/10.1186/s13071-017-2028-5] [PMID: 28202044]

[11]   Sunter J, Gull K. Shape, form, function and *Leishmania* pathogenicity: from textbook descriptions to biological understanding. Open Biol 2017; 7(9) : 170165.
[http://dx.doi.org/10.1098/rsob.170165] [PMID: 28903998]

[12]   Pace D. Leishmaniasis. J Infect 2014; 1-9.

[13]   Burza S, Croft S L, Boelaert M. Leishmaniasis. The Lancet 2018.
[http://dx.doi.org/10.1016/s0140-6736(18)31204-2]

[14]   Reimão JQ, Coser EM, Lee MR, Coelho AC. Laboratory diagnosis of cutaneous and visceral leishmaniasis: current and future methods. Microorganisms 2020; 8(11) : E1632.
[http://dx.doi.org/10.3390/microorganisms8111632] [PMID: 33105784]

[15]   Adrienne J. Showler& Andrea K. Boggild. Cutaneous leishmaniasis in travellers: a focus on epidemiology and treatment in 2015. Curr Infect Dis Rep 2015; 17: 37.
[http://dx.doi.org/10.1007/s11908-015-0489-2]

[16]   Zijlstra EE, Musa AM, Khalil E A G, el-Hassan IM, el-Hassan AM. Post-kala-azar dermal leishmaniasis. Lancet Infect Dis 2003; 3(2): 87-98.
[http://dx.doi.org/10.1016/S1473-3099(03)00517-6] [PMID: 12560194]

[17]   Ganguly S, Mukhopadhyay D, Das NK, *et al.* Enhanced lesional Foxp3 expression and peripheral anergic lymphocytes indicate a role for regulatory T cells in Indian post-kala-azar dermal leishmaniasis. J Invest Dermatol 2010; 130(4): 1013-22.
[http://dx.doi.org/10.1038/jid.2009.393] [PMID: 20032994]

[18]   Katara GK, Ansari NA, Verma S, Ramesh V, Salotra P. Foxp3 and IL-10 expression correlates with parasite burden in lesional tissues of post kala azar dermal leishmaniasis (PKDL) patients. PLoS Negl Trop Dis 2011; 5(5) : e1171.
[http://dx.doi.org/10.1371/journal.pntd.0001171] [PMID: 21655313]

[19] Mukhopadhyay D, Mukherjee S, Roy S, *et al.* M2 polarization of monocytes-macrophages is a hallmark of indian post kala-azar dermal leishmaniasis. PLoS Negl Trop Dis 2015; 9(10) : e0004145.
[http://dx.doi.org/10.1371/journal.pntd.0004145] [PMID: 26496711]

[20] Desjeux P, Ghosh RS, Dhalaria P, Strub-Wourgaft N. Report of the post kala-azar dermal leishmaniasis (PKDL) consortium meeting, New Delhi, India. Parasit Vectors 2012; 6: 196.

[21] Control of the leishmaniases. WHO Technical Report Series. 2010. Available at: http://apps.who.int/iris/bitstream/ 10665/44412/1/WHO_TRS_949_eng.pdf

[22] National Organization for Rare Disorders. https://rarediseases.org/rare-diseases/leishmaniasis /#symptoms

[23] Laskay T, Mikó TL, Negesse Y, Solbach W, Röllinghoff M, Frommel D. Detection of cutaneous Leishmania infection in paraffin-embedded skin biopsies using the polymerase chain reaction. Trans R Soc Trop Med Hyg 1995; 89(3): 273-5.
[http://dx.doi.org/10.1016/0035-9203(95)90537-5] [PMID: 7660431]

[24] Sreenivas G, Raju BV, Singh R, *et al.* DNA polymorphism assay distinguishes isolates of Leishmania donovani that cause kala-azar from those that cause post-kala-azar dermal Leishmaniasis in humans. J Clin Microbiol 2004; 42(4): 1739-41.
[http://dx.doi.org/10.1128/JCM.42.4.1739-1741.2004] [PMID: 15071036]

[25] Sreenivas G, Ansari NA, Singh R, *et al.* Diagnosis of visceral leishmaniasis: Comparative potential of amastigote antigen, recombinant antigen and PCR. Br J Biomed Sci 2002; 59: 218-22.
[http://dx.doi.org/10.1080/09674845.2002.11783663]

[26] Kumar R, Bumb RA, Ansari NA, Mehta RD, Salotra P. Cutaneous leishmaniasis caused by *Leishmania tropica* in Bikaner, India: parasite identification and characterization using molecular and immunologic tools. Am J Trop Med Hyg 2007; 76(5): 896-901.
[http://dx.doi.org/10.4269/ajtmh.2007.76.896] [PMID: 17488912]

[27] Sundar S, Singh OP. Molecular diagnosis of visceral leishmaniasis. Mol Diagn Ther 2018; 22(4): 443-57.
[http://dx.doi.org/10.1007/s40291-018-0343-y] [PMID: 29922885]

[28] Maurya R, Mehrotra S, Prajapati VK, Nylén S, Sacks D, Sundar S. Evaluation of blood agar microtiter plates for culturing leishmania parasites to titrate parasite burden in spleen and peripheral blood of patients with visceral leishmaniasis. J Clin Microbiol 2010; 48(5): 1932-4.
[http://dx.doi.org/10.1128/JCM.01733-09] [PMID: 20335419]

[29] Salotra P, Sreenivas G, Pogue GP, *et al.* Development of a species-specific PCR assay for detection of *Leishmania donovani* in clinical samples from patients with kala-azar and post-kala-azar dermal leishmaniasis. J Clin Microbiol 2001; 39(3): 849-54.
[http://dx.doi.org/10.1128/JCM.39.3.849-854.2001] [PMID: 11230394]

[30] el Tai NO, Osman OF, el Fari M, Presber W, Schönian G. Genetic heterogeneity of ribosomal internal transcribed spacer in clinical samples of *Leishmania donovani* spotted on filter paper as revealed by single-strand conformation polymorphisms and sequencing. Trans R Soc Trop Med Hyg 2000; 94(5): 575-9.
[http://dx.doi.org/10.1016/S0035-9203(00)90093-2] [PMID: 11132393]

[31] Rotureau B, Ravel C, Couppié P, *et al.* Use of PCR-restriction fragment length polymorphism analysis to identify the main new world Leishmania species and analyze their taxonomic properties and polymorphism by application of the assay to clinical samples. J Clin Microbiol 2006; 44(2): 459-67.
[http://dx.doi.org/10.1128/JCM.44.2.459-467.2006] [PMID: 16455899]

[32] Zampieri RA, Laranjeira-Silva MF, Muxel SM, Stocco de Lima AC, Shaw JJ, Floeter-Winter LM. High resolution melting analysis targeting hsp70 as a fast and efficient method for the discrimination of *Leishmania* species. PLoS Negl Trop Dis 2016; 10(2) : e0004485.
[http://dx.doi.org/10.1371/journal.pntd.0004485] [PMID: 26928050]

[33] Ferreira SdeA, Almeida GG, Silva SdeO, *et al.* Nasal, oral and ear swabs for canine visceral leishmaniasis diagnosis: new practical approaches for detection of *Leishmania infantum* DNA. PLoS Negl Trop Dis 2013; 7(4) : e2150.
[http://dx.doi.org/10.1371/journal.pntd.0002150] [PMID: 23593518]

[34] Castilho TM, Camargo LMA, McMahon-Pratt D, Shaw JJ, Floeter-Winter LM. A real-time polymerase chain reaction assay for the identification and quantification of American Leishmania species on the basis of glucose-6-phosphate dehydrogenase. Am J Trop Med Hyg 2008; 78(1): 122-32.
[http://dx.doi.org/10.4269/ajtmh.2008.78.122] [PMID: 18187795]

[35] Wortmann G, Hochberg L, Houng H-H, *et al.* Rapid identification of *Leishmania* complexes by a real-time PCR assay. Am J Trop Med Hyg 2005; 73(6): 999-1004.
[http://dx.doi.org/10.4269/ajtmh.2005.73.999] [PMID: 16354801]

[36] Khosravi S, Hejazi SH, Hashemzadeh M, Eslami G, Darani HY. Molecular diagnosis of Old World leishmaniasis: real-time PCR based on tryparedoxin peroxidase gene for the detection and identification of *Leishmania* spp. J Vector Borne Dis 2012; 49(1): 15-8.
[PMID: 22585237]

[37] Cortes S. PCR as a rapid and sensitive tool in the diagnosis of human and canine leishmaniasis using Leishmania donovani -specific kinetoplastid primers. Trans R Soc Trop Med Hyg 2004; 1(): 12-7.
[PMID: 14702834]

[38] Hassan MQ, Ghosh A, Ghosh SS, *et al.* Enzymatic amplification of mini-exon-derived RNA gene spacers of *Leishmania donovani*: primers and probes for DNA diagnosis. Parasitology 1993; 107(Pt 5): 509-17.
[http://dx.doi.org/10.1017/S0031182000068086] [PMID: 8295790]

[39] Mugasa CM, Laurent T, Schoone GJ, *et al.* Simplified molecular detection of Leishmania parasites in various clinical samples from patients with leishmaniasis. Parasit Vectors 2010; 3(1): 13. [PubMed: 20196849].
[http://dx.doi.org/10.1186/1756-3305-3-13] [PMID: 20196849]

[40] Verma S, Avishek K, Sharma V, Negi NS, Ramesh V, Salotra P. Application of loop-mediated isothermal amplification assay for the sensitive and rapid diagnosis of visceral leishmaniasis and post-kala-azar dermal leishmaniasis. Diagn Microbiol Infect Dis 2013; 75(4): 390-5. [PubMed: 23433714].
[http://dx.doi.org/10.1016/j.diagmicrobio.2013.01.011] [PMID: 23433714]

[41] Sukphattanaudomchoke C, Siripattanapipong S, Thita T, *et al.* Simplified closed tube loop mediated isothermal amplification (LAMP) assay for visual diagnosis of Leishmania infection. Acta Trop 2020; 212 : 105651.
[http://dx.doi.org/10.1016/j.actatropica.2020.105651] [PMID: 32763231]

[42] Chappuis F, Rijal S, Soto A, Menten J, Boelaert M. A meta-analysis of the diagnostic performance of the direct agglutination test and rK39 dipstick for visceral leishmaniasis. BMJ 2006; 333(7571): 723.
[http://dx.doi.org/10.1136/bmj.38917.503056.7C] [PMID: 16882683]

[43] Cunningham J, Hasker E, Das P, *et al.* A global comparative evaluation of commercial immunochromatographic rapid diagnostic tests for visceral leishmaniasis. Clin Infect Dis 2012; 55(10): 1312-9.
[http://dx.doi.org/10.1093/cid/cis716] [PMID: 22942208]

[44] Jacquet D, Boelaert M, Seaman J, *et al.* Comparative evaluation of freeze-dried and liquid antigens in the direct agglutination test for serodiagnosis of visceral leishmaniasis (ITMA-DAT/VL). Trop Med Int Health 2006; 11(12): 1777-84.
[http://dx.doi.org/10.1111/j.1365-3156.2006.01743.x] [PMID: 17176341]

[45] Costs of medicines in current use for the treatment of leishmaniasis. https://www.who.int/

[46] Singh OP, Singh B, Chakravarty J, Sundar S. Current challenges in treatment options for visceral leishmaniasis in India: a public health perspective. Infect Dis Poverty 2016; 5: 19.

[http://dx.doi.org/10.1186/s40249-016-0112-2] [PMID: 26951132]

[47]   Pinto-Martinez AK, Rodriguez-Durán J, Serrano-Martin X, Hernandez-Rodriguez V, Benaim G. Mechanism of action of miltefosine on leishmania donovani involves the impairment of acidocalcisome function and the activation of the sphingosine-dependent plasma membrane Ca^{2+} channel. Antimicrob Agents Chemother 2017; 62(1): e01614-7.
[http://dx.doi.org/10.1128/AAC.01614-17] [PMID: 29061745]

[48]   Chattopadhyay A, Jafurulla M. A novel mechanism for an old drug: amphotericin B in the treatment of visceral leishmaniasis. Biochem Biophys Res Commun 2011; 416(1-2): 7-12.
[http://dx.doi.org/10.1016/j.bbrc.2011.11.023] [PMID: 22100811]

[49]   Bern C, Adler-Moore J, Berenguer J, *et al.* Liposomal amphotericin B for the treatment of visceral leishmaniasis. Clin Infect Dis 2006; 43(7): 917-24.
[http://dx.doi.org/10.1086/507530] [PMID: 16941377]

[50]   Nagle AS, Khare S, Kumar AB, *et al.* Recent developments in drug discovery for leishmaniasis and human African trypanosomiasis. Chem Rev 2014; 114(22): 11305-47.
[http://dx.doi.org/10.1021/cr500365f] [PMID: 25365529]

[51]   Diro E, Blesson S, Edwards T, *et al.* A randomized trial of AmBisome monotherapy and AmBisome and miltefosine combination to treat visceral leishmaniasis in HIV co-infected patients in Ethiopia. PLoS Negl Trop Dis 2019; 13(1) : c0006988.
[http://dx.doi.org/10.1371/journal.pntd.0006988] [PMID: 30653490]

[52]   Mahajan R, Das P, Isaakidis P, *et al.* Combination treatment for visceral leishmaniasis patients coinfected with Human Immunodeficiency Virus in India. Clin Infect Dis 2015; 61(8): 1255-62.
[http://dx.doi.org/10.1093/cid/civ530] [PMID: 26129756]

[53]   Stone NR, Bicanic T, Salim R, Hope W. Liposomal Amphotericin B (AmBisome®C): A review of the pharmacokinetics, pharmacodynamics, clinical experience and future directions. Drugs 2016; 76(4): 485-500.
[http://dx.doi.org/10.1007/s40265-016-0538-7] [PMID: 26818726]

[54]   de Menezes JP, Guedes CE, Petersen AL, Fraga DB, Veras PS. Advances in development of new treatment for leishmaniasis. BioMed Res Int 2015; 2015 : 815023.
[http://dx.doi.org/10.1155/2015/815023] [PMID: 26078965]

[55]   Wiwanitkit V. Interest in paromomycin for the treatment of visceral leishmaniasis (kala-azar). Ther Clin Risk Manag 2012; 8: 323-8.
[http://dx.doi.org/10.2147/TCRM.S30139] [PMID: 22802694]

[56]   Sundar S, Jha TK, Thakur CP, Sinha PK, Bhattacharya SK. Injectable paromomycin for Visceral leishmaniasis in India. N Engl J Med 2007; 356(25): 2571-81.
[http://dx.doi.org/10.1056/NEJMoa066536] [PMID: 17582067]

[57]   Chawla B, Jhingran A, Panigrahi A, Stuart KD, Madhubala R. Paromomycin affects translation and vesicle-mediated trafficking as revealed by proteomics of paromomycin -susceptible -resistant *Leishmania donovani.* PLoS One 2011; 6(10) : e26660.
[http://dx.doi.org/10.1371/journal.pone.0026660] [PMID: 22046323]

[58]   Ritmeijer K, Dejenie A, Assefa Y, *et al.* A comparison of miltefosine and sodium stibogluconate for treatment of visceral leishmaniasis in an Ethiopian population with high prevalence of HIV infection. Clin Infect Dis 2006; 43(3): 357-64.
[http://dx.doi.org/10.1086/505217] [PMID: 16804852]

[59]   Ritmeijer K, ter Horst R, Chane S, *et al.* Limited effectiveness of high-dose liposomal amphotericin B (AmBisome) for treatment of visceral leishmaniasis in an Ethiopian population with high HIV prevalence. Clin Infect Dis 2011; 53(12): e152-8.
[http://dx.doi.org/10.1093/cid/cir674] [PMID: 22016502]

[60]   Sundar S, Rai M. Advances in the treatment of leishmaniasis. Curr Opin Infect Dis 2002; 15(6): 593-8.

[http://dx.doi.org/10.1097/00001432-200212000-00007] [PMID: 12821836]

[61]   Berman JD, Gallalee JV, Best JM. Sodium stibogluconate (Pentostam) inhibition of glucose catabolism *via* the glycolytic pathway, and fatty acid beta-oxidation in *Leishmania mexicana* amastigotes. Biochem Pharmacol 1987; 36(2): 197-201.
[http://dx.doi.org/10.1016/0006-2952(87)90689-7] [PMID: 3028425]

[62]   Demicheli C, Frézard F, Lecouvey M, Garnier-Suillerot A. Antimony(V) complex formation with adenine nucleosides in aqueous solution. Biochim Biophys Acta 2002; 1570(3): 192-8.
[http://dx.doi.org/10.1016/S0304-4165(02)00198-8] [PMID: 12020809]

[63]   Moreira VR, de Jesus LCL, Soares RP, *et al.* Meglumine antimoniate (glucantime) causes oxidative stress-derived DNA damage in BALB/c mice infected by leishmania (leishmania) infantum. Antimicrob Agents Chemother 2017; 61(6): e02360-16.
[http://dx.doi.org/10.1128/AAC.02360-16] [PMID: 28320726]

[64]   Priscila M. De Andrade, Daiana C. De Melo, Ana Elisa T. Alcoba, Walnir G., Ferreira Júnior, Mariana C. Pagotti, Lizandra G. Magalhães, Tainá C.L. Dos Santos, Antônio E.M. Crotti, Cassia C.F. Alves and Mayker L.D. Miranda. Chemical composition and evaluation of anti-leishmanial and cytotoxic activities of the essential oil from leaves *of Cryptocarya aschersoniana Mez.* (*Lauraceae Juss.*). Annals of the Brazilian Academy of Sciences 2018; 90(3): 2671-8.

[65]   Bouyahya A, Et-Touys A, Dakka N, Fellah H, Abrini J, Bakri Y. Antileishmanial potential of medicinal plant extracts from the North-West of Morocco. Beni-Suef University J Basic Appl Sci 2018; 7: 50-4.
[http://dx.doi.org/10.1016/j.bjbas.2017.06.003]

[66]   Pereira IAG, Mendonça DVC, Tavares GSV, *et al.* Parasitological and immunological evaluation of a novel chemotherapeutic agent against visceral leishmaniasis. Parasite Immunol 2020; 42(12) : e12784.
[http://dx.doi.org/10.1111/pim.12784] [PMID: 32772379]

[67]   Ebtesam M. Alolayan, Dina M. Metwally, Mohamed F. Serag El-Din, Sara S. Alobud, Nour I. Alsultan, Sarah S. Alsaif, Manal A. Awad and Ahmed E. Abdel Moneim. Clinical efficacy associated with enhanced antioxidant enzyme activities of silver nanoparticles biosynthesized using *Moringa oleifera* leaf extract, against cutaneous leishmaniasis in a murine model of *Leishmania major.* Int J Environ Res Public Health 2018; 15: 1037.

[68]   Mendonça DVC, Lage DP, Calixto SL, *et al.* Antileishmanial activity of a naphthoquinone derivate against promastigote and amastigote stages of *Leishmania infantum* and *Leishmania amazonensis* and its mechanism of action against *L. amazonensis* species. Parasitol Res 2018; 117(2): 391-403.
[http://dx.doi.org/10.1007/s00436-017-5713-6] [PMID: 29248978]

[69]   Spavieri J, Allmendinger A, Kaiser M, *et al.* Antimycobacterial, antiprotozoal and cytotoxic potential of twenty-one brown algae (Phaeophyceae) from British and Irish waters. Phytother Res 2010; 24(11): 1724-9.
[http://dx.doi.org/10.1002/ptr.3208] [PMID: 20564461]

[70]   Lauve Rachel Tchokouaha Yamthe. Regina appiah-opong, patrick valere tsouh fokou, nole tsabang, fabrice fekam boyom, alexander kwadwo nyarko and michael david wilson. marine algae as source of novel anti-leishmanial drugs: a review. Mar Drugs 2017; 15: 323.
[http://dx.doi.org/10.3390/md15110323]

[71]   Sabrin RM. Ibrahim, Hossam M Abdallah, Gamal A Mohamed, Samir A Ross. Integracides H-J: New tetracyclic triterpenoids from the endophytic fungus *Fusarium sp.* Fitoterapia 2016; 112: 161-7.
[http://dx.doi.org/10.1016/j.fitote.2016.06.002]

[72]   Toghueo RMK. Anti-leishmanial and Anti-inflammatory Agents from Endophytes: A Review. Nat Prod Bioprospect 2019; 9(5): 311-28.
[http://dx.doi.org/10.1007/s13659-019-00220-5] [PMID: 31564050]

[73]   Ehab S. Elkhayat, Sabrin R M Ibrahim, Gamal A Mohamed, Samir A Ross. Terrenolide S, a new anti-leishmanial butenolide from the endophytic fungus *Aspergillus terreus.* Nat Prod Res 2016; 30(7):

814-20.
[http://dx.doi.org/10.1080/14786419.2015.1072711] [PMID: 26299734]

[74]   Martínez-Luis S, Della-Togna G, Coley PD, Kursar TA, Gerwick WH, Cubilla-Rios L. Antileishmanial constituents of the Panamanian endophytic fungus Edenia sp. J Nat Prod 2008; 71(12): 2011-4.
[http://dx.doi.org/10.1021/np800472q] [PMID: 19007286]

## CHAPTER 5

Dengue Hemorrhagic Fever: The Potential Repurposing Drugs

Wattana Leowattana[1,*], **Pathomthep Leowattana**[2] and **Tawithep Leowattana**[3]

[1] *Department of Clinical Tropical Medicine, Faculty of Tropical Medicine, Mahidol University, 420/6 Rajavithi road, Rachatawee, Bangkok 10400, Thailand*

[2] *Tivanon Medical Clinics, 99 Tivanon Road, Muang, Nonthaburi 11000, Thailand*

[3] *Department of Medicine, Faculty of Medicine, Srinakharinwirot University, 114 Sukhumvit 23, Wattana District, Bangkok 10110, Thailand*

Abstract: Dengue is the most significant arthropod-borne viral infection of humans. More than 3.8 billion people live in endemic areas. Dengue virus infection (DVI) results in more than 500,000 hospitalizations every year, with increased threats of dengue hemorrhagic fever (DHF) and dengue shock syndrome (DSS) during secondary infections. In spite of the high disease burden of the dengue virus, there are no specific antiviral drugs available, and the approved vaccine is harmful in the naïve population with respect to the initiation of primary dengue infection. Several clinically approved drugs have entered human clinical trials. This review addresses the repurposing drug targets that have been investigated in DHF and DSS patients. Furthermore, their essential antiviral action and specific classes of clinically approved drugs have been clarified. These clinical trials' outcomes can enhance our understanding of the antiviral activities of these repurposing drugs to alleviate the clinical severity of dengue viral infection.

Keywords: Antiviral treatment, Balapiravir, Celgosivir, Chloroquine, Clinically approved drugs, Cromolyn, Dengue hemorrhagic fever antibiotics, Doxycycline, Ivermectin, Ketotifen, Montelukast, Repurposing drugs, Ribavirin, Rupatadine, Sofosbuvir, UV-4B.

INTRODUCTION

The Flaviviridae is a family of viruses that use humans and other mammals as natural hosts. This family is primarily spread through arthropod vectors. The common viruses of this family are yellow fever virus (YFV), West Nile virus (WNV), Japanese encephalitis virus (JEV), and dengue virus (DENV) [1]. DENV

* **Corresponding author Wattana Leowattana:** Department of Clinical Tropical Medicine, Faculty of Tropical Medicine, Mahidol University, 420/6 Rajavithi road, Rachatawee, Bangkok 10400, Thailand; Tel: +6623549100; E-mail: wattana.leo@mahidol.ac.th

Atta-ur-Rahman, *FRS* and M. Iqbal Choudhary (Eds.)

is becoming one of the worst mosquito-borne human pathogens globally. Approximately 400 million people in more than 100 countries are infected each year, leading to 25,000 deaths [2 - 4]. *Aedes aegypti*, which is usually found in tropical areas, and *Aedes albopictus*, commonly found in subtropical areas, are the important vectors of DENV [5]. These mosquitoes are the reservoirs of DENV that could transmit it after infection. Due to the expansion of these vector species, global warming, failure to control the vectors, and urbanization mostly stimulate the drastic increase of DVI worldwide. During 2010-2020, the virus has dramatically re-emerged with significant outbreaks in Africa, South-East Asia, South America, Australia, North America, and Europe [6 - 10]. In endemic areas, most DHF patients are in the younger population, causing a high disease severity. Although DVI is almost asymptomatic and self-limiting, dengue fever (DF) could progress to severe dengue diseases [dengue hemorrhagic fever (DHF) and dengue shock syndrome (DSS)]. They usually manifest as retro-orbital pain, severe headaches, muscle pain, bone pain, joint pain, nausea, vomiting, and rash. In the absence of effective prevention by a reliable safe and efficacious vaccine and specific treatment against DVI, patient management is involved in symptomatic treatment and the limitation of transmission progression. Regarding the geographical region, symptomatic patients' mortality rate varies from 1.2% to 3.5%. Hence, effective antiviral drugs to treat DVI are urgently needed [11, 12].

DENV REPLICATION

DENV is a positive-sense, single-stranded RNA virus within an envelope. There are 4 antigenically definite serotypes (DENV 1-4). The first step in infection is the virus particle interaction with the host cell receptors with envelope (E) glycoprotein. There are several host cell receptors such as glycosaminoglycans (GAGs), dendritic cell-specific intercellular adhesion molecule 3-grabbing non-integrin (DC-SIGN), and T-cell immunoglobulin-mucin domain (TIM). After that, the virus penetrates the host cells by endocytosis [13]. The conformational modifications in the E glycoprotein are induced by low pH within the endosomal vesicle causing the fusion of membrane, and the nucleocapsid is released into the cytoplasm. Moreover, the viral RNA is translated into 1 polyprotein and then is spliced into three structural proteins; capsid (C), membrane (M), envelop (E), and seven non-structural (NS) proteins (NS1, NS2A, NS2B, NS3, NS4A, NS4B, and NS5). The NS proteins utilize lipid metabolism in that cell and produce a re-organization of the endoplasmic reticulum (ER) membrane where viral RNA is replicated inside. Many enzymes in cells, such as kinases and α-glucosidases, serve to replicate RNA, translation, and folding of that protein. Several copies of the C protein package newly initiated genomic RNA and the nucleocapsid and then bud into the lumen of ER to create an enveloped immature virion. Hence, virions are transported *via* the secretory pathway where the E and M proteins encounter post-translational adaptations and conformational changes, comprising the breakdown of precursor M to its mature form by protease furin of the host cell. Progeny virus release occurs through exocytosis and can infect another cell [14]. Molecular study of DENV life cycle and the interaction between virus and host have warranted finding out the small-molecule and peptide antagonists against the interaction of virus and the host cell, the processing of RNA, the genome replication, and the assembly and budding of the mature virus [15 - 17].

The key challenge to dengue therapeutics' success is the rapid decrease in viremia of the patient during a febrile phase, especially in secondary DVI. Hence, the ideal drug that could inhibit DENV should be rapid, active against the four DENV serotypes, possess a good safety window and minimal drug interaction. Many drug candidates have been developed which inhibit either a host or viral protein essential for entry, translation of polyprotein by a proteolytic process, RNA replication, the packaging of the viral genome, and the release of the virion from affected cells. However, all of the candidates have not proved to be better than the placebo in a clinical trial. The discrepancy between pre-clinical and clinical outcomes is the fundamental factor of the study designed. The most common factors included the indefinite and broad spectrum clinical manifestations, the lack of animal models, the limitation of a biological parameter that correlates with clinical outcomes, and the limited financial support for the clinical trials.

Drug repositioning or repurposing can be taken into account as a primary objective and is urgently needed. The repurposing drugs may be authorized or currently used against several clinical situations, or they can be alternatives that have not been successful in any stage of the clinical studies for different purposes. Notably, repurposing drugs are the revelation of new investigations for authorized or unsuccessful agents. The drug repurposing strategy's significance is a quicker and more secure pathway to create new drugs for DHF and DSS management for which a specific treatment is still unavailable. Drug repurposing provides the potentiality to decrease duration and hazards intrinsic to the process of discovery of any drug and urgently advance a candidate drug to the final stage of development [18 - 20]. Moreover, drug repurposing provides an opportunity to develop multi-target drugs able to interfere with several pathways concerned in the pathophysiology of the specific diseases. Multi-target drugs have many advantages such as a synergistic effect, acting on different targets, simplified pharmacokinetics and pharmacodynamics profile, good compliance, and a lower opportunity of drug interferences [21, 22].

DRUG REPURPOSING FOR DENGUE

RdRp Inhibitors

Balapiravir

Balapiravir is a precursor of a nucleoside analogue (NA) named R1479 and was designed for Hepatitis C Virus (HCV) infection by Hoffmann-La Roche [23, 24]. Balapiravir 1,500 mg twice daily for 14 days could decrease plasma concentrations of HCV in a time and dose-dependent fashion. Moreover, adult patients were tolerated very well at 3,000 mg per day of balapiravir [25]. However, clinical safety evidence was reported in the patients receiving extended treatments (a few months) of balapiravir combined with ribavirin and pegylated interferon. Hence, the clinical study of balapiravir for HCV treatment was stopped. Because HCV and DENV have RdRp with a similar overall architecture, balapiravir was subsequently studied in DENV [26]. Nguyen et al. conducted an RCT to study the effect of balapiravir in 32 adult dengue patients (10 = 1,500 mg, 22 = 3,000 mg orally every 12 hours for 5 days) <48 hours of fever compared with 32 adult dengue patients with placebo. They reported that the two-time per day assessment of viremia and one-time per day monitoring of serum NS1 antigen in the balapiravir group did not change the virological markers' kinetics decrease in the fever clearance time with the placebo group. Moreover, the cytokine levels kinetics in plasma and the whole blood transcription profile were also not reduced in the patients treated with balapiravir [27]. The placebo group and the balapiravir group experienced the same mild side effects with good compliance. The patients treated with 3,000 mg balapiravir showed the drug level in plasma of the first twelfth hours, similar to the sufficient level of balapiravir *in vitro*. In 2014, *in vivo* efficacy of balapiravir was clarified in many aspects to show differences in *in vivo* and *in vitro* actions. They reported that early R1479 treatment demonstrated a potent inhibitory effect on DENV polymerase in peripheral blood mononuclear cells (PBMC), which were infected, but delayed treatment reduced the powerful inhibitory effect by 125-fold after added R1479 twenty-four hours post-infection [28]. This outcome relies on the inhibitory effect of cytokines on the alteration of R1479 to R1479-triphosphate. The pretreatment of PBMC with cytokines will decrease the powerful inhibitory effect of R1479 by 6.3- to 19.2-fold. They concluded that the viral infection-induced cytokine reaction could affect the transformation of R1479 to its triphosphate form, resulting in decreased powerful inhibitory effect in the delayed treatment. These results demonstrated why the balapiravir study was not successful in the clinical trial.

Sofosbuvir

Sofosbuvir was developed in 2007 by Michael Sofia, a Pharmasset scientist; however, it was first evaluated in humans in 2010 [29]. Sofosbuvir inhibits the hepatitis C NS5B protein. It is metabolized to the active drug GS-461203 (2'-deoxy-2'-α-fluoro-β-C-methyluridine-5'-triphosphate). Hence, GS-461203 is an incomplete substrate for the NS5B protein, RNA polymerase of the virus, and a viral RNA synthesis inhibiter. The U.S. Food and Drug Administration (FDA) approved sofosbuvir to treat chronic HCV infection on December 6, 2013. Sofosbuvir's effectiveness was studied in 6 clinical trials comprising 1,947 patients who had not been formerly treated for their disease or had not responded to prior treatment, including patients co-infected with HIV and HCV. The trials were designed to evaluate whether the HCV was no longer identified in the blood at least 12 weeks after stopping the treatment, suggesting that a patient with HCV infection has been cured [30, 31]. Since the NS5 catalytic domain region of the Flavivirus and HCV share remarkable similarities, sofosbuvir may be used as a repurposing drug for DHF treatment [26]. In 2018, Gan and colleagues demonstrated the potential effects of sofosbuvir as an anti-dengue agent *in vitro* and *in silico* models. They found that sofosbuvir triphosphate was docked into the active site of DENV2 polymerase and showed a -6.9 kcal/mol binding affinity. Moreover, *in vitro* plaque assay further validated sofosbuvir's hypothesis as a potential DENV2 polymerase blocker with an EC90 = 0.4 μM [32]. Xu and colleagues evaluated sofosbuvir for decisive inhibitory action against DENV replication. They used biochemical assays and cell-based assay with purified full-length NS5 enzymes of DENV. The virus yields reduction assays and cytopathic effect protection demonstrated that sofosbuvir had an inhibitory effect on DENV in cell culture with EC50 of 4.9 μM and 1.4 μM, respectively. Furthermore, Real-time RT-PCR confirmed that sofosbuvir inhibits the replication of DENV RNA with an EC50 of 9.9 μM. They concluded that sofosbuvir has anti-DENV replication activity [33]. Hence, sofosbuvir should be studied in more detail to reveal its efficacy against DENV and its potential action as a DENV polymerase blocker.

Ribavirin

Ribavirin is an antiviral drug used to treat respiratory syncytial virus (RSV) infection, chronic hepatitis C (CHC) infection, and some viral hemorrhagic fevers. The combination of ribavirin and sofosbuvir, simeprevir, peg-interferon α-2b, or peg-interferon α-2a was applied for CHC treatment [34 - 36]. It is also used to treat Crimean–Congo hemorrhagic fever, Lassa fever, and Hantavirus infection but could not treat Ebola or Marburg infections. Ribavirin is available in oral or inhaled form. It was approved for human use in 1986. In 1982, Koff and colleagues studied the inhibitory effects of ribavirin against DENV *in vitro*. They found that ribavirin could reduce the growth of DENV types 1-4 in monkey kidney (LLC-MK2) cells below the cytotoxic concentrations [37]. In 2004, Benarroch and colleagues demonstrated that ribavirin inhibited the action of the DENV 2'-O-methyltransferase NS5 domain by evaluating the crystal structure of a tertiary complex of it [38]. Two years after that, Takhampunya and colleagues studied the effects of ribavirin on DENV replication in LLC-MK2 cells. They reported that the ribavirin has IC50 equal to 50.9 ± 18 µM in inhibiting DENV2 replication [39]. Moreover, Rattanaburee and colleagues investigated the effects of ribavirin on replicating DENV and the transcription of cytokine in the epithelial carcinoma cells of the human lung (A549). They found that when DENV-infected cells were treated with ribavirin, the replication of DENV and the transcription of cytokine (IL-6 and TNF-α) and chemokine (IP-10 and RANTES) were significantly decreased [40]. The available information indicates that ribavirin administered alone is ineffective for clinical use, especially in treatment against CHC, and may also be in DHF. In contrast, animal model studies' unavailability, a phase II clinical trial of ribavirin combined with synergistic drugs is urgently needed for DENV infection.

Antibiotic

Doxycycline

Doxycycline is a broad-spectrum tetracycline-class antibiotic used to treat infections caused by bacteria or parasites. Doxycycline is developed by removing a hydroxyl group from the tetracyclines. It increased fluid and tissue penetration, lipophilic activity, and half-life, increasing activity against bacteria that resisted tetracycline [41, 42]. Doxycycline inhibits protein synthesis by binding to the 30S ribosomal messenger RNA. It is bacteriostatic. These properties prevent the aminoacyl transfer RNA from binding with the messenger RNA-ribosome complex and interrupting the creation of the initiation complex necessary for amino acid protein synthesis. In 2013, Rothan and colleagues conducted an *in vitro* study to evaluate the doxycycline's potential action against DENV replication. They found that doxycycline could inhibit the DENV serine protease with Ki values 55 ± 5 µM [43]. They also reported the sufficient cytotoxic levels of 50% (CC50) against Vero cells of doxycycline as 125 ± 4 µM. Levels below CC50 were used for testing the doxycycline inhibition against DENV2 replication in Vero cells. The results demonstrated a significant decrease in viral load after doxycycline treatment in a concentration-dependent pattern. Moreover, doxycycline could reduce viral RNA at EC50 of 40 ± 3 µM. In 2014, Rothan *et al.* studied doxycycline's potential activity against DENV replication *in vitro* again. They demonstrated that doxycycline inhibited the DENV2 NS2B-NS3pro with an

IC50 value of 52.3 ± 6.2 µM at 37°C and 26.7 ± 5.3 µM at 40°C. The inhibitory effect of doxycycline was evaluated using different concentrations against DENV2 and measured with an assay of plaque formation. They found that the virus titers reduced significantly after adding doxycycline at concentrations lower than its 50% cytotoxic level (CC50, 100 µM), demonstrating concentration-dependent inhibition with an EC50 of 50 µM. Doxycycline substantially inhibited post-infection replication of the four dengue serotypes and viral entry. This inhibition was serotype-specific inhibition (potent activity against DENV2 and DENV4 compared to DENV1 and DENV3) [44]. They concluded that doxycycline's anti-dengue activity and its anti-inflammatory actions might decrease the severity of clinical outcomes such as severe DHF and DSS. Since there is a limitation of the animal model available for DVI at that time, they suggested that clinical trials would be needed to reveal conclusive evidence of the anti-dengue activities of doxycycline (Table **1**).

Iminosugars

Deoxynojirimycin (DNJ) and castanospermine (Cast) are iminosugars that inhibit ER α-glucosidases I and II of the host. This host enzyme-inhibitory activity can affect morphogenesis by misfolding several viruses' glycoproteins, including DENVs, and reducing viral titers. Accordingly, iminosugars can use as a broad-spectrum antiviral drug. A derivative of Cast, Celgosivir, and UV-4, derived from DNJ, are 2 iminosugar drugs evaluated for DENV inhibitors in clinical studies [19].

Celgosivir

A water-soluble prodrug of the alkaloid Cast is called Celgosivir. It is produced from the Moreton Bay chestnut tree (*Castanospermum australae*). Migenix developed it to treat HCV infection. Celgosivir crosses cell membranes and is expeditiously converted to Cast [45]. Celgosivir has a new action mechanism by blocking the host glycosylation of viral proteins [46]. It inhibits the catalytic action of α-glucosidase I and II (ER-resident enzymes), which plays a crucial role in the correct folding of glycoproteins. The viral protein folding was affected by Cast treatment due to removing terminal glucose residue from N-linked glycans [47]. Lack of transformation of the high mannose sugar on viral proteins resulted in misfolding and protein assembling, causing cellular ER stress. The expression of unfolded protein response (UPR) genes from ER stress induces various signaling pathways regarded as cell death [48]. In 2007, Schul and colleagues conducted celgosivir oral administration in a DF viremia model in mice. They demonstrated that celgosivir significantly decreased circulating DENV in a dose-dependent fashion, although it reduced splenomegaly and proinflammatory cytokine concentrations after delayed therapy. They concluded that the circulating DENV in a mouse model was a useful tool for evaluating anti-DENV drugs and indicated that early antiviral therapy in the acute phase of DHF could decrease the disease severity [49].

Furthermore, Rathore and colleagues reported celgosivir's effectiveness in mouse models that could re-issue the primary or secondary antibody-dependent enhanced DVI. Mice treated with celgosivir demonstrated decreased viremia, improved immune response, and enhanced survival, as reflected by the analysis of the cytokines in serum. The survival was increased even after delayed treatment. They suggested that celgosivir may be a potential candidate drug for the clinical trial in DHF patients [50]. In 2012, Watanabe et al. showed that celgosivir protection is schedule and dose-dependent, and a twice-daily dose of 50, 25, or 10 mg/kg is better than 100 mg/kg one time per day. These results impacted the dose regimen selection for celgosivir clinical trial as a treatment against DHF [51]. A phase 1b RCT proof-of-concept trial (CELADEN) was conducted in one center in Singapore. Low et al. used the effective doses of celgosivir in animals and used the effective dose in previous large clinical trials for CHC and HIV infection. The patients who were confirmed with dengue fever were included. Twenty-four patients with primary or secondary DENV1–3 infections were treated with celgosivir 400 mg per day on the 1st day of fever. Then they received 200 mg 2 times a day for maintenance doses. Twenty-six comparable patients received a matched placebo. Mean virologically log reduction in the celgosivir group was slightly higher than in the placebo group but no statistically significant. The area under the curve (AUC) of fever was also no significant difference. However, serum NS1 concentration's clearance time was shorter in the celgosivir group than the placebo group significantly [52]. This finding seems to impact celgosivir's application to treat more severe vascular permeability syndrome [53]. They reported similar incidences of side effects between groups. They concluded that celgosivir is well-tolerated and safe. However, it does not decrease the viral load or fever clearance time in DHF patients. In 2016, Watanabe *et al.* try to modify the therapeutic regimen for celgosivir in animal models of DVI serotypes 1 and 2. They studied a regimen of four-time daily treatment instead of two times daily and found that the four-time daily regimen significantly decreased viremia, demonstrating that the same regimen could be useful in future clinical trials [54].

UV-4B

In 2013, Perry and colleagues conducted *in vivo* study of the UV-4, iminosugar drug, to protect from lethal DENV challenge by utilizing a well-established model of DHF and DSS-like lethal condition in type I and II interferon receptors lacking mice (AG129).

Table 1. The RNA-dependent RNA polymerase (RdRp) inhibitors and antibiotic drugs are repurposed as DENV inhibitors.

Drug Name	Chemical Structure	Drug Class	Pre-clinical Data	Clinical Data
Balapiravir		RdRp inhibitors	-Reduction in viral replication *in vitro*	-RCT (n = 64) could not show the improvement in viremia, clinical outcomes, and disease severity
Sofosbuvir		RdRp inhibitors	-Reduction in viral replication *in vitro*	-None
Ribavirin		RdRp inhibitors	-Reduction in viral replication *in vitro*	-None
Doxycycline		Antibiotic	-Reduction in viral replication *in vitro*	-None

They found that UV-4 was a powerful iminosugar for treating DVI in this mouse model. Specifically, the treatment with UV-4 could decrease viremia, mortality, and cytokine storm in critical tissues. Besides, UV-4 treatment can be delayed, and the anti-DENV antibody response was also not changed [55]. In 2016, Warfield and colleagues studied the therapeutic window and minimal effective dose of UV-4B in a severe DENV2 infection mouse model with an antibody-dependent enhancement (ADE) which types I and II interferon receptors depletion. They found that 10-20 mg/kg of UV-4B treated three times per day for seven days with started 48 h after the infection has a significant survival benefit. Moreover, UV-4B also decreased viral particles *in vitro* with DENV serotypes 1, 2, 3, and 4. They concluded that UV-4B is suitable for phases 1 and 2 clinical trials in human DHF and DSS [56]. Plummer and colleagues demonstrated that mice treated with UV-4B resulted in both nonselective and selective effects. More specific positive selection was observed as predicted in glycosylated proteins and unpredictably in NS5, which showed that UV-4B has a broad impact on viral replication. Despite continuous forced drug pressure over 18 cycles of replication resulting in increased accumulation of mutations, a virus with increased fitness was not observed. They concluded that it is unlikely that UV-4B drug resistance by DENV will create in humans [57] (Table **2**).

Anti-parasitic drugs

Chloroquine (CQ)

CQ is a widely used drug for malaria and rheumatoid arthritis treatment for over 70 years. It acts as an anti-inflammatory drug with a weak base that tends to accumulate in cells' acidic organelles. Moreover, it also interferes with the endosome-mediated endocytosis of the virus. The pretreatment of mammalian cells with CQ can decrease the efficiency of DVI. Apart from directly affecting DENV, CQ also modulates antigen presentation in dendritic cells and downregulates proinflammatory cytokines [58 - 60]. Moreover, CQ could be implicated in stimulating proinflammatory cytokine pathways in severe DHF. In human macrophage cells (U937) and African green monkey kidney cells (Vero), CQ was reported to block DENV-2 replication in a dose-dependent fashion at non-toxic levels [61, 62]. CQ decreased the expression levels of proinflammatory cytokines (TNF-α, IFN-α, IL-6, IL-12, IFN-β, and IFN-γ in DENV-infected U937 cells. Furthermore, CQ could inhibit IFN-α expression in plasmacytoid dendritic cells infected with DENV, meaning that CQ could stimulate the cytokine activity against DENV [63].

Table 2. The iminosugars drugs are repurposed as DENV inhibitors.

Drug Name	Chemical Structure	Drug Class	Pre-Clinical Data	Clinical Data
Celgosivir		Iminosugars	-Reduced viral replication *in vitro* -Provided protection against lethal DENV challenge in a mouse model	-RCTs (n=50) could not show improvement in the viremia and clinical outcomes. -Acknowledging the possibility of failing to achieve a therapeutic dose.
UV-4B		Iminosugars	-Reduced viral replication *in vitro* -Reduced mortality and viremia in the animal model	-None

Although CQ appears to achieve beneficial effects in DVI *in vitro*, it seems to be least capable of combatting DHF in clinical settings (64, 65). Tricou and colleagues found that a 3-day CQ treatment had no favorable effect on circulating NS1, viremia, fever clearance time, cytokine, and T-cell response. However,

fewer patients who developed DHF were reported for the CQ treated group than the placebo group with no significant difference. Another clinical trial was conducted in Brazil in 2013 by Borges and colleagues. They randomly administered CQ or placebo for three days to 129 DHF patients. There were 37 confirmed DHF and completed the study (19 treated with CQ and 18 treated with placebo). They found no statistically significant difference in the disease duration or the fever clearance time. However, 12 confirmed dengue patients (63%) reported a significant reduction in the intensity of pain and a substantial improvement in their quality of life (QoL) (p = 0.0004) during the CQ treatment. Moreover, the symptoms of them returned abruptly after these patients stopped CQ treatment. They concluded that CQ is not powerful enough in DHF therapy and had no significant effect on the disease duration of DHF. By the way, CQ may improve the QoL [66].

Ivermectin

In 1973, the Kitasato Institute in Japan collaborated with the Merck Sharpe & Dohme Research Laboratories (MSDRL) in the US to explore new and innovative antibiotics. They discovered the avermectin-producing micro-organism, *Streptomyces avermectinius*. Ivermectin binds tightly to glutamate-gated chloride channels, which were found in muscle and nerve cells of invertebrates by increasing the permeability of the cell membrane to chloride ions. The parasite will be paralyzed and death by the direct effect or by causing them to be starved, resulting from the hyperpolarization [67]. Ivermectin is an anti-parasitic drug with broad-spectrum used to treat microfilariae of *Onchocerca volvulus* in humans. Moreover, it could be used for scabies and lice therapy [68, 69]. Ivermectin was evaluated as an anti-DENV by *in silico* docking studies on an undeveloped site of the NS3 protein [70]. Due to the NS3 DENV-helicase complex structure was not available, the crystal of the NS3 helicase of the Kunjin virus was used as a template for the docking. They reported that ivermectin could block DENV helicase in a FRET-based helicase assay with an IC50 of 500±70 nM and could not block the helicase domain of DENV polymerase activity or ATPase activity at a level of 1,000 nM. Furthermore, the mutation of helicases was developed to evaluate the crucial interactions of this enzyme with ivermectin. They found that ivermectin could not inhibit the prepared mutants, meaning that the catalytic site mutations are deleterious for ivermectin to bind to the helicase. In Vero-B cells CPE reduction assays, ivermectin demonstrated an EC50 > 1 µM and in a qRT-PCR assay, an EC50 of 0.7 µM. Moreover, the kinetics of helicase and the inhibition tests demonstrated that RNA's availability was needed to bind ivermectin with protein efficiently. It acts as a non-competitive antagonist, and the effect should be better within 14 h after treatment. Ivermectin can also block DVI by interfering with the NS5 interaction with the importin [71, 72]. Importin

(Impα/ß1) is significant for recognizing and subsequent movement of proteins between the nucleus and cytoplasm. They used a protein-protein binding assay and found that ivermectin can block the interaction of Impα/ß1 and NS5 with an IC50 of 17 µM, but not the interaction of NS5 with Impß1 (IC50 > 22 mM). This result demonstrated that ivermectin is specific for one of the several nuclear import mechanisms. Additionally, at a concentration of 25 µM, ivermectin inhibits the virus production in Vero cells. These data showed that nuclear import inhibitors could be considered a potent and specific antiviral agent [73, 74]. An RCT is currently being studied to evaluate ivermectin efficacy against DHF (Table **3**).

Table 3. The anti-parasitic drugs are repurposed as DENV inhibitors.

Drug Name	Chemical Structure	Drug Class	Pre-Clinical Data	Clinical Data
Chloroquine		Anti-parasitic	-Reduced viral replication *in vitro*. -Reduced the cytokine response *in vitro*	-RCT (n=307) could not show improvement in viremia and clinical outcomes -RCT (n=37) could not show improvement in viremia and clinical outcomes
Ivermectin		Anti-parasitic	-Reduced viral replication *in vitro*.	-None

Mast Cell Stabilizers

Cromolyn and Ketotifen

Many studies reported the implication of mast cells (MCs) and their products released in severe DHF [75 - 77]. MCs are immune cells that inhabit all tissues closely and usually surround the capillaries [78]. MCs are reacted to DVI after a mosquito bite. They responded by releasing the granules, including the liberation of pre-formed mediators comprising anti-coagulants and proteases and cytokine synthesis and lipid mediators at the site of the skin infection [79]. They also reacted with T cells to increase the viral eradication at the point of cutaneous infection [80]. However, MCs' beneficial effect in removing DENV with the uncontrolled release was increased vascular leakage in an animal model [81]. The escalation in serum concentrations of the MC-specific chymase and protease occurred in DHF patients and increased to the highest levels in severe DHF or DSS compared to the DHF patients without severity [82]. Furthermore, the increased vascular permeability in an animal model of DVI was not detected in a mouse with MC deficient and when cromolyn and ketotifen inhibited MC activation [77, 83]. Cromolyn is an MC stabilizer that inhibits the liberation of inflammatory mediators like the other antihistamine. It is usually used to treat asthma, allergic conjunctivitis, allergic rhinitis, and ulcerative colitis. Ketotifen is an MC stabilizer and an uncompetitive H1-antihistamine. It is mostly used in allergic conjunctivitis caused by allergens and used to prevent asthmatic attacks. Cromolyn and ketotifen stabilize the MC membrane, preventing the liberation of the inflammation mediators. The use of these drugs could reduce vascular leakage in mouse models of DVI, especially wild-type and immune-compromised [84]. These data demonstrated that MC stabilizers could be considered the candidate drugs in clinical trials shortly.

Leukotriene Inhibitor and Platelet-activating Factor (PAF) Inhibitor

Montelukast and Rupatadine

Several vasoactive lipid mediators are liberated by MC activation, composing leukotriene and PAF, and besides MCs, these are released by the activation of endothelium and other immune cells. A leukotriene inhibitor effectively reduced DENV influenced vascular permeability, as was a PAF-inhibitor, in mice. PAF had formerly been involved in DENV-induced vascular leakage in an animal model [85]. Montelukast is an inhibitor of leukotriene receptor used to treat asthma, bronchospasm, and seasonal allergies. It inhibits MC activity, blocking mediators like the leukotriene. Rupatadine is a second-generation, non-sedating, long-acting antihistamine with selective peripheral anti-H1 receptor action. It further blocks the PAF receptors base on *in vitro* and *in vivo* studies [86, 87]. The rupatadine effects were evaluated *in vitro* and in an animal model, which demonstrated significantly decreased endothelium's permeability by the serum of DVI and significantly blocked the increased hematocrit in the mice with DVI in a dose-dependence fashion [88].

Recently, Malavige and colleagues conducted an RCT in 183 adult patients to evaluate rupatadine efficacy for treating acute dengue infection [89]. They found that rupatadine 40 mg per day showed a well-tolerated and safe outcome with a similar percentage of side effects with rupatadine compared with placebo. However, they did not show the primary endpoint of the ascites or pleural effusions reduction. Moreover, post hoc analysis demonstrated significantly higher platelet counts and lower liver enzyme concentrations. Rupatadine treatment indicates minimal tissue damage and a little pleural effusion, meaning that further investigation is needed to study the drug's utility against dengue vascular damage thoroughly. Furthermore, Park and colleagues reported that montelukast was only one of the specific drugs that demonstrated the DENV inhibitory activity *in vitro* and *in vivo* by directly blocking DENV replication and relieving related symptoms [90] (Table **4**).

Table 4. The mast cell stabilizers, a leukotriene inhibitor, and platelet-activating factor (PAF)-inhibitor drugs are repurposed as DENV inhibitors.

Drug Name	Chemical Structure	Drug Class	Pre-Clinical Data	Clinical Data
Cromolyn		-Mast cell stabilizers	-Reduction of vascular leakage in the animal model	-None
Ketotifen		-Mast cell stabilizers -H1-antihistamine	-Reduction of vascular leakage in the animal model	-None
Montelukast		-Mast cell stabilizers -Leukotriene inhibitor	-Reduction of vascular leakage in the animal model	-None
Rupatadine		-Mast cell stabilizers -PAF-inhibitor	-Reduction of vascular leakage in the animal model	-RCT (n=183) could not show improvement in vasculopathy and clinical outcomes

CONCLUDING REMARKS

The current standard therapies for DVI remain symptomatic and supportive treatment. It is hard to guess the dengue disease severity because the warning signs usually show in the late state. Therefore, DHF patients' hospitalization can improve the clinical outcome by closely monitoring clinical manifestation and applying the appropriate interventions. Ideally, the drugs that can reduce the viremia of DENV could decrease the risk of disease severity and dramatically improve the clinical outcomes of DHF patients. However, the studies to develop the targeted therapeutics drugs remain limited, and the hindrance is comprised of virus-intrinsic factors and the factors from host response. Furthermore, the precise understanding of the disease's pathophysiology will identify new targets for the intervention. Due to an extended period, several phases of the studies, and costly process for the classical drug-discovery, identifying new indications for currently used drugs, drug repurposing could improve and strengthen several new drugs for DHF. An effective timesaver to newly available drugs could serve as a life-saving strategy for thousands of patients because DHF is endemic in the world's poorest countries. We have explored many approved drugs in different pharmacological classes that were repurposed for treating DVI. Although some of the drugs did not illustrate actual effectiveness against DVI, a consistent number of those drugs could be regarded as an appropriate and advanced starting point to develop new treatment guidelines. These demonstrated the significance of the repurposing strategy in finding a new DHF therapy.

CONSENT FOR PUBLICATION

Not applicable.

CONFLICT OF INTEREST

The author declares no conflict of interest, financial or otherwise.

ACKNOWLEDGEMENTS

Declared none.

REFERENCES

[1]   Mukhopadhyay S, Kuhn RJ, Rossmann MG. A structural perspective of the flavivirus life cycle. Nat Rev Microbiol 2005; 3(1): 13-22.
[http://dx.doi.org/10.1038/nrmicro1067] [PMID: 15608696]

[2]   Bhatt S, Gething PW, Brady OJ, *et al.* The global distribution and burden of dengue. Nature 2013; 496(7446): 504-7.
[http://dx.doi.org/10.1038/nature12060] [PMID: 23563266]

[3]   Cucunawangsih Lugito NPH. Trends of dengue disease epidemiology. Virology (Auckl) 2017; 8:

1178122X17695836.
[http://dx.doi.org/10.1177/1178122X17695836] [PMID: 28579763]

[4] Guo C, Zhou Z, Wen Z, *et al.* Global epidemiology of dengue outbreaks in 1990-2015: A systematic review and meta-analysis. Front Cell Infect Microbiol 2017; 7: 317.
[http://dx.doi.org/10.3389/fcimb.2017.00317] [PMID: 28748176]

[5] Higa Y. Dengue Vectors and their Spatial Distribution. Trop Med Health 2011; 39(4) (Suppl.): 17-27.
[http://dx.doi.org/10.2149/tmh.2011-S04] [PMID: 22500133]

[6] Rezza G. Dengue and chikungunya: long-distance spread and outbreaks in naïve areas. Pathog Glob Health 2014; 108(8): 349-55.
[http://dx.doi.org/10.1179/2047773214Y.0000000163] [PMID: 25491436]

[7] Liu K, Hou X, Ren Z, *et al.* Climate factors and the East Asian summer monsoon may drive large outbreaks of dengue in China. Environ Res 2020; 183: 109190.
[http://dx.doi.org/10.1016/j.envres.2020.109190] [PMID: 32311903]

[8] Faria NR, da Costa AC, Lourenço J, *et al.* Genomic and epidemiological characterisation of a dengue virus outbreak among blood donors in Brazil. Sci Rep 2017; 7(1): 15216.
[http://dx.doi.org/10.1038/s41598-017-15152-8] [PMID: 29123142]

[9] Dumre SP, Bhandari R, Shakya G, *et al.* Dengue virus serotypes 1 and 2 responsible for major dengue outbreaks in Nepal: Clinical, laboratory, and epidemiological features. Am J Trop Med Hyg 2017; 97(4): 1062-9.
[http://dx.doi.org/10.4269/ajtmh.17-0221] [PMID: 29031282]

[10] Barzon L. Ongoing and emerging arbovirus threats in Europe. J Clin Virol 2018; 107: 38-47.
[http://dx.doi.org/10.1016/j.jcv.2018.08.007] [PMID: 30176404]

[11] Hadinegoro SR, Arredondo-García JL, Capeding MR, *et al.* Efficacy and long-term safety of a dengue vaccine in regions of endemic disease. N Engl J Med 2015; 373(13): 1195-206.
[http://dx.doi.org/10.1056/NEJMoa1506223] [PMID: 26214039]

[12] McFee RB. Selected mosquito borne illnesses - Dengue. Dis Mon 2018; 64(5): 246-74.
[http://dx.doi.org/10.1016/j.disamonth.2018.01.011] [PMID: 29566984]

[13] Lescar J, Soh S, Lee LT, Vasudevan SG, Kang C, Lim SP. The dengue virus replication complex: From RNA replication to protein-protein interactions to evasion of innate immunity. Adv Exp Med Biol 2018; 1062: 115-29.
[http://dx.doi.org/10.1007/978-981-10-8727-1_9] [PMID: 29845529]

[14] Guzman MG, Gubler DJ, Izquierdo A, Martinez E, Halstead SB. Dengue infection. Nat Rev Dis Primers 2016; 2: 16055.
[http://dx.doi.org/10.1038/nrdp.2016.55] [PMID: 27534439]

[15] Botting C, Kuhn RJ. Novel approaches to flavivirus drug discovery. Expert Opin Drug Discov 2012; 7(5): 417-28.
[http://dx.doi.org/10.1517/17460441.2012.673579] [PMID: 22439769]

[16] Lim SP, Wang QY, Noble CG, *et al.* Ten years of dengue drug discovery: progress and prospects. Antiviral Res 2013; 100(2): 500-19.
[http://dx.doi.org/10.1016/j.antiviral.2013.09.013] [PMID: 24076358]

[17] Kok WM. New developments in flavivirus drug discovery. Expert Opin Drug Discov 2016; 11(5): 433-45.
[http://dx.doi.org/10.1517/17460441.2016.1160887] [PMID: 26966889]

[18] Botta L, Rivara M, Zuliani V, Radi M. Drug repurposing approaches to fight Dengue virus infection and related diseases. Front Biosci 2018; 23: 997-1019.
[http://dx.doi.org/10.2741/4630] [PMID: 28930586]

[19] Lo YC, Huang IH, Ho TC, Chien YW, Perng GC. Antiviral drugs and other therapeutic options for

dengue virus infection. Curr Treat Options Infect Dis 2017; 9: 185-93.
[http://dx.doi.org/10.1007/s40506-017-0122-z]

[20] Wang Q, Xu R. DenguePredict: An integrated drug repositioning approach towards drug discovery for dengue. AMIA Annu Symp Proc 2015; 2015: 1279-88.
[PMID: 26958268]

[21] Troost B, Smit JM. Recent advances in antiviral drug development towards dengue virus. Curr Opin Virol 2020; 43: 9-21.
[http://dx.doi.org/10.1016/j.coviro.2020.07.009] [PMID: 32795907]

[22] Silva NM, Santos NC, Martins IC. Dengue and zika viruses: epidemiological history, potential therapies, and promising vaccines. Trop Med Infect Dis 2020; 5(4): 150.
[http://dx.doi.org/10.3390/tropicalmed5040150] [PMID: 32977703]

[23] Klumpp K, Lévêque V, Le Pogam S, *et al.* The novel nucleoside analog R1479 (4′-azidocytidine) is a potent inhibitor of NS5B-dependent RNA synthesis and hepatitis C virus replication in cell culture. J Biol Chem 2006; 281(7): 3793-9.
[http://dx.doi.org/10.1074/jbc.M510195200] [PMID: 16316989]

[24] Toniutto P, Fabris C, Bitetto D, *et al.* Antiviral treatment in patients with hepatitis C virus-related cirrhosis awaiting liver transplantation. Ther Clin Risk Manag 2008; 4(3): 599-603.
[http://dx.doi.org/10.2147/TCRM.S2661] [PMID: 18827855]

[25] Roberts SK, Cooksley G, Dore GJ, *et al.* Robust antiviral activity of R1626, a novel nucleoside analog: a randomized, placebo-controlled study in patients with chronic hepatitis C. Hepatology 2008; 48(2): 398-406.
[http://dx.doi.org/10.1002/hep.22321] [PMID: 18553458]

[26] Yap TL, Xu T, Chen YL, *et al.* Crystal structure of the dengue virus RNA-dependent RNA polymerase catalytic domain at 1.85-angstrom resolution. J Virol 2007; 81(9): 4753-65.
[http://dx.doi.org/10.1128/JVI.02283-06] [PMID: 17301146]

[27] Nguyen NM, Tran CN, Phung LK, *et al.* A randomized, double-blind placebo controlled trial of balapiravir, a polymerase inhibitor, in adult dengue patients. J Infect Dis 2013; 207(9): 1442-50.
[http://dx.doi.org/10.1093/infdis/jis470] [PMID: 22807519]

[28] Chen YL, Abdul Ghafar N, Karuna R, *et al.* Activation of peripheral blood mononuclear cells by dengue virus infection depotentiates balapiravir. J Virol 2014; 88(3): 1740-7.
[http://dx.doi.org/10.1128/JVI.02841-13] [PMID: 24257621]

[29] Sofia MJ, Bao D, Chang W, *et al.* Discovery of a β-d-2′-deoxy-2′-α-fluoro-2′-β-C-methyluridine nucleotide prodrug (PSI-7977) for the treatment of hepatitis C virus. J Med Chem 2010; 53(19): 7202-18.
[http://dx.doi.org/10.1021/jm100863x] [PMID: 20845908]

[30] Nakamura M, Kanda T, Haga Y, *et al.* Sofosbuvir treatment and hepatitis C virus infection. World J Hepatol 2016; 8(3): 183-90.
[http://dx.doi.org/10.4254/wjh.v8.i3.183] [PMID: 26839641]

[31] Kattakuzhy S, Levy R, Kottilil S. Sofosbuvir for treatment of chronic hepatitis C. Hepatol Int 2015; 9(2): 161-73.
[http://dx.doi.org/10.1007/s12072-014-9606-9] [PMID: 25788194]

[32] Gan CS, Lim SK, Chee CF, Yusof R, Heh CH. Sofosbuvir as treatment against dengue? Chem Biol Drug Des 2018; 91(2): 448-55.
[http://dx.doi.org/10.1111/cbdd.13091] [PMID: 28834304]

[33] Xu HT, Colby-Germinario SP, Hassounah SA, *et al.* Evaluation of Sofosbuvir (β-D-2′-deoxy-2′-α-fluoro-2′-β-C-methyluridine) as an inhibitor of Dengue virus replication. Sci Rep 2017; 7(1): 6345.
[http://dx.doi.org/10.1038/s41598-017-06612-2] [PMID: 28740124]

[34]   Paeshuyse J, Dallmeier K, Neyts J. Ribavirin for the treatment of chronic hepatitis C virus infection: a review of the proposed mechanisms of action. Curr Opin Virol 2011; 1(6): 590-8.
[http://dx.doi.org/10.1016/j.coviro.2011.10.030] [PMID: 22440916]

[35]   Flori N, Funakoshi N, Duny Y, *et al.* Pegylated interferon-α2a and ribavirin versus pegylated interferon-α2b and ribavirin in chronic hepatitis C : a meta-analysis. Drugs 2013; 73(3): 263-77.
[http://dx.doi.org/10.1007/s40265-013-0027-1] [PMID: 23436591]

[36]   Zeuzem S, Poordad F. Pegylated-interferon plus ribavirin therapy in the treatment of CHC: individualization of treatment duration according to on-treatment virologic response. Curr Med Res Opin 2010; 26(7): 1733-43.
[http://dx.doi.org/10.1185/03007995.2010.487038] [PMID: 20482242]

[37]   Koff WC, Elm JL Jr, Halstead SB. Antiviral effects if ribavirin and 6-mercapto-9-tetrahyd-o-2-furylpurine against dengue viruses *in vitro.* Antiviral Res 1982; 2(1-2): 69-79.
[http://dx.doi.org/10.1016/0166-3542(82)90027-4] [PMID: 7201778]

[38]   Benarroch D, Egloff MP, Mulard L, Guerreiro C, Romette JL, Canard B. A structural basis for the inhibition of the NS5 dengue virus mRNA 2'-O-methyltransferase domain by ribavirin 5'-triphosphate. J Biol Chem 2004; 279(34): 35638-43.
[http://dx.doi.org/10.1074/jbc.M400460200] [PMID: 15152003]

[39]   Takhampunya R, Ubol S, Houng HS, Cameron CE, Padmanabhan R. Inhibition of dengue virus replication by mycophenolic acid and ribavirin. J Gen Virol 2006; 87(Pt 7): 1947-52.
[http://dx.doi.org/10.1099/vir.0.81655-0] [PMID: 16760396]

[40]   Rattanaburee T, Junking M, Panya A, *et al.* Inhibition of dengue virus production and cytokine/chemokine expression by ribavirin and compound A. Antiviral Res 2015; 124: 83-92.
[http://dx.doi.org/10.1016/j.antiviral.2015.10.005] [PMID: 26542647]

[41]   Joshi N, Miller DQ. Doxycycline revisited. Arch Intern Med 1997; 157(13): 1421-8.
[http://dx.doi.org/10.1001/archinte.1997.00440340035003] [PMID: 9224219]

[42]   Cunha BA. Doxycycline re-revisited. Arch Intern Med 1999; 159(9): 1006-7.
[http://dx.doi.org/10.1001/archinte.159.9.1006] [PMID: 10326943]

[43]   Rothan HA, Buckle MJ, Ammar YA, *et al.* Study the antiviral activity of some derivatives of tetracycline and non-steroid anti inflammatory drugs towards dengue virus. Trop Biomed 2013; 30(4): 681-90.
[PMID: 24522138]

[44]   Rothan HA, Mohamed Z, Paydar M, Rahman NA, Yusof R. Inhibitory effect of doxycycline against dengue virus replication *in vitro.* Arch Virol 2014; 159(4): 711-8.
[http://dx.doi.org/10.1007/s00705-013-1880-7] [PMID: 24142271]

[45]   Kang MS. Uptake and metabolism of BuCast: a glycoprotein processing inhibitor and a potential anti-HIV drug. Glycobiology 1996; 6(2): 209-16.
[http://dx.doi.org/10.1093/glycob/6.2.209] [PMID: 8727792]

[46]   Durantel D. Celgosivir, an alpha-glucosidase I inhibitor for the potential treatment of HCV infection. Curr Opin Investig Drugs 2009; 10(8): 860-70.
[PMID: 19649930]

[47]   Taylor DL, Sunkara PS, Liu PS, Kang MS, Bowlin TL, Tyms AS. 6-0-butanoylcastanospermine (MDL 28,574) inhibits glycoprotein processing and the growth of HIVs. AIDS 1991; 5(6): 693-8.
[http://dx.doi.org/10.1097/00002030-199106000-00008] [PMID: 1652979]

[48]   Schröder M, Kaufman RJ. ER stress and the unfolded protein response. Mutat Res 2005; 569(1-2): 29-63.
[http://dx.doi.org/10.1016/j.mrfmmm.2004.06.056] [PMID: 15603751]

[49]   Schul W, Liu W, Xu HY, Flamand M, Vasudevan SG. A dengue fever viremia model in mice shows

reduction in viral replication and suppression of the inflammatory response after treatment with antiviral drugs. J Infect Dis 2007; 195(5): 665-74.
[http://dx.doi.org/10.1086/511310] [PMID: 17262707]

[50] Rathore AP, Paradkar PN, Watanabe S, *et al.* Celgosivir treatment misfolds dengue virus NS1 protein, induces cellular pro-survival genes and protects against lethal challenge mouse model. Antiviral Res 2011; 92(3): 453-60.
[http://dx.doi.org/10.1016/j.antiviral.2011.10.002] [PMID: 22020302]

[51] Watanabe S, Rathore AP, Sung C, *et al.* Dose- and schedule-dependent protective efficacy of celgosivir in a lethal mouse model for dengue virus infection informs dosing regimen for a proof of concept clinical trial. Antiviral Res 2012; 96(1): 32-5.
[http://dx.doi.org/10.1016/j.antiviral.2012.07.008] [PMID: 22867971]

[52] Low JG, Sung C, Wijaya L, *et al.* Efficacy and safety of celgosivir in patients with dengue fever (CELADEN): a phase 1b, randomised, double-blind, placebo-controlled, proof-of-concept trial. Lancet Infect Dis 2014; 14(8): 706-15.
[http://dx.doi.org/10.1016/S1473-3099(14)70730-3] [PMID: 24877997]

[53] Halstead SB. Stumbles on the path to dengue control. Lancet Infect Dis 2014; 14(8): 661-2.
[http://dx.doi.org/10.1016/S1473-3099(14)70770-4] [PMID: 24877998]

[54] Watanabe S, Chan KW, Dow G, Ooi EE, Low JG, Vasudevan SG. Optimizing celgosivir therapy in mouse models of dengue virus infection of serotypes 1 and 2: The search for a window for potential therapeutic efficacy. Antiviral Res 2016; 127: 10-9.
[http://dx.doi.org/10.1016/j.antiviral.2015.12.008] [PMID: 26794905]

[55] Perry ST, Buck MD, Plummer EM, *et al.* An iminosugar with potent inhibition of dengue virus infection *in vivo.* Antiviral Res 2013; 98(1): 35-43.
[http://dx.doi.org/10.1016/j.antiviral.2013.01.004] [PMID: 23376501]

[56] Warfield KL, Plummer EM, Sayce AC, *et al.* Inhibition of endoplasmic reticulum glucosidases is required for *in vitro* and *in vivo* dengue antiviral activity by the iminosugar UV-4. Antiviral Res 2016; 129: 93-8.
[http://dx.doi.org/10.1016/j.antiviral.2016.03.001] [PMID: 26946111]

[57] Plummer E, Buck MD, Sanchez M, *et al.* Dengue virus evolution under a host-targeted antiviral. J Virol 2015; 89(10): 5592-601.
[http://dx.doi.org/10.1128/JVI.00028-15] [PMID: 25762732]

[58] Navarro-Sanchez E, Altmeyer R, Amara A, *et al.* Dendritic-cell-specific ICAM3-grabbing non-integrin is essential for the productive infection of human dendritic cells by mosquito-cell-derived dengue viruses. EMBO Rep 2003; 4(7): 723-8.
[http://dx.doi.org/10.1038/sj.embor.embor866] [PMID: 12783086]

[59] Randolph VB, Stollar V. Low pH-induced cell fusion in flavivirus-infected Aedes albopictus cell cultures. J Gen Virol 1990; 71(Pt 8): 1845-50.
[http://dx.doi.org/10.1099/0022-1317-71-8-1845] [PMID: 2167941]

[60] Accapezzato D, Visco V, Francavilla V, *et al.* Chloroquine enhances human CD8+ T cell responses against soluble antigens *in vivo.* J Exp Med 2005; 202(6): 817-28.
[http://dx.doi.org/10.1084/jem.20051106] [PMID: 16157687]

[61] Farias KJ, Machado PR, da Fonseca BA. Chloroquine inhibits dengue virus type 2 replication in Vero cells but not in C6/36 cells. ScientificWorldJournal 2013; 2013: 282734.
[http://dx.doi.org/10.1155/2013/282734] [PMID: 23431254]

[62] Farias KJ, Machado PR, de Almeida Junior RF, de Aquino AA, da Fonseca BA. Chloroquine interferes with dengue-2 virus replication in U937 cells. Microbiol Immunol 2014; 58(6): 318-26.
[http://dx.doi.org/10.1111/1348-0421.12154] [PMID: 24773578]

[63] Gandini M, Gras C, Azeredo EL, *et al.* Dengue virus activates membrane TRAIL relocalization and

IFN-α production by human plasmacytoid dendritic cells *in vitro* and *in vivo*. PLoS Negl Trop Dis 2013; 7(6): e2257.
[http://dx.doi.org/10.1371/journal.pntd.0002257] [PMID: 23755314]

[64]   Tricou V, Minh NN, Van TP, *et al.* A randomized controlled trial of chloroquine for the treatment of dengue in Vietnamese adults. PLoS Negl Trop Dis 2010; 4(8): e785.
[http://dx.doi.org/10.1371/journal.pntd.0000785] [PMID: 20706626]

[65]   Tricou V, Minh NN, Farrar J, Tran HT, Simmons CP. Kinetics of viremia and NS1 antigenemia are shaped by immune status and virus serotype in adults with dengue. PLoS Negl Trop Dis 2011; 5(9): e1309.
[http://dx.doi.org/10.1371/journal.pntd.0001309] [PMID: 21909448]

[66]   Borges MC, Castro LA, Fonseca BA. Chloroquine use improves dengue-related symptoms. Mem Inst Oswaldo Cruz 2013; 108(5): 596-9.
[http://dx.doi.org/10.1590/S0074-02762013000500010] [PMID: 23903975]

[67]   Pemberton DJ, Franks CJ, Walker RJ, Holden-Dye L. Characterization of glutamate-gated chloride channels in the pharynx of wild-type and mutant Caenorhabditis elegans delineates the role of the subunit GluCl-alpha2 in the function of the native receptor. Mol Pharmacol 2001; 59(5): 1037-43.
[http://dx.doi.org/10.1124/mol.59.5.1037] [PMID: 11306685]

[68]   Babalola OE. Ocular onchocerciasis: current management and future prospects. Clin Ophthalmol 2011; 5: 1479-91.
[http://dx.doi.org/10.2147/OPTH.S8372] [PMID: 22069350]

[69]   Strycharz JP, Yoon KS, Clark JM. A new ivermectin formulation topically kills permethrin-resistant human head lice (Anoplura: Pediculidae). J Med Entomol 2008; 45(1): 75-81.
[http://dx.doi.org/10.1093/jmedent/45.1.75] [PMID: 18283945]

[70]   Mastrangelo E, Pezzullo M, De Burghgraeve T, *et al.* Ivermectin is a potent inhibitor of flavivirus replication specifically targeting NS3 helicase activity: new prospects for an old drug. J Antimicrob Chemother 2012; 67(8): 1884-94.
[http://dx.doi.org/10.1093/jac/dks147] [PMID: 22535622]

[71]   Wagstaff KM, Sivakumaran H, Heaton SM, Harrich D, Jans DA. Ivermectin is a specific inhibitor of importin α/β-mediated nuclear import able to inhibit replication of HIV-1 and dengue virus. Biochem J 2012; 443(3): 851-6.
[http://dx.doi.org/10.1042/BJ20120150] [PMID: 22417684]

[72]   Jans DA, Wagstaff KM. Ivermectin as a broad-spectrum host-directed antiviral: the real deal? Cells 2020; 9(9): 2100.
[http://dx.doi.org/10.3390/cells9092100] [PMID: 32942671]

[73]   Tay MY, Fraser JE, Chan WK, *et al.* Nuclear localization of dengue virus (DENV) 1-4 non-structural protein 5; protection against all 4 DENV serotypes by the inhibitor Ivermectin. Antiviral Res 2013; 99(3): 301-6.
[http://dx.doi.org/10.1016/j.antiviral.2013.06.002] [PMID: 23769930]

[74]   Yang SNY, Atkinson SC, Wang C, *et al.* The broad spectrum antiviral ivermectin targets the host nuclear transport importin α/β1 heterodimer. Antiviral Res 2020; 177: 104760.
[http://dx.doi.org/10.1016/j.antiviral.2020.104760] [PMID: 32135219]

[75]   Rajapakse S. Dengue shock. J Emerg Trauma Shock 2011; 4(1): 120-7.
[http://dx.doi.org/10.4103/0974-2700.76835] [PMID: 21633580]

[76]   St John AL. Influence of mast cells on dengue protective immunity and immune pathology. PLoS Pathog 2013; 9(12): e1003783.
[http://dx.doi.org/10.1371/journal.ppat.1003783] [PMID: 24367254]

[77]   Morrison J, Rathore APS, Mantri CK, Aman SAB, Nishida A, St John AL. Transcriptional profiling confirms the therapeutic effects of mast cell stabilization in a dengue disease model. J Virol 2017;

91(18): e00617-17.
[http://dx.doi.org/10.1128/JVI.00617-17] [PMID: 28659489]

[78]   Kunder CA, St John AL, Abraham SN. Mast cell modulation of the vascular and lymphatic endothelium. Blood 2011; 118(20): 5383-93.
[http://dx.doi.org/10.1182/blood-2011-07-358432] [PMID: 21908429]

[79]   Rathore APS, St John AL. Immune responses to dengue virus in the skin. Open Biol 2018; 8(8): 180087.
[http://dx.doi.org/10.1098/rsob.180087] [PMID: 30135238]

[80]   Mantri CK, St John AL. Immune synapses between mast cells and γδ T cells limit viral infection. J Clin Invest 2019; 129(3): 1094-108.
[http://dx.doi.org/10.1172/JCI122530] [PMID: 30561384]

[81]   Syenina A, Jagaraj CJ, Aman SA, Sridharan A, St John AL. Dengue vascular leakage is augmented by mast cell degranulation mediated by immunoglobulin Fcγ receptors. eLife 2015; 4: e05291.
[http://dx.doi.org/10.7554/eLife.05291] [PMID: 25783751]

[82]   Tissera H, Rathore APS, Leong WY, *et al.* Chymase Level Is a Predictive Biomarker of Dengue Hemorrhagic Fever in Pediatric and Adult Patients. J Infect Dis 2017; 216(9): 1112-21.
[http://dx.doi.org/10.1093/infdis/jix447] [PMID: 28968807]

[83]   Avirutnan P, Matangkasombut P. Unmasking the role of mast cells in dengue. eLife 2013; 2: e00767.
[http://dx.doi.org/10.7554/eLife.00767] [PMID: 23638302]

[84]   St John AL, Rathore AP, Raghavan B, Ng ML, Abraham SN. Contributions of mast cells and vasoactive products, leukotrienes and chymase, to dengue virus-induced vascular leakage. eLife 2013; 2: e00481.
[http://dx.doi.org/10.7554/eLife.00481] [PMID: 23638300]

[85]   Souza DG, Fagundes CT, Sousa LP, *et al.* Essential role of platelet-activating factor receptor in the pathogenesis of Dengue virus infection. Proc Natl Acad Sci USA 2009; 106(33): 14138-43.
[http://dx.doi.org/10.1073/pnas.0906467106] [PMID: 19666557]

[86]   Merlos M, Giral M, Balsa D, *et al.* Rupatadine, a new potent, orally active dual antagonist of histamine and platelet-activating factor (PAF). J Pharmacol Exp Ther 1997; 280(1): 114-21.
[PMID: 8996188]

[87]   Picado C. Rupatadine: pharmacological profile and its use in the treatment of allergic disorders. Expert Opin Pharmacother 2006; 7(14): 1989-2001.
[http://dx.doi.org/10.1517/14656566.7.14.1989] [PMID: 17020424]

[88]   Jeewandara C, Gomes L, Wickramasinghe N, *et al.* Platelet activating factor contributes to vascular leak in acute dengue infection. PLoS Negl Trop Dis 2015; 9(2): e0003459.
[http://dx.doi.org/10.1371/journal.pntd.0003459] [PMID: 25646838]

[89]   Malavige GN, Wijewickrama A, Fernando S, *et al.* A preliminary study on efficacy of rupatadine for the treatment of acute dengue infection. Sci Rep 2018; 8(1): 3857.
[http://dx.doi.org/10.1038/s41598-018-22285-x] [PMID: 29497121]

[90]   Park SJ, Kim J, Kang S, *et al.* Discovery of direct acting antiviral agents with a graphene-based fluorescent nanosensor. Sci Adv 2020; 6(22): eaaz8201.
[http://dx.doi.org/10.1126/sciadv.aaz8201] [PMID: 32523995]

SUBJECT INDEX

A

Abdominal cramps 55
ACE2 receptor 68
Acetylation 27, 32
  levels 32
Acetyltransferase 35, 39, 85
Acid(s) 56, 57, 69, 80, 81, 82, 131, 142, 150,
    167, 170
  anacardic 150
  carboxylic 142
  dehydroamino 80, 81, 82
  fatty 69, 170
  nonulosonate sugar legionaminic 57
  nucleic 167
  oxalic 131
  pseudaminic 56
  transferring glutamic 81
Acinetobacter baumannii 141
Active transport system 170, 176
Activity 13, 35, 37, 38, 39, 40, 43, 44, 45, 47,
    48, 49, 50, 58, 59, 60, 61, 62, 69, 70, 80,
    84, 85, 129, 130, 139, 140, 165, 173,
    177, 187, 196
  acyltransferase 44
  antituberculosis 130
  antiviral 139, 187
  cytokine 196
  deamidase 44, 48
  enzymatic 35, 37, 38, 39, 45, 50, 85
  fungicidal 173
  glucosyltransferase 60
  glycosyltransferase 58, 59
  haemolytic 140
  hemopoietic 165
  leishmanicidal 177
  phosphatase 40
  proteolytic 80
  synergistic 47
Adaptive immunity 28, 30, 32, 84, 85
ADP-ribosylation 26, 28, 44, 46, 47, 63, 65
  factor 44

  signaling 46
  transferases 46
Akt protein kinase 52
Amastigotes 156, 160, 161, 162, 163, 165,
    167, 178, 179
  axenic 178
  intracellular 179
Amino acid protein synthesis 192
Amphotericin B (AmB) 156, 158, 168, 169,
    170, 171, 172, 173, 174, 176
Andean sickness 159
Anemia 163, 165
Antibody-dependent enhancement (ADE) 195
Antifungal activities 123, 125, 133, 135, 140,
    143, 147
Anti-leishmanial 167, 177, 178, 179, 180
  activity 177, 178, 179, 180
  medicines 167
Antimicrobial activities 77, 79, 83, 86, 125,
    128, 132, 134, 135, 136, 137, 138, 139,
    146, 147, 148, 149, 150
  broad-spectrum 137
  of hydrazones 134, 135, 137
  of quinoline derivatives 132
Antiviral drugs 26, 86, 187, 191, 193
  broad-spectrum 193
Apoptosis 32, 40, 48, 61
  chemotherapeutic-induced 40
Assay 167, 193, 198
  enzyme-linked immunosorbent 167
  protein-protein binding 198
Assembly 56, 80
  flagellar filament 56
  ribosomal 80
ATPase activity 197
ATP-dependent lactam synthase 79
Autoproteolysis 48

B

Bacillus subtilis 75

www.ingramcontent.com/pod-product-compliance
Lightning Source LLC
Chambersburg PA
CBHW050838220326
41598CB00006B/392